Hypertension

Editor

EDWARD D. FROHLICH

MEDICAL CLINICS
OF NORTH AMERICA

www.medical.theclinics.com

Consulting Editor
BIMAL H. ASHAR

January 2017 • Volume 101 • Number 1

ELSEVIER

1600 John F. Kennedy Boulevard • Suite 1800 • Philadelphia, Pennsylvania, 19103-2899

http://www.theclinics.com

MEDICAL CLINICS OF NORTH AMERICA Volume 101, Number 1
January 2017 ISSN 0025-7125, ISBN-13: 978-0-323-48263-9

Editor: Jessica McCool
Developmental Editor: Alison Swety

Medical Clinics of North America (ISSN 0025-7125) is published bimonthly by Elsevier Inc., 360 Park Avenue South, New York, NY 10010-1710. Months of publication are January, March, May, July, September, and November. Business and editorial offices: 1600 John F. Kennedy Boulevard, Suite 1800, Philadelphia, PA 19103-2899. Periodicals postage paid at New York, NY, and additional mailing offices. Subscription prices are USD $268.00 per year (US individuals), $563.00 per year (US institutions), $100.00 per year (US Students), $330.00 per year (Canadian individuals), $731.00 per year (Canadian institutions), $200.00 per year (Canadian and foreign students), $402.00 per year (foreign individuals), and $731.00 per year (foreign institutions). To receive student/resident rate, orders must be accompanied by name of affiliated institution, date of term, and the signature of program/residency coordinator on institution letterhead. Orders will be billed at individual rate until proof of status is received. Foreign air speed delivery is included in all Clinics' subscription prices. All prices are subject to change without notice. **POSTMASTER:** Send address changes to *Medical Clinics of North America*, Elsevier Health Sciences Division, Subscription Customer Service, 3251 Riverport Lane, Maryland Heights, MO 63043. **Customer Service: Telephone: 1-800-654-2452** (U.S. and Canada); **1-314-447-8871** (outside U.S. and Canada). **Fax: 314-447-8029. E-mail: journalscustomerserviceusa@elsevier.com** (for print support); **journalsonlinesupport-usa@elsevier.com** (for online support).

Reprints. For copies of 100 or more of articles in this publication, please contact the Commercial Reprints Department, Elsevier Inc., 360 Park Avenue South, New York, NY 10010-1710. Tel.: 212-633-3874; Fax: 212-633-3820; E-mail: reprints@elsevier.com.

Medical Clinics of North America is also published in Spanish by McGraw-Hill Interamericana Editores S. A., P.O. Box 5-237, 06500 Mexico, D.F., Mexico.

Medical Clinics of North America is covered in *MEDLINE/PubMed (Index Medicus), Current Contents, ASCA, Excerpta Medica, Science Citation Index,* and *ISI/BIOMED.*

PROGRAM OBJECTIVE
The goal of the *Medical Clinics of North America* is to keep practicing physicians up to date with current clinical practice by providing timely articles reviewing the state of the art in patient care.

TARGET AUDIENCE
All practicing physicians and other healthcare professionals.

LEARNING OBJECTIVES
Upon completion of this activity, participants will be able to:
1. Review the effects of hypertension on the kidneys, myocardium, and other organ systems.
2. Discuss treatment approaches to hypertension with comorbidities such as obesity, renal artery disease, and cardiac transplantation.
3. Recognize guidelines and future challenges in the management of hypertension.

ACCREDITATION
The Elsevier Office of Continuing Medical Education (EOCME) is accredited by the Accreditation Council for Continuing Medical Education (ACCME) to provide continuing medical education for physicians.

The EOCME designates this enduring material for a maximum of 15 *AMA PRA Category 1 Credit*(s)™. Physicians should claim only the credit commensurate with the extent of their participation in the activity.

All other health care professionals requesting continuing education credit for this enduring material will be issued a certificate of participation.

DISCLOSURE OF CONFLICTS OF INTEREST
The EOCME assesses conflict of interest with its instructors, faculty, planners, and other individuals who are in a position to control the content of CME activities. All relevant conflicts of interest that are identified are thoroughly vetted by EOCME for fair balance, scientific objectivity, and patient care recommendations. EOCME is committed to providing its learners with CME activities that promote improvements or quality in healthcare and not a specific proprietary business or a commercial interest.

The planning committee, staff, authors and editors listed below have identified no financial relationships or relationships to products or devices they or their spouse/life partner have with commercial interest related to the content of this CME activity:
Majd AlGhatrif, MD; Bimal H. Ashar, MD, MBA, FACP; Alexei Y. Bagrov, MD, PhD; George L. Bakris, MD, FASN, FAHA, FASH; Javier Beaumont, PhD; Amanda L. Bennett, MD; Peminda K. Cabandugama, MD; Aram V. Chobanian, MD; Walmor C. De Mello, MD, PhD; Javier Díez, MD, PhD; Francis G. Dunn, MBChB, FRCP, FACC; Rocío Eiros, MD; Olga V. Fedorova, PhD; Edward D. Frohlich, MD, MACP, FACC; Anjali Fortna; Catalina Gallego, MD; Michael J. Gardner, MD; Juan J. Gavira, MD, PhD; Arantxa González, PhD; David G. Harrison, MD; Marie Krousel-Wood, MD, MSPH; Edward G. Lakatta, MD; Roxana Loperena, BSc; Begoña López, PhD; Friedrich C. Luft, MD; Jessica McCool; María U. Moreno, PhD; Wilson Nadruz, MD, PhD; Premkumar Nandhakumar; Erin Peacock, PhD, MPH; Athanase D. Protogerou, MD, PhD; Susana Ravassa, PhD; Richard N. Re, MD; Michel E. Safar, MD; Gorka San José, PhD; Amil M. Shah, MD, MPH; Scott D. Solomon, MD; James R. Sowers, MD; Tony Stanton, MBChB, PhD, FCSANZ, FESC, FRCP, FRACP; Hillel Sternlicht, MD; Dinko Susic, MD, PhD; Stephen C. Textor, MD; Jasmina Varagic, MD, PhD; Hector O. Ventura, MD; Mingyi Wang, MD, PhD.

The planning committee, staff, authors and editors listed below have identified financial relationships or relationships to products or devices they or their spouse/life partner have with commercial interest related to the content of this CME activity:
Jacques Blacher, MD, PhD is on the speakers' bureau for Servier; Sanofi; Amgen Inc; Boehringer Ingelheim GmbH; PharmAlliance; Novartis AG; and Astra Zeneca, and is a consultant/advisor for Sanofi.
Marc A. Pfeffer, MD, PhD is a consultant/advisor for Bayer AG; Boehringer Ingelheim GmbH; DalCor Pharmaceuticals; Gilead; GSK group of companies; Janssen Global Services, LLC, a division of Johnson & Johnson; Eli Lilly and Company; The Medicines Company; Merck & Co., Inc; Novartis AG; Novo Nordisk A/S; Relypsa Inc; Salix Pharmaceuticals; Sanofi; Teva Pharmaceutical Industries Ltd; Thrasos therapeutics; and Vericel Corporation, has research support from Novartis AG; Sanofi; Brigham and Women's Hospital; has stock ownership in DalCor Pharmaceuticals, and receives royalties/patents from Brigham and Women's Hospital and Novartis AG.

UNAPPROVED/OFF-LABEL USE DISCLOSURE

The EOCME requires CME faculty to disclose to the participants:

1. When products or procedures being discussed are off-label, unlabelled, experimental, and/or investigational (not US Food and Drug Administration [FDA] approved); and
2. Any limitations on the information presented, such as data that are preliminary or that represent ongoing research, interim analyses, and/or unsupported opinions. Faculty may discuss information about pharmaceutical agents that is outside of FDA-approved labelling. This information is intended solely for CME and is not intended to promote off-label use of these medications. If you have any questions, contact the medical affairs department of the manufacturer for the most recent prescribing information.

TO ENROLL

To enroll in the *Medical Clinics of North America* Continuing Medical Education program, call customer service at 1-800-654-2452 or sign up online at http://www.theclinics.com/home/cme. The CME program is available to subscribers for an additional annual fee of USD $295.

METHOD OF PARTICIPATION

In order to claim credit, participants must complete the following:

1. Complete enrolment as indicated above.
2. Read the activity.
3. Complete the CME Test and Evaluation. Participants must achieve a score of 70% on the test. All CME Tests and Evaluations must be completed online.

CME INQUIRIES/SPECIAL NEEDS

For all CME inquiries or special needs, please contact elsevierCME@elsevier.com.

MEDICAL CLINICS OF NORTH AMERICA

RELATED INTEREST

Cardiology Clinics, August 2016 (Vol. 34, Issue 3)
Pulmonary Hypertension
Ronald J. Oudiz, *Editor*
http://www.cardiology.theclinics.com

THE CLINICS ARE AVAILABLE ONLINE!
Access your subscription at:
www.theclinics.com

Contributors

CONSULTING EDITOR

BIMAL H. ASHAR, MD, MBA, FACP
Associate Professor of Medicine, Division of General Internal Medicine, Johns Hopkins University School of Medicine, Baltimore, Maryland

EDITOR

EDWARD D. FROHLICH, MD, MACP, FACC
Alton Ochsner Distinguished Scientist, Ochsner Clinic Foundation, New Orleans, Louisiana

AUTHORS

MAJD AIGHATRIF, MD
Laboratory of Cardiovascular Science, NIA, NIH; Department of Medicine, Johns Hopkins Bayview Medical Center, Johns Hopkins School of Medicine, Baltimore, Maryland

ALEXEI Y. BAGROV, MD, PhD
Laboratory of Cardiovascular Science, NIA, NIH, Baltimore, Maryland

GEORGE L. BAKRIS, MD, FASN, FAHA, FASH
Section of Endocrinology, Diabetes and Metabolism, Department of Medicine, ASH Comprehensive Hypertension Center, The University of Chicago Medicine, Chicago, Illinois

JAVIER BEAUMONT, PhD
Programme of Cardiovascular Diseases, Center of Applied Medical Research, University of Navarra; IdiSNA, Navarra Institute for Health Research, Pamplona, Spain

AMANDA L. BENNETT, MD
Department of Internal Medicine, Ochsner Clinic Foundation, New Orleans, Louisiana

JACQUES BLACHER, MD, PhD
Centre de Diagnostic et de Thérapeutique, Hôpital Hôtel Dieu, Paris, France

PEMINDA K. CABANDUGAMA, MD
Endocrinology Fellow, Division of Endocrinology, Diabetes and Cardiovascular Center, University of Missouri, Columbia, Missouri

ARAM V. CHOBANIAN, MD
Dean Emeritus, Department of Medicine, Boston University School of Medicine; President Emeritus, Boston University, Boston, Massachusetts

WALMOR C. DE MELLO, MD, PhD
Department of Pharmacology, School of Medicine, Medical Sciences Campus, UPR, San Juan, Puerto Rico

JAVIER DÍEZ, MD, PhD
Programme of Cardiovascular Diseases, Center of Applied Medical Research; Department of Cardiology and Cardiac Surgery, University Clinic, University of Navarra; IdiSNA, Navarra Institute for Health Research, Pamplona, Spain

FRANCIS G. DUNN, MBChB, FRCP, FACC
Consultant Cardiologist, Honorary Professor, Division of Cardiovascular Sciences, Stobhill Hospital, University of Glasgow, Glasgow, Scotland

ROCÍO EIROS, MD
Department of Cardiology and Cardiac Surgery, University Clinic, University of Navarra, Pamplona, Spain

OLGA V. FEDOROVA, PhD
Laboratory of Cardiovascular Science, NIA, NIH, Baltimore, Maryland

EDWARD D. FROHLICH, MD, MACP, FACC
Alton Ochsner Distinguished Scientist, Ochsner Clinic Foundation, New Orleans, Louisiana

CATALINA GALLEGO, MD
Programme of Cardiovascular Diseases, Center of Applied Medical Research, University of Navarra, Pamplona, Spain; Programa de Cardiología Clínica, Clínica CardioVID, Universidad Pontificia Bolivariana, Medellín, Colombia

MICHAEL J. GARDNER, MD
Associate Professor of Clinical Medicine, Division of Endocrinology, Diabetes and Cardiovascular Center, University of Missouri, Columbia, Missouri

JUAN J. GAVIRA, MD, PhD
Department of Cardiology and Cardiac Surgery, University Clinic, University of Navarra; IdiSNA, Navarra Institute for Health Research, Pamplona, Spain

ARANTXA GONZÁLEZ, PhD
Programme of Cardiovascular Diseases, Center of Applied Medical Research, University of Navarra; IdiSNA, Navarra Institute for Health Research, Pamplona, Spain

DAVID G. HARRISON, MD
Betty and Jack Bailey Professor of Medicine, Pharmacology and Physiology, Director of Clinical Pharmacology, Division of Clinical Pharmacology, Department of Medicine, Vanderbilt University Medical Center, Vanderbilt University, Nashville, Tennessee

MARIE KROUSEL-WOOD, MD, MSPH
Professor of Medicine and Epidemiology; Tulane University School of Medicine; Tulane University School of Public Health and Tropical Medicine; Ochsner Clinic Foundation, New Orleans, Louisiana

EDWARD G. LAKATTA, MD
Laboratory of Cardiovascular Science, NIA, NIH, Baltimore, Maryland

ROXANA LOPERENA, BSc
Department of Molecular Physiology and Biophysics, Vanderbilt University School of Medicine, Nashville, Tennessee

BEGOÑA LÓPEZ, PhD
Programme of Cardiovascular Diseases, Center of Applied Medical Research, University of Navarra; IdiSNA, Navarra Institute for Health Research, Pamplona, Spain

FRIEDRICH C. LUFT, MD
Professor of Medicine, Charité Medical Faculty, Experimental and Clinical Research Center, Max-Delbrück Center for Molecular Medicine, Berlin, Germany

MARÍA U. MORENO, PhD
Programme of Cardiovascular Diseases, Center of Applied Medical Research, University of Navarra; IdiSNA, Navarra Institute for Health Research, Pamplona, Spain

WILSON NADRUZ, MD, PhD
Cardiovascular Division, Brigham and Women's Hospital, Boston, Massachusetts; Department of Internal Medicine, University of Campinas, Campinas, Brazil

ERIN PEACOCK, PhD, MPH
Research Scientist, Tulane University School of Medicine, New Orleans, Louisiana

MARC A. PFEFFER, MD, PhD
Division of Cardiology, Department of Medicine, Brigham and Women's Hospital; Dzau Professor of Medicine, Harvard Medical School, Boston, Massachusetts

ATHANASE D. PROTOGEROU, MD, PhD
Hypertension Center and Cardiovascular Research Laboratory, 1st Department of Propaedeutic Medicine, Laiko Hospital, Medical School, National and Kapodistrian University of Athens, Athens, Greece

SUSANA RAVASSA, PhD
Programme of Cardiovascular Diseases, Center of Applied Medical Research, University of Navarra; IdiSNA, Navarra Institute for Health Research, Pamplona, Spain

RICHARD N. RE, MD
Scientific Director, Ochsner Health System; Clinical Professor of Medicine, Professor of Physiology, Tulane University School of Medicine, New Orleans, Louisiana

MICHEL E. SAFAR, MD
Centre de Diagnostic et de Thérapeutique, Hôpital Hôtel Dieu, Paris, France

GORKA SAN JOSÉ, PhD
Programme of Cardiovascular Diseases, Center of Applied Medical Research, University of Navarra; IdiSNA, Navarra Institute for Health Research, Pamplona, Spain

AMIL M. SHAH, MD, MPH
Cardiovascular Division, Brigham and Women's Hospital, Boston, Massachusetts

SCOTT D. SOLOMON, MD
Cardiovascular Division, Brigham and Women's Hospital, Boston, Massachusetts

JAMES R. SOWERS, MD
Professor of Medicine and Medical Pharmacology and Physiology; Division of Endocrinology, Diabetes and Cardiovascular Center; Department of Physiology and Pharmacology, University of Missouri; Harry S. Truman VA Hospital, Columbia, Missouri

TONY STANTON, MBChB, PhD, FCSANZ, FESC, FRCP, FRACP
Consultant Cardiologist, Associate Professor of Medicine, Nambour Hospital, School of Medicine, University of Queensland, Nambour, Queensland, Australia

HILLEL STERNLICHT, MD
Section of Endocrinology, Diabetes and Metabolism, Department of Medicine, ASH Comprehensive Hypertension Center, The University of Chicago Medicine, Chicago, Illinois

DINKO SUSIC, MD, PhD
Retired Senior Staff Scientist, Hypertension Research Laboratory, Ochsner Clinic Foundation, New Orleans, Louisiana

STEPHEN C. TEXTOR, MD
Professor of Medicine; Division of Nephrology and Hypertension, Mayo Clinic, Rochester, Minnesota

JASMINA VARAGIC, MD, PhD
Associate Professor, Hypertension & Vascular Research, Department of Surgery; Department of Physiology and Pharmacology, Wake Forest School of Medicine, Medical Center Boulevard, Winston-Salem, North Carolina

HECTOR O. VENTURA, MD
Department of Cardiomyopathy & Heart Transplantation, John Ochsner Heart and Vascular Institute, New Orleans, Louisiana

MINGYI WANG, MD, PhD
Laboratory of Cardiovascular Science, NIA, NIH, Baltimore, Maryland

Contents

> This article provides a preview to the forthcoming articles in this issue, which are written by well-known and authoritative authors for the readers' pleasure and reference. This article hopes to provide a general overview that stimulates interest, better understanding, and continued joint commitment to the important subject of hypertension.

> Left ventricular (LV) diastolic dysfunction (LVDD) is characterized by alterations in LV diastolic filling, and is a strong predictor of cardiovascular events and heart failure. Hypertension is the most important risk factor for LVDD in the community and promotes LVDD through several mechanisms, including hemodynamic overload and myocardial ischemia. Associated factors such as age, ethnicity, dietary sodium, obesity, diabetes mellitus, and chronic kidney disease also contribute to LVDD in hypertensive individuals. Blood pressure lowering using antihypertensive medications can improve LVDD; however, it remains unclear whether this improvement in LV diastolic function can improve cardiovascular outcomes.

> This article discusses the role of hypertension in heart failure. Elevated blood pressure has the greatest population attributable risk for the development of heart failure. The mortality rates following the clinical recognition of heart failure is increased multifold. The treatment of hypertension with antihypertensive agents is particularly effective in preventing heart failure, which makes it the most effective therapy for heart failure.

> The risks associated with hypertension emerge through a series of complex interactions. Myocardial ischemia is the major contributor to this

risk. The mechanisms driving ischemia reflect many of the key factors in hypertension, including endothelial and neurohumoral factors, fibrosis, and hemodynamics. Left ventricular hypertrophy and fibrosis are of fundamental importance and together with hemodynamics provide an optimal template for myocardial ischemia. Understanding the pathophysiology has aided a more rational management approach but challenges remain which, if surmounted, will have an impact on the morbidity and mortality caused by myocardial ischemia in patients with hypertension.

The chronic hemodynamic load imposed by hypertension on the left ventricle leads to lesions in the myocardium that result in structural remodeling, which provides support for alterations in cardiac function, perfusion, and electrical activity that adversely influence the clinical evolution of hypertensive heart disease. Management must include detecting, reducing, and reversing left ventricular hypertrophy, as well as the detection and repair of microscopic lesions responsible for myocardial remodeling. Reducing the burden associated with hypertensive heart disease can be targeted using personalized treatment. The noninvasive, biomarker-mediated identification of subsets of patients with hypertensive heart disease is essential to provide personalized treatment.

Hypertension is a common complication among post cardiac transplant recipients affecting more than 95% of patients. Increased blood pressure poses a significant cardiovascular morbidity and mortality in these patients; it should be identified quickly and needs to be managed appropriately. Understanding the pathophysiology and contributing factors to this disease in these complex and unique patients is the key to appropriate treatment selection.

Renal artery disease produces a spectrum of progressive clinical manifestations ranging from minor degrees of hypertension to circulatory congestion and kidney failure. Moderate reductions in renal blood flow do not induce tissue hypoxia or damage, making medical therapy for renovascular hypertension feasible. Several prospective trials indicate that optimized medical therapy using agents that block the renin-angiotensin system should be the initial management. Evidence of progressive disease and/or treatment failure should allow recognition of high-risk subsets that benefit from renal revascularization. Severe reductions in kidney blood flow ultimately activate inflammatory pathways that do not reverse with restoring blood flow alone.

resistance. Several pathophysiologic factors participate in the link between hypertension and CRS. This article updates recent literature with
a focus on the function of insulin resistance, obesity, and renin angiotensin
aldosterone system-mediated oxidative stress on endothelial dysfunction
and the pathogenesis of hypertension.

pathways contributing to hypertension over (presumably) dietary salt intake or directly through increased peripheral vascular resistance. The Mendelian mutations exercise large effects on blood pressure. Inversely, studying the entire human genome for sources signaling blood pressure has yielded many signals with small effects. Thus far, few loci have been validated or translated into targets. Both genetic strategies are necessary, and much remains to be done.

Hypertension is the second most common cause of chronic kidney disease (CKD) and is a potentiator of kidney failure when accompanying disease. CKD is a common cause of resistant hypertension. Nephropathy progression has dramatically slowed over the past 3 decades from an average of 8 to between 2–3 mL/min per year regardless of diabetes status. The incidence of very high albuminuria as well as progression from high albuminuria very high albuminuria has substantially decreased over the past 3 decades. This improvement relates to better blood pressure control using agents that slow nephropathy as well as better glycemic and cholesterol control.

This article summarizes pertinent data from clinical trials on the effects of antihypertensive therapy on cardiovascular complications. Prior definitions of hypertension and blood pressure goals of therapy are discussed, and differences between national and international guidelines on such goals are summarized. The results of the SPRINT study are summarized, and the impact of this study on future goals of treatment is discussed. New recommendations are provided on blood pressure goals, and the effects such goals might have on clinical practice are discussed.

Adherence to antihypertensive medication remains a key modifiable factor in the management of hypertension. The multidimensional nature of adherence and blood pressure (BP) control call for multicomponent, patient-centered interventions to improve adherence. Promising strategies to improve antihypertensive medication adherence and BP control include regimen simplification, reduction of out-of-pocket costs, use of allied health professionals for intervention delivery, and self-monitoring of BP. Research to understand the effects of technology-mediated interventions, mechanisms underlying adherence behavior, and sex-race differences in determinants of low adherence and intervention effectiveness may enhance patient-specific approaches to improve adherence and disease control.

Foreword

The Sounds of Progress

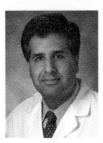

Bimal H. Ashar, MD, MBA, FACP
Consulting Editor

In 1905, Dr Nikolai Korotkoff developed a technique for measuring blood pressure by applying a cuff with an inflatable bladder around the patient's arm and using a stethoscope to listen to sounds in the brachial artery. The identification of these "Korotkoff sounds" marked the emergence of hypertension as a medical condition that could be measured in an ongoing fashion. Despite the advances that have been made over the last century in better understanding the epidemiology, pathophysiology, and therapeutic approaches to controlling blood pressure, diseases attributable to hypertension remain the leading cause of death in the world. In the United States, one in every three adults has high blood pressure. Only about half of those patients have their values under control. The Centers for Disease Control and Prevention estimates that by adding up the cost of health care services, medications, and missed days of work, high blood pressure costs the nation almost $50 billion each year.

In this issue of the *Medical Clinics of North America*, Dr Edward D. Frohlich and his colleagues provide an in-depth review of the pathophysiology of hypertension and the impact that this condition has on inducing coronary disease, heart failure, and kidney disease. The authors further highlight the complexity of controlling high blood pressure and the importance of tailoring treatment approaches to specific populations of patients (eg, diabetics, cardiac transplant patients, elderly patients). No review of hypertension would be complete without a description of the current therapeutic guidelines. Dr Chobanian examines the Eighth Joint National Committee guidelines while identifying where controversies may exist.

It is been over 110 years since Dr Korotkoff described the sounds that would so significantly impact the fight against cardiovascular disease. Since 1950, age-adjusted death rates from cardiovascular disease have declined 60%, partially due to the identification and treatment of hypertension. Yet, much still needs to be accomplished. We

Med Clin N Am 101 (2017) xvii–xviii
http://dx.doi.org/10.1016/j.mcna.2016.10.003
0025-7125/17/© 2016 Published by Elsevier Inc.

medical.theclinics.com

hope that the articles in this issue provide the framework to assist clinicians in assessing and managing this very important clinical entity.

Bimal H. Ashar, MD, MBA, FACP
Division of General Internal Medicine
Johns Hopkins University School of Medicine
601 North Caroline Street
#7143
Baltimore, MD 21287, USA

E-mail address:
Bashar1@jhmi.edu

Preface

Continuing Challenges and Unresolved Problems in Hypertensive Diseases

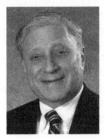

Edward D. Frohlich, MD, MACP, FACC
Editor

This is the sixth issue of the *Medical Clinics of North America* that I have edited and dedicated to current thinking about hypertension. These issues are dedicated to the continuing history of innovative concepts about the hypertensive diseases, our pathophysiologic understanding of their underlying mechanisms of the related clinical problems, current concepts of their treatment, and alliterations by the selected contributors' personal comprehension of their subjects about which each of them have expressed. Fortunately, I have continued to invite them on the basis of my personal and long-standing knowledge and experience with them and the subject material they discuss for us. I have a continuing and deep appreciation of them for their willingness to join with me in our respective articles of our fundamental material. Each was written with great familiarity and deep conviction.

The earlier issues of the *Medical Clinics of North America* that I edited were focused exclusively on hypertension and outlived two prior medical publishers. The first two were the publishers of highly reputable authoritative medical literature. The third and current publisher, Elsevier, succeeded them after they retired into their historically highly merited bibliographic positions. Each had been the publisher of several of my other contributions and was led by leaders whom I consider among my best academic friends. The current publisher, Elsevier, introduces this edition during the 101st anniversary of the *Medical Clinics*. Finally, I add my personal comment that the first publisher, Mr. Lewis Reines, related closely with me in our joint endeavors ever since 1969.

The importance of the subject of hypertension is highly regarded by my coauthors in the "cutting edge" of medical knowledge and practice over the years. In the early years of these *Medical Clinics*, the treatment of hypertensive diseases was only beginning.

Med Clin N Am 101 (2017) xix–xxi
http://dx.doi.org/10.1016/j.mcna.2016.10.002
0025-7125/17/© 2016 Published by Elsevier Inc.

medical.theclinics.com

Over the years, public, corporate pharmaceutical industry, and academic overview maintained the necessary continuing expertise in the subject and remained unabated and sustained by the National High Blood Pressure Education Program (of the National Institutes of Health, NIH). This latter and highly esteemed Program was born from the deep commitment of Dr Theodore Cooper, former Director of the National Heart, Lung, and Blood Institute (NHLBI) and, later, Secretary of the Department of Education (of the Department of Health, Education, and Welfare) and its long-standing and most recent staff, which was headed by Dr Edward Roccella and the NHLBI Directorships of Drs Robert Levy and Claude Lenfant. Without their respective commitment to this Program, our constantly growing knowledge of hypertension would not have been possible. I have enjoyed each of the 32 years that I remained in its service as a contributing member representing either the American Medical Association, the American Heart Association and its Council for High Blood Pressure Research, or the American College of Cardiology over successive years of my tenure. Hence, these six editions of the *Medical Clinics of North America* are dedicated to all of the contributing authors who have participated in prior issues (some as well cited leaders of their respective representative institutions). They have all supported their respected academic institutions and the knowledge promulgated through their support.

Finally, I want to also express my deep appreciation to my dear friends, teachers, and role models throughout the years. The inspiration, knowledge, and stimulation from each of the following listed below have contributed to the excitement, joy, and utmost satisfaction that I have treasured over the years:

Theodore E. Woodward, MD, Professor and Chairman, Department of Medicine, University of Maryland School of Medicine.

Hugh H. Hussey, MD, Professor of Medicine and Dean, Georgetown University School of Medicine, and Editor-in-Chief of the *Journal of the American Medical Association*.

Edward D. Freis, MD, Professor of Medicine, Georgetown University School of Medicine and Senior Medical Investigator and Founder, and Director of the Veterans Administration Cooperative Study on Hypertension.

William E. Middleton, MD, Medical Director, Veterans Administration, Washington, DC, and former Chair of Medicine and Dean of the University of Wisconsin.

Irvine H. Page, MD, Head of Research Division, Cleveland Clinic, Cleveland, Ohio, discoverer of Angiotensin and of Serotonin, and the concept of the Mosaic Theory of Hypertension.

Harriet P. Dustan, MD, Former President, American Heart Association, and past member of the staff of Research Division of Cleveland Clinic, and later, Senior Physician of the University of Alabama Veterans Administration Hospital, Past Member Advisory Boards of National Heart, Lung, and Blood Institute (NIH) and American College of Physicians.

Solomon Papper, MD, Professor of Medicine and Head of the Department of Medicine, University of Oklahoma School of Medicine, Oklahoma City, Oklahoma.

My many research fellows, colleagues, patients, and institutions from whom I learned much over my many years in academic medicine at my several "home" institutions.

And, my wife of over 57 years, Sherry Frohlich, my children (Margie, Bruce, and Lara), and my parents, May and William Frohlich, who stimulated my ongoing commitment to life, learning, family love, and much more.

None the least, to my office assistant, Caramia Fairchild, for over 27 years of faithful commitment.

Edward D. Frohlich, MD, MACP, FACC
Alton Ochsner Distinguished Scientist
Ochsner Clinic Foundation
1514 Jefferson Highway
New Orleans, LA 70121, USA

E-mail address:
efrohlich@ochsner.org

Hypertension

New and Future Challenges

Edward D. Frohlich, MD, MACP, FACC

KEYWORDS

- Hypertension • Cardiac failure • Systolic function • Cardiovascular

KEY POINTS

- This article provides a preview to the articles in this issue, which are written by well-known and authoritative authors for the readers' pleasure and reference.
- This article hopes to provide a general overview that stimulate interests, better understanding, and continued joint commitment to the important subject of hypertension.

Most general textbooks of medicine generally lack any discussion of cardiac failure dealing with preserved systolic function (ie, diastolic dysfunction). This subject, however, is among the most frequent causes of hospitalization of patients in the United States and other industrialized nations. It is frequently encountered among women, more frequently in the elderly of both genders, is common among patients with hypertension, and is currently included in most cardiovascular teaching programs. It is especially included in this hypertension issue, specifically to emphasize for hypertensionologists that impaired diastolic function occurs commonly in patients with hypertension, in particular those with left ventricular hypertrophy, frequently those with left bundle branch block, and those with a left ventricular ejection rate of less than 30 mL/s to 40 mL/s (see Wilson Nadruz Junior and colleagues' article, "Diastolic Dysfunction and Hypertension," in this issue). These patients have been shown to merit particular attention for ventricular pacing and careful follow-up.

This article presents an introduction to each article in this issue of the *Medical Clinics of North America* (*MCNA*), providing reflections and overview of the present and an inkling of the newer developments for the field of hypertension. To begin, "Diastolic Dysfunction and Hypertension" is discussed by Wilson Nadruz Junior and Amil M. Shah of the Cardiovascular Division, Brigham and Women's Hospital (Boston), and Dr Scott D. Solomon, Professor of Medicine and honoree of The Edward D. Frohlich Cardiovascular Pathophysiology Chair. It emphasizes that exceedingly common cardiac problem that is not usually included in discussions concerning impaired cardiac function, predisposing hypertensive patients to subsequent left ventricular failure.

Alton Ochsner Distinguished Scientist, Ochsner Clinic Foundation, 1514 Jefferson Highway, New Orleans, LA 70121, USA
E-mail address: efrohlich@ochsner.org

Med Clin N Am 101 (2017) 1–6
http://dx.doi.org/10.1016/j.mcna.2016.08.018
0025-7125/17/© 2016 Elsevier Inc. All rights reserved.

Dr Marc A. Pfeffer of Brigham and Women's Hospital begins with his overview of old and new challenges involving therapeutic trials dealing with cardiac failure. It was his large survival and vascular enlargement (SAVE) multicenter trial in which he and his colleagues first identified those patients who, after myocardial infarction, were treated with the first renin-angiotensin inhibiting agent in that classic study (see Marc A. Pfeffer's article, "Heart Failure and Hypertension: Importance of Prevention," in this issue). Of special interest, this class of antihypertensive agents was initially considered for patients with left ventricular failure. Fortunately, modern cardiovascular medicine considers these drugs among those generally considered to be included among the major agents for use in the treatment of left ventricular failure.

In his article, dealing with heart failure from hypertension and its prevention with his supporting selected references, Dr Pfeffer details the exciting history of the tremendous number of well-designed clinical studies that carefully document the efficacy of antihypertensive therapy in preventing morbidity and mortality from cardiac failure (see Marc A. Pfeffer's article, "Heart Failure and Hypertension: Importance of Prevention," in this issue). I believe that no one would doubt that the Veterans Administration (VA) Cooperative Study Group reported the first controlled, double-blinded, multicenter series of studies conceived, conducted, and directed by Dr Edward D. Freis. This series of VA studies first demonstrated the efficacy of antihypertensive therapy and its significant reduction in mortality from cardiac failure. Thereafter, as outlined by Dr Pfeffer, over the remainder of the twentieth century and into the twenty-first century, the many well-conceived and well-conducted studies confirmed and extended the necessary details (see Marc A. Pfeffer's article, "Heart Failure and Hypertension: Importance of Prevention," in this issue). Their key features should be credited to Dr Freis, his colleagues, the initial centers, the volunteer patients, and the VA Cooperative Study.

Dr Francis G. Dunn (Honorary Professor in Cardiovascular Sciences at the University of Glasgow) and his colleague Dr Tony Stanton (Consultant Cardiologist at the School of Medicine, Nambour Hospital, Nambour, Australia) discuss the frequent coexistence of ischemic coronary vascular disease and hypertension (see Tony Stanton and Francis G. Dunn's article, "Hypertension, Left Ventricular Hypertrophy, and Myocardial Ischemia," in this issue). This cardiac problem frequently affects the coronary circulation in patients with arteriolar constriction throughout resistance vessels of both ventricles and is also commonly associated with occlusive atherosclerosis of the larger coronary arteries. Drs Dunn and Stanton, in their lucid presentation, also include a clear discussion of ischemic cardiac changes that are complexly related to both hemodynamic and nonhemodynamic complications of myocardial fibrosis, arterial stiffness, endothelial dysfunction, and extracellular inflammation. These considerations are discussed carefully with respect to the wide variety of diagnostic procedures that are available for the clinical assessment and management of the hypertensive patient (see Tony Stanton and Francis G. Dunn's article, "Hypertension, Left Ventricular Hypertrophy, and Myocardial Ischemia," in this issue). This scholarly work from Glasgow has been recognized by the medical community provides evidence of Dr Dunn's recent leadership and his appointment as President of the Royal College of Physicians and Surgeons of Glasgow.

María U. Moreno and colleagues' article, "The Hypertensive Myocardium: from Microscopic Lesions to Clinical Complications and Outcomes," in this issue focuses on the microscopic myocardial lesions in hypertensive heart disease and its clinical outcomes. For far too long, clinicians have considered that coronary vascular disease complicating hypertension is the major complication of atherosclerotic coronary arterial occlusive disease. In recent years, however, the cardiac changes that involve the microcirculation of both ventricles have come to be appreciated. The many studies of Dr Diez and his colleagues concern the sequential microbiological changes that result in the cardinal cardiac lesions evolving in the development of the myriad of factors promoting ischemia and hypertensive heart disease. These important vascular concerns are cogently discussed in the light of recent awareness of their tremendous complexity.

Exploration of the many clinical problems associated with hypertensive cardiac, vascular, and renal diseases are involved with the discipline of cardiac transplantation (see Amanda L. Bennett and Hector O. Ventura's article, "Hypertension in Patients with Cardiac Transplantation," in this issue). Many of these patients may have coexisting renal and other challenges that add to the existing concerns about their management not only by their experienced surgeons but also by the many cardiologists and other physicians, nurses, and technical personnel who belong to the hard-working teams continuously available for the management of their patients. This difficult subject is discussed (see Amanda L. Bennett and Hector O. Ventura's article, "Hypertension in Patients with Cardiac Transplantation," in this issue).

Another area that has stimulated much interest and controversy relates to the management of those hypertensive patients with either unilateral or bilateral renal arterial disease. They frequently relate to vascular disease involving atherosclerotic or fibrosing renal arterial lesions of these arteries, whether unilateral or bilateral. This difficult clinical problem has been discussed in an earlier *MCNA* issue by Dr Stephen C. Textor of the Mayo Clinic, Rochester, Minnesota, and is now considered in his update (see Stephen C. Textor's article, "Renal Arterial Diseases and Hypertension," in this issue).

One major as-yet incompletely understood problem of the medical profession, the general public, and the media relates to the subject of aging and how it impinges on the enlarging list of the many aspects of medicine and society included among the hypertensive, vascular, renal, brain, and other diseases. This is a tremendously complicated subject relating to the aging process. These major and perhaps still ill-defined problems involve many aspects that must be considered adding to the unresolved complexity of the overall problem of aging — as is in normotensive individuals who are generally considered free of many comorbid factors (see Majd AlGhatrif and colleagues' article, "The pressure of Aging," in this issue). They include a tremendous number of medical and societal issues as well as an increasing list of disease mechanisms that include the large number of neurologic and dementing illnesses, including Alzheimer disease. This problem is further complicated when cardiovascular, renal, endocrine, and many other diseases are included. These and other considerations, are briefly raised by Dr Edward G. Lakatta and his colleagues of the National Institute on Aging and the Johns Hopkins University School of Medicine. Their discussion includes many factors requiring a host of important and novel concerns that provide this tremendously insightful article with necessary consideration (see Majd AlGhatrif and colleagues' article, "The pressure of Aging," in this issue).

My colleague, Dr Richard N. Re, at the Ochsner Clinic Foundation, has introduced an extremely important investigative concept dealing with his exciting exposition of independent renin-angiotensin systems that involve the various target organs of hypertensive cardiovascular disease. In doing so, he introduces the provocative concept of specific autocrine, paracrine, and intracrine biological aspects of the cardiovascular, renal, and brain circulatory changes involving these organs that promote their further development of structural and functional alterations (see Richard N. Re's article, "A Reassessment of the Pathophysiology of Progressive Cardiorenal Disorders," in this issue).[1] Following this line of thinking presented by Dr Re, Professor Walmor C. De Mello of the University of Puerto Rico, discusses his ongoing studies that provide insight into the importance of the local cardiac renin-angiotensin system and its relevant clinical relationships (see Walmor C. De Mello's article, "Local Renin Angiotensin Aldosterone Systems and Cardiovascular Diseases," in this issue). Thus, Professor De Mello refers primarily to the role of this local system in the development of abnormal cardiac rhythm and myocardial functions.

Dr James R. Sowers and his coworkers at the University of Missouri School of Medicine follow with their discussion related to the many aspects associated with hypertension and the cardiorenal syndrome. Dr Sowers is editor in chief of *Cardiorenal Medicine* and shares current thinking about some of the myriad problems (see Peminda K. Cabandugama and colleagues' article, "The Renin Angiotensin Aldosterone System in Obesity and Hypertension: Roles in Cardiorenal Metabolic Syndrome," in this issue). This concise and pertinent discussion of these issues includes hypertension, the hyperlipidemias, diabetes mellitus, certain other endocrine-related diseases, and, of course, exogenous obesity.

This frequent coexistence of hypertension with the problem of exogenous obesity clearly involves several other competing factors, including gout, hyperuricemia, and other associated microbiological factors, which were under current areas of investigation in our laboratory at the Ochsner Institutions with my former colleagues Dr Dinko Susic (who had joined the program from his former University of Belgrade Department of Physiology [Belgrade, Serbia]) and invited Dr Jasmina Varagic (currently with the Hypertension and Vascular Disease Center, Division of Surgical Sciences, Wake Forest School of Medicine [Winston-Salem, North Carolina]) (see Dinko Susic and Jasmina Varagic's article, "Obesity: A Perspective from Hypertension," in this issue). After spending 20 years at Ochsner, Dr Susic retired to his former home in Belgrade and shortly thereafter returned to Ochsner for a brief visit (to review his present article with me and Dr Varagic). On returning to Belgrade, however, Dr Susic suddenly died (see Dinko Susic and Jasmina Varagic's article, "Obesity: A Perspective from Hypertension," in this issue). As editor of this issue, I wish to express my deep and sincere regrets to his family. I am particularly grateful to Dr Varagic, who masterfully carried through their editorial responsibilities with only 2 weeks of time to submit their work. Personally, I am most grateful to both of these hard-working and committed colleagues for more than 20 years of joint collaboration (see Dinko Susic and Jasmina Varagic's article, "Obesity: A Perspective from Hypertension," in this issue).

Another aspect to a clearer understanding of the pathophysiology of hypertension relates to those hypertensive patients having coexistent diabetes mellitus and the necessity for the clear understanding of the complex selection of antihypertensive agents from the large number of drugs having varied mechanisms (see Michel E. Safar and colleagues' article, "Patient Management of Hypertensive Subjects Without and with Diabetes Mellitus Type II," in this issue). This subject is covered by Dr Michel E. Safar of the Hôpital Hôtel-Dieu (Paris, France), who is a world-class hypertension leader and a long-standing friend. His thoughtful contribution to this important subject is a meaningful and a particularly important forum. I am pleased once again that we are participating together with his present contribution on the coexistence of diabetes mellitus and hypertension (see Michel E. Safar and colleagues' article, "Patient Management of Hypertensive Subjects Without and with Diabetes Mellitus Type II," in this issue).

The next article by Roxana Loperena and Dr David G. Harrison of Vanderbilt University contributes new information about oxidative metabolic mechanisms underlying the pathophysiology of cardiovascular disease development and its still enigmatic elaboration and involvement throughout the circulation and target organs. These considerations are of important concern relating to the development of cardiovascular, renal, and brain oxidative metabolic events in the elaboration of the pathophysiology of hypertension (see Roxana Loperena and David G. Harrison's article, "Oxidative Stress and Hypertensive Diseases," in this issue). (Parenthetically, I must also reflect on the years that David Harrison and I shared at the University of Oklahoma while he was in medical school and where I was involved introducing a new course on pathophysiology, exploring many clinical problems and their disease mechanisms.)

Discussion of the many issues that are associated genetically with understanding of the extremely important (but often unresolved) mechanisms are related to certain hypertensive diseases. They include many associated with underlying biological and genetic mechanisms, often involving controversial academic issues. Providing his personal thoughts on this difficult subject is Dr Friedrich C. Luft of the Experimental and Clinical Research Center, MDC/Charité (Berlin, Germany), who is an important leader in this exciting area of genetic concepts involving the clinical investigation of hypertension (see Friedrich C. Luft's article, "What Have We Learned from the "Genetics of Hypertension"?," in this issue).

The important role of the kidney in hypertension is a broad and common subject, indeed. One leading clinician and investigative leader in the nephrological understanding about hypertension is Dr George L. Bakris of the University of Chicago School of Medicine (see Hillel Sternlicht and George L. Bakris' article, "The Kidney in Hypertension," in this issue). He has been a long-time contributor to the MCNA series and a consultant with the Food and Drug Administration dealing with the antihypertensive drugs and many current therapeutic antihypertensive guidelines as well as with several pharmaceutical, governmental, and other organizations concerned with the role of the kidney in hypertension. In their article on the kidney in hypertension, Dr Bakris and Dr Hillel Sternlicht clearly present several important issues dealing with frequent clinical aspects of hypertension and cardiovascular-renal diseases and related therapeutic issues (see Hillel Sternlicht and George L. Bakris' article, "The Kidney in Hypertension," in this issue).

Currently, the controversial subject concerning introduction of antihypertensive therapy for elderly hypertensive patients and the recommended guidelines for therapy are discussed by Dr Aram V. Chobanian (see Aram V. Chobanian's article, "Guidelines for the Management of Hypertension," in this issue). In this regard, he deals with a key area related to the selection of drugs among the large number of agents and their varied guidelines for implementation of treatment. Thus, exceedingly important issues have remained topics of great discussion by the general public, the lay and professional media, physicians in general, and specialized areas of medical practice. Some of the important questions that have been raised include the choice of drug or therapeutic class of agents for patients with specific organ involvement from hypertension. These issues involve the patient's age, gender, and race and consider which therapeutic agent should be prescribed for selected comorbid indications, potential drug interactions, and so forth. To help guide clinicians in these (and other) important key decisions in a concise and expert fashion is the article written by Dr Aram V. Chobanian (President Emeritus of Boston University and Dean Emeritus of Boston University School of Medicine, who is my dear friend of many years) (see Aram V. Chobanian's article, "Guidelines for the Management of Hypertension," in this issue).

And, lastly (but not least by any means), are important considerations that are presented by Dr Marie Krousel-Wood and her colleague, Dr Erin Peacock, at the Ochsner Clinic Foundation and the Tulane University School of Medicine (New Orleans), concerning the major problems faced by all patients and their physicians relating adherence to all (including antihypertensive) therapies (see Erin Peacock and Marie Krousel-Wood's article, "Adherence to Antihypertensive Therapy," in this issue). These issues concerning maintenance of prescribed drug treatments are highly complex and not only include those concerns related to cost of therapy prescribed. They also related to problems dealing with whether the actually prescribed agent or its generic equivalent is ascribed, other frequent comorbid problems (including depression),[2] and other drugs prescribed by all physician(s) involving medical care. This important article involving necessary incompletely appreciated and complicated problems relating to adherence to prescribed treatment is placed as a concluding article in this issue as food for thought in the daily practice of medicine.

At this point in this introductory article, I cannot help but reflect and comment briefly on one of my important lifetime mentors and role models, Dr Irvine H. Page. I am confident that his thinking must have emerged from the varied areas contributed to this issue without the reader pausing to think about Dr Page's multifactorial Mosaic Theory of Hypertension[3] and his major discoveries of angiotensin and serotonin for the world of medicine.[4,5] In my personal reveries about my former colleagues and mentors, I paused to consider this outstanding leader's legion of clinical and investigative contributions to medicine. Perhaps a personal expression of my gratitude for his support, friendship, and thinking may be sufficient herein, but I cannot help but ask myself just what he might say at this intervening time by posing a question. I would ask him for his comment considering the present state of knowledge about this tremendously complex subject of hypertension after so many years. I might simply answer briefly for him, "Ed, you guessed it; I am positively overwhelmed!"

In conclusion, this introductory article provides a preview to the articles in this issue, which are written by well-known and authoritative authors for the readers' pleasure and reference. Hopefully, it provides a general overview that stimulates interest, better understanding, and continued joint commitment to a most important subject of this extremely vital subject. Finally, I want to express my deep and heartfelt appreciation to each of my many close friends, colleagues, coworkers, mentors, and role models who stimulated and contributed to this issue. For these and the many other contributions and meetings shared with each other, I express my sincere thanks for the many relationships and the overall understanding about hypertension and its related thinking.

REFERENCES

1. Re RN. Tissue renin angiotensin systems. Med Clin North Am 2004;88:19–38.
2. Krousel-Wood M, Frohlich ED. Hypertension and depression: coexisting barriers to medication adherence. J Clin Hypertens (Greenwich) 2010;12:481–6.
3. Page IH. Pathogenesis of arterial hypertension. JAMA 1949;140:455–7.
4. Page IH. Mosaic Hemerom: a crystalline pressor substance (angiotonin) resulting from the action between renin and renin-activator. J Exp Med 1940;71:29–42.
5. Turirog BM, Page IH. Serotonin content of some mammalian tissues and urine and a method for its determination. Am J Physiol 1953;175:157–61.

Diastolic Dysfunction and Hypertension

Wilson Nadruz, MD, PhD[a,b], Amil M. Shah, MD, MPH[a], Scott D. Solomon, MD[a],*

KEYWORDS

- Hypertension • Diastolic dysfunction • Heart failure • Left ventricular hypertrophy

KEY POINTS

- Hypertension is the leading etiology for diastolic dysfunction, which is ubiquitous in elderly individuals and contributes to the development of heart failure.
- In addition to hypertension, diabetes, renal function, salt intake, and others contribute to the development and progression of diastolic dysfunction in hypertensive individuals.
- Lowering blood pressure improves diastolic dysfunction, but it is uncertain whether this improvement is translated into better cardiovascular outcome in hypertensive patients.

INTRODUCTION

Left ventricular (LV) diastolic dysfunction (LVDD) is characterized by alterations in LV diastolic filling, which may include impairments in myocardial relaxation and abnormal distensibility of the myocardium.[1,2] It is commonly seen in community settings, especially among elderly individuals, and is a strong predictor of cardiovascular events and incident heart failure (HF).[2] Several risk factors, including hypertension, coronary artery disease, obesity, and diabetes mellitus, are implicated in the development of LVDD.[2] Hypertension has been reported as the most important risk factor for LVDD in the community and a major contributor to the development of HF.[3,4] Importantly, LVDD is considered a critical link between hypertension and HF, particularly in individuals with HF and preserved ejection fraction (HFpEF),[1] which is quite prevalent, accounting for up to one-half of patients with HF, and is associated with substantial morbidity and mortality.[5] The prevalence of HFpEF has progressively increased over the last decades, but death rates have not changed substantially.[6] Even though various therapies improve survival in patients with HF and a reduced ejection fraction, no pharmacologic therapy has been shown to effectively reduce mortality in HFpEF patients.[5] These trends highlight the importance of understanding the pathophysiologic alterations that precede the development HFpEF, particularly hypertension-induced LVDD.

Conflicts of Interest: None.
[a] Cardiovascular Division, Brigham and Women's Hospital, 75 Francis Street, Boston, MA 02115, USA; [b] Department of Internal Medicine, University of Campinas, Campinas, Brazil
* Corresponding author.
E-mail address: ssolomon@bwh.harvard.edu

Med Clin N Am 101 (2017) 7–17
http://dx.doi.org/10.1016/j.mcna.2016.08.013
0025-7125/17/© 2016 Elsevier Inc. All rights reserved.
medical.theclinics.com

MECHANISMS OF LEFT VENTRICULAR DIASTOLIC DYSFUNCTION IN HYPERTENSION

Diastole includes isovolumic relaxation and the 3 filling phases (rapid filling, diastasis, and atrial contraction) of the cardiac cycle. Diastolic dysfunction refers to slow or delayed relaxation, abnormal LV diastolic distensibility, and impaired filling of the myocardium.[1,2] In LVDD, the LV cannot fill with enough blood at low pressures and the chamber filling is slow or incomplete in the absence of increases in the left atrial pressure. Consequently, LV filling becomes more dependent on left atrial contraction and higher atrial pressures.[7] Impairment in relaxation may result from any mechanism that influences the removal of calcium from the cytosol and actin–myosin cross-bridge detachment,[8] whereas reduced LV chamber compliance may be related to alterations in myocardial composition, including interstitial fibrosis, alterations in titin phosphorylation, and increases in microtubules content in cardiomyocytes.[2,5]

Hemodynamic and Nonhemodynamic Factors

Hypertension may induce LVDD through several potential mechanisms, including hemodynamic and nonhemodynamic factors, and myocardial ischemia (**Fig. 1**). The strong association between hypertension and LVDD[3,9] supports the notion that pressure overload plays a major role in the development of LVDD. Indeed, casual blood pressure measurements are consistently associated with markers of impaired diastolic function.[3,9] In addition, 24-hour blood pressure measurements, which are more representative of the hemodynamic load imposed by hypertension, show a stronger association with LVDD than casual blood pressure.[10] The use of ambulatory blood pressure monitoring is particularly useful to identify individuals with masked hypertension, among whom the prevalence of LVDD is similar to those with sustained hypertension.[11]

Hypertension induces stiffening of larger arteries and hemodynamic influences derived from these vascular alterations have also been suggested to influence LV diastolic function.[12] Stiffening of the aorta produces an earlier return of wave reflection from the periphery to the proximal aorta with consequent augmentation of aortic systolic pressure, and reductions in diastolic blood pressure. These events result in increases in LV afterload during systole and reductions in LV coronary perfusion during diastole, which may favor the development of LVDD.[13] Several studies have

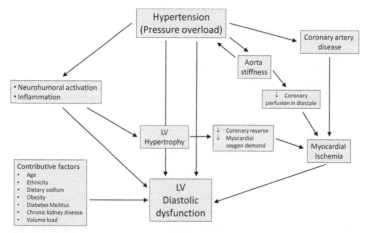

Fig. 1. Pathways of left ventricular (LV) diastolic dysfunction secondary to hypertension.

shown that pulse wave velocity, a measure of aortic stiffness, and central blood pressure measurements have greater relationship with LVDD as compared with brachial blood pressure measurements, underscoring the importance of large artery stiffening in the pathogenesis of impaired diastolic function.[13–15]

Other hemodynamic and nonhemodynamic factors have also been suggested to influence LVDD in hypertensive subjects. Volume overload seems to contribute to LVDD in some hypertensive subgroups, particularly in those with primary aldosteronism, obesity, and end-stage renal disease.[16–18] In addition, alterations in neurohumoral activity and inflammation have been related to impairments in LV relaxation and distensibility.[5,7,19] Notably, the activation of the renin–angiotensin–aldosterone system is suggested to exert an important role in LVDD by modulating the development of fibrosis.[19]

Myocardial Ischemia

Myocardial ischemia impairs LV relaxation and may promote reductions in LV compliance.[19] Hypertension is a major risk factor for coronary atherosclerosis and LVDD is aggravated in hypertensive subjects with coronary artery disease.[20] Additionally, hypertensive patients, especially those with LV hypertrophy, are reported to have reduced coronary reserve and increased myocardial oxygen demand, which may contribute to impaired LV relaxation and increased LV filling pressure.[21] Potential mechanisms involved in hypertension-associated reduction of coronary reserve include remodeling of coronary arteries, endothelial dysfunction, and increased resistance at microvascular level.[21]

ASSESSMENT OF LEFT VENTRICULAR DIASTOLIC FUNCTION

The LV end-diastolic pressure measured during cardiac catheterization has been considered as a gold standard for evaluation of LV filling pressure.[1] However, this procedure is invasive and unfeasible for daily practice. In the last decades, Doppler echocardiography has emerged as the most commonly used tool to identify LVDD in clinical grounds.[1] Several echocardiographic measurements have been used to estimate LV diastolic function, which include: mitral valve peak E-wave (E) and A-wave (A) velocities, the E/A ratio, mitral valve deceleration time, tissue Doppler imaging e' velocity (e'), the E/e' ratio, left atrial volume index, pulmonary vein systolic and diastolic wave velocities, tricuspid regurgitation systolic jet velocity, and isovolumic relaxation time.[22] As a result, there has been great variability in the criteria used to define LVDD. As an attempt to standardize the definition of LVDD, recent guidelines from the American Society of Echocardiography and the European Association of Cardiovascular Imaging recommended that, in the presence of normal LV ejection fraction ($\geq$50%) and no myocardial disease, 4 echocardiographic variables should be used to evaluate LV diastolic function: e' velocity, E/e' ratio, left atrium maximum volume index, and tricuspid regurgitation systolic jet velocity (**Fig. 2**).[22] These guidelines also suggest that the presence of a reduced ejection fraction or the presence of myocardial disease (eg, pathologic LV hypertrophy) in subjects with preserved ejection fraction are consistent with LVDD. Nevertheless, the authors recognize that this latter recommendation was based on expert consensus and, therefore, still needs to be validated.

LEFT VENTRICULAR HYPERTROPHY AND GEOMETRY

LV hypertrophy is commonly seen in hypertensive patients and is considered as a response to the hemodynamic overload imposed by hypertension.[23] LV mass and LV hypertrophy are strongly associated with impaired relaxation and increased LV

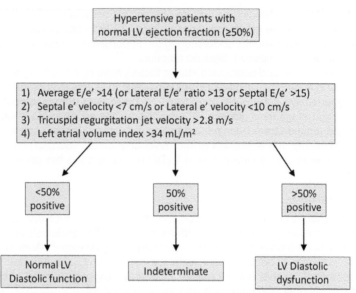

Fig. 2. Algorithm for diagnosis of left ventricular (LV) diastolic dysfunction in individuals with normal LV ejection fraction and no myocardial disease suggested by the American Society of Echocardiography and the European Association of Cardiovascular Imaging. (*Adapted from* Nagueh SF, Smiseth OA, Appleton CP, et al. Recommendations for the evaluation of left ventricular diastolic function by echocardiography: an update from the American Society of Echocardiography and the European Association of Cardiovascular Imaging. J Am Soc Echocardiogr 2016;29:290.)

filling pressure,[24,25] and LVDD may be seen in up to 84% of hypertensive individuals with LV hypertrophy.[26] Conversely, it has been estimated that 11% to 20% of hypertensive patients have LVDD without exhibiting LV hypertrophy.[24,27] Variation in LV geometry is also associated with impairments in LV diastolic function. Concentric hypertrophy, which is associated with increased myocardial stiffness owing to a low LV volume–mass ratio and fibrosis[19] is the geometric pattern most commonly associated with LVDD.[24,28,29] In contrast, concentric remodeling does not seem to be associated with a greater prevalence of LVDD when compared with normal LV geometry.[28,29]

CLINICAL FACTORS INFLUENCING LEFT VENTRICULAR DIASTOLIC FUNCTION IN HYPERTENSION
Age

Aging is an independent contributor to the deterioration of diastolic function. Mechanisms involved in aging-associated cardiac alterations include ventricular–arterial stiffening, impaired $[Ca^{2+}]i$ regulation, physical deconditioning, and vascular dysfunction.[30] LV stiffness increases with normal aging, regardless of adequate blood pressure control and LV mass reductions.[31] The prevalence of hypertension increases with age, and more than 50% of individuals with age between 60 and 69 years of age and approximately 75% of those with age 70 years or older are affected.[4] As a result, aging and hypertension are remarkably related and interact with each other to cause LVDD.[24]

Ethnicity

Data from the ASCOT (Anglo-Scandinavian Cardiac Outcomes Trial) showed that, among hypertensive subjects, blacks had worse diastolic function than whites.[32] These differences were not explained by variation in blood pressure and LV mass, suggesting that blacks may have an increased susceptibility to cardiac dysfunction in response similar blood pressure levels. Likewise, analysis of the community-based population of the CARDIA study (Coronary Artery Risk Development in Young Adults) demonstrated that blacks have worse diastolic function compared with whites, which remained significant after adjustment for major cardiovascular risk factors and antihypertensive medications.[33]

Dietary Sodium Intake

Salt intake, measured from 24-hour urinary sodium excretion, was reported to be related to impaired diastolic function independent of LV mass in hypertensive but not normotensive individuals.[34] Additionally, low-sodium DASH (Dietary Approaches to Stop Hypertension) diet interventions were associated with favorable changes in diastolic function in a small sample of hypertensive subjects with LVDD.[35] Mechanisms underlying the association between high dietary sodium and LVDD may include sodium-induced increases in blood pressure parameters and large artery stiffness, which would ultimately lead to increases in the hemodynamic load to the heart.[36] In addition, salt intake seems to induce cardiac fibrosis independent of changes in hemodynamic load, suggesting that dietary sodium may exert direct effects on the myocardium.[37]

Obesity

Obesity exerts a substantial impact on cardiac structure and function and is associated with LVDD independent of blood pressure levels and hypertension. In response to excessive fat mass, obese individuals exhibit increases in total and central blood volume, which may result in eccentric hypertrophy and LVDD.[17] In addition, nonhemodynamic factors, including adipokines, inflammation, insulin resistance, sympathetic overdrive, and activation of the renin–angiotensin–aldosterone system may also contribute to obesity-associated LV dysfunction and remodeling.[5,38] Even though usually related to increases in LV mass, obesity-associated diastolic dysfunction may also occur in the absence of LV hypertrophy.

Obesity is a major risk factor for hypertension, and hypertension and obesity often coexist.[4] When hypertension occurs in obese subjects, pressure overload ensues, thus exerting an additional deleterious effect on LV function. Studies evaluating hypertensive populations have consistently shown impaired LV diastolic function in obese individuals relative to lean individuals, and the magnitude of LVDD is directly related to increases in body mass index.[39,40]

Diabetes Mellitus

Diabetes mellitus promotes structural and functional changes in the heart, independent of coronary heart disease and hypertension.[23,41] Biopsies of the diabetic heart usually reveal interstitial fibrosis and cardiomyocyte hypertrophy, and proposed mechanisms underlying these alterations include activation of the renin–angiotensin–aldosterone system, inflammation, hyperinsulinemia, hyperglycemia, and oxidative stress.[5,23,41] Impaired diastolic function is an earliest functional abnormality in diabetes-associated cardiomyopathy and is related to LV fibrosis and hypertrophy.[41] The coexistence of diabetes mellitus and systemic hypertension results in a negative synergistic effect on LV diastolic function and is related to higher filling pressures than in either condition alone.[42]

Chronic Kidney Disease

Patients with chronic kidney disease frequently have impaired diastolic function and the presence of LVDD inversely correlates with glomerular filtration rate levels.[18,43] Potential explanations for the greater prevalence of LVDD include the increased aortic stiffness often observed in chronic kidney disease and volume overload, which is particularly seen in end-stage renal disease.[18] In hypertensive subjects, the presence of chronic kidney disease is associated with worse diastolic function, independent of LV mass and brachial blood pressure measurements.[43,44]

PREVALENCE OF LEFT VENTRICULAR DIASTOLIC DYSFUNCTION IN HYPERTENSION

Extensive evidence has demonstrated that the prevalence of LVDD is substantial in hypertensive patients.[9,24,26,45–49] However, the precise estimation of the frequency of LVDD among hypertensive individuals is a difficult task, given that different imaging techniques and criteria have been used to define LVDD. Furthermore, marked differences in clinical characteristics may also influence the prevalence of LVDD among the studied populations. This is particularly challenging given the well-recognized age-related changes in tissue Doppler–based early myocardial relaxation (e') velocities, which makes the interpretation of noninvasive diastolic measures in the elderly challenging. As a result, great heterogeneity in the frequency of LVDD has been reported in hypertensive cohorts, with values ranging from 18% to 84% (**Table 1**).

LEFT VENTRICULAR DIASTOLIC DYSFUNCTION AND LEFT VENTRICULAR SYSTOLIC FUNCTION IN HYPERTENSIVE SUBJECTS

Several studies using measures of systolic function other than LV ejection fraction have demonstrated that a substantial proportion of hypertensive individuals with LVDD and preserved ejection fraction show subtle impairments in systolic function.[24,48,49] In particular, longitudinal strain, which is a more sensitive measure of LV systolic function than ejection fraction,[50] is impaired in hypertensive subjects with LVDD compared with those with normal diastolic function.[49] Longitudinal strain has been reported to be a powerful predictor of cardiovascular outcomes in patients with HFpEF, suggesting that decreases in systolic function may have important prognostic value in individuals with LVDD.[51] Systolic dysfunction and diastolic dysfunction are interrelated because of alterations in myocyte calcium cycling.[52] Furthermore, fibrosis not only impairs LV filling, but also limits the transduction of cardiac myocyte contraction into LV force development.[53] This body of evidence suggests a complex interplay between systolic and diastolic function, thus arguing against the concept that individuals with LVDD and normal ejection fraction have "isolated" diastolic dysfunction and challenging the perception of systolic abnormalities as a late alteration in the natural history of hypertension.[25,49]

PROGNOSIS AND TREATMENT

LVDD is a strong predictor of cardiovascular events[54–57] and HF[57,58] in hypertensive individuals, independent of blood pressure levels and LV mass. The greater risk associated with LVDD might be explained by the presence of subclinical coronary artery disease, which impairs LV diastolic function and is associated with higher rate of cardiovascular events. It is also possible that impairments in diastolic function are

Table 1
Prevalence of LV diastolic dysfunction in hypertensive populations

Study, Reference, Year	N	Women (%)	Mean Age, y	Prevalence of LVDD (%)	Echocardiographic Variables Used to Define LVDD	Prevalence of LVH (%)
Verdechia et al,[45] 1990	145	47	52	46	A/E ratio	15
Wachtell et al,[26] 2000	750	44	65	84	IVRT, E/A ratio and E-wave deceleration time	100[a]
De Simone et al,[46] 2005	1384	53	54	20	IVRT, E/A ratio and E-wave deceleration time	27
Zanchetti et al,[47] 2007	2545	51	70	46	IVRT, E/A ratio and E-wave deceleration time, pulmonary vein systolic/diastolic velocities ratio, and pulmonary vein peak A flow velocity	46
Sciarretta et al,[48] 2009	1073	48	59	66	E-wave deceleration time, E/A ratio, E/e' ratio and left atrial volume index.	N/A
Dini et al,[24] 2013	1556	52	66	18	E/e' ratio and left atrial volume index.	29
Ballo et al,[49] 2014	509	48	64	28	E/e' ratio, Ar–Ad duration, change in E/A ratio with the Valsalva maneuver, IVRT, pulmonary artery systolic pressure, and left atrial volume index	40
Santos et al,[9] 2016	3001	62	76	67	E-wave deceleration time, E/A ratio, E/e' ratio	N/A

Abbreviations: A, mitral peak A-wave velocity; Ar–Ad, difference between the atrial reversal waveform duration and mitral A-wave duration; E, mitral peak E-wave velocity; e', tissue Doppler imaging e' velocity; IVRT, isovolumic relaxation time; LV, left ventricular; LVDD, left ventricular diastolic dysfunction; LVH, left ventricular hypertrophy; N/A, not available.
  [a] LVH was defined by electrocardiography.

proportionate to the degree of hypertensive associated target organ damage. Therefore, LVDD may be acting as a marker of the deleterious effects of hypertension.[56]

Several studies have demonstrated consistently that lowering blood pressure with antihypertensive medications improves LV diastolic function.[57,59–62] This effect was seen with several antihypertensive classes, indicating that blood pressure reduction, rather than the use of specific antihypertensive agents, is important to improve LV diastolic function. Furthermore, the control of associated factors, including dietary sodium intake, obesity, and coronary artery disease, may further contribute to improve LVDD in hypertensive patients.[35,63,64] However, it is uncertain whether improvements in LVDD are translated into better cardiovascular outcome in hypertensive patients. Data from the LIFE study (Losartan Intervention for End Point Reduction in Hypertension) showed that antihypertensive treatment improved LV diastolic function, but such improvements were not associated with reductions in the composite endpoint of cardiovascular mortality, myocardial infarction, or stroke.[57] Likewise, large clinical trials testing different antihypertensive agents have failed to show improvements in mortality in patients with HFpEF, even though the impact on diastolic function, and whether this could identify particularly responsive subgroups, was not assessed.[5] Therefore, it remains unclear whether LVDD may be a target for therapy to prevent cardiovascular outcomes in hypertensive patients.

SUMMARY

Hypertension is the most important risk factor for LVDD in the community, and promotes LVDD through several mechanisms, including hemodynamic overload and myocardial ischemia. LVDD is a powerful predictor of cardiovascular events and HF, and blood pressure–lowering using antihypertensive medications improves LVDD. Nevertheless, it is uncertain whether improvements in LVDD may be translated into better cardiovascular outcome in hypertensive patients.

REFERENCES

1. Verma A, Solomon SD. Diastolic dysfunction as a link between hypertension and heart failure. Med Clin North Am 2009;93:647–64.
2. Wan SH, Vogel MW, Chen HH. Pre-clinical diastolic dysfunction. J Am Coll Cardiol 2014;63:407–16.
3. Redfield MM, Jacobsen SJ, Burnett JC Jr, et al. Burden of systolic and diastolic ventricular dysfunction in the community: appreciating the scope of the heart failure epidemic. JAMA 2003;289:194–202.
4. Chobanian AV, Bakris GL, Black HR, et al. Seventh report of the Joint National Committee on Prevention, Detection, Evaluation, and Treatment of High Blood Pressure. Hypertension 2003;42:1206–52.
5. Shah SJ, Kitzman DW, Borlaug BA, et al. Phenotype-specific treatment of heart failure with preserved ejection fraction: a multiorgan roadmap. Circulation 2016;134:73–90.
6. Owan TE, Hodge DO, Herges RM, et al. Trends in prevalence and outcome of heart failure with preserved ejection fraction. N Engl J Med 2006;355:251–9.
7. Gaasch WH, Zile MR. Left ventricular diastolic dysfunction and diastolic heart failure. Annu Rev Med 2004;55:373–94.
8. Kass DA, Bronzwaer JG, Paulus WJ. What mechanisms underlie diastolic dysfunction in heart failure? Circ Res 2004;94:1533–42.
9. Santos AB, Gupta DK, Bello NA, et al. Prehypertension is associated with abnormalities of cardiac structure and function in the atherosclerosis risk in communities study. Am J Hypertens 2016;29:568–74.
10. Galderisi M, Petrocelli A, Alfieri A, et al. Impact of ambulatory blood pressure on left ventricular diastolic dysfunction in uncomplicated arterial systemic hypertension. Am J Cardiol 1996;77:597–601.
11. Oe Y, Shimbo D, Ishikawa J, et al. Alterations in diastolic function in masked hypertension: findings from the masked hypertension study. Am J Hypertens 2013; 26:808–15.
12. Laurent S, Boutouyrie P. The structural factor of hypertension: large and small artery alterations. Circ Res 2015;116:1007–21.

13. Abhayaratna WP, Srikusalanukul W, Budge MM. Aortic stiffness for the detection of preclinical left ventricular diastolic dysfunction: pulse wave velocity versus pulse pressure. J Hypertens 2008;26:758–64.
14. Zhang Y, Li Y, Ding FH, et al. Cardiac structure and function in relation to central blood pressure components in Chinese. J Hypertens 2011;29:2462–8.
15. Zhang Y, Kollias G, Argyris AA, et al. Association of left ventricular diastolic dysfunction with 24-h aortic ambulatory blood pressure: the SAFAR study. J Hum Hypertens 2015;29:442–8.
16. Rossi GP, Cesari M, Cuspidi C, et al. Long-term control of arterial hypertension and regression of left ventricular hypertrophy with treatment of primary aldosteronism. Hypertension 2013;62:62–9.
17. Alpert MA, Omran J, Mehra A, et al. Impact of obesity and weight loss on cardiac performance and morphology in adults. Prog Cardiovasc Dis 2014;56:391–400.
18. London GM. Cardiovascular disease in chronic renal failure: pathophysiologic aspects. Semin Dial 2003;16:85–94.
19. Janardhanan R, Desai AS, Solomon SD. Therapeutic approaches to diastolic dysfunction. Curr Hypertens Rep 2009;11:283–91.
20. Vlasseros I, Katsi V, Vyssoulis G, et al. Aggravation of left ventricular diastolic dysfunction in hypertensives with coronary artery disease. Hypertens Res 2013;36:885–8.
21. Escobar E. Hypertension and coronary heart disease. J Hum Hypertens 2002;16: S61–3.
22. Nagueh SF, Smiseth OA, Appleton CP, et al. Recommendations for the evaluation of left ventricular diastolic function by echocardiography: an update from the American Society of Echocardiography and the European Association of Cardiovascular Imaging. J Am Soc Echocardiogr 2016;29:277–314.
23. Nadruz W. Myocardial remodeling in hypertension. J Hum Hypertens 2015;29: 1–6.
24. Dini FL, Galderisi M, Nistri S, et al. Abnormal left ventricular longitudinal function assessed by echocardiographic and tissue Doppler imaging is a powerful predictor of diastolic dysfunction in hypertensive patients: the SPHERE study. Int J Cardiol 2013;168:3351–8.
25. Santos M, Shah AM. Alterations in cardiac structure and function in hypertension. Curr Hypertens Rep 2014;16:428.
26. Wachtell K, Smith G, Gerdts E, et al. Left ventricular filling patterns in patients with systemic hypertension and left ventricular hypertrophy (the LIFE study). Losartan Intervention For Endpoint. Am J Cardiol 2000;85:466–72.
27. Phillips RA, Goldman ME, Ardeljan M, et al. Determinants of abnormal left ventricular filling in early hypertension. J Am Coll Cardiol 1989;14:979–85.
28. Fox ER, Taylor J, Taylor H, et al. Left ventricular geometric patterns in the Jackson cohort of the Atherosclerotic Risk in Communities (ARIC) study: clinical correlates and influences on systolic and diastolic dysfunction. Am Heart J 2007;153: 238–44.
29. Chahal NS, Lim TK, Jain P, et al. New insights into the relationship of left ventricular geometry and left ventricular mass with cardiac function: a population study of hypertensive subjects. Eur Heart J 2010;31:588–94.
30. Upadhya B, Taffet GE, Cheng CP, et al. Heart failure with preserved ejection fraction in the elderly: scope of the problem. J Mol Cell Cardiol 2015;83:73–87.
31. Borlaug B, Redfield M, Melenovsky V, et al. Longitudinal changes in left ventricular stiffness: a community-based study. Circ Heart Fail 2013;6:944–52.

32. Sharp A, Tapp R, Francis DP, et al. Ethnicity and left ventricular diastolic function in hypertension an ASCOT (Anglo-Scandinavian Cardiac Outcomes Trial) sub-study. J Am Coll Cardiol 2008;52:1015–21.

33. Kishi S, Reis JP, Venkatesh BA, et al. Race-ethnic and sex differences in left ventricular structure and function: the Coronary Artery Risk Development in Young Adults (CARDIA) Study. J Am Heart Assoc 2015;4:e001264.

34. Langenfeld MR, Schobel H, Veelken R, et al. Impact of dietary sodium intake on left ventricular diastolic filling in early essential hypertension. Eur Heart J 1998;19: 951–8.

35. Hummel SL, Seymour EM, Brook RD, et al. Low-sodium DASH diet improves diastolic function and ventricular-arterial coupling in hypertensive heart failure with preserved ejection fraction. Circ Heart Fail 2013;6:1165–71.

36. Cwynar M, Gąsowski J, Stompór T, et al. Blood pressure and arterial stiffness in patients with high sodium intake in relation to sodium handling and left ventricular diastolic dysfunction status. J Hum Hypertens 2015;29:583–91.

37. Frohlich ED, Varagic J. Sodium directly impairs target organ function in hypertension. Curr Opin Cardiol 2005;20:424–9.

38. de Simone G, Izzo R, De Luca N, et al. Left ventricular geometry in obesity: is it what we expect? Nutr Metab Cardiovasc Dis 2013;23:905–12.

39. Grandi AM, Zanzi P, Fachinetti A, et al. Insulin and diastolic dysfunction in lean and obese hypertensives: genetic influence. Hypertension 1999;34:1208–14.

40. Leggio M, Cruciani G, Sgorbini L, et al. Obesity-related adjunctive systo-diastolic ventricular dysfunction in patients with hypertension: echocardiographic assessment with tissue Doppler velocity and strain imaging. Hypertens Res 2011;34: 468–73.

41. Murarka S, Movahed MR. Diabetic cardiomyopathy. J Card Fail 2010;16:971–9.

42. Russo C, Jin Z, Homma S, et al. Effect of diabetes and hypertension on left ventricular diastolic function in a high-risk population without evidence of heart disease. Eur J Heart Fail 2010;12:454–61.

43. Yang Y, Wang Y, Shi ZW, et al. Association of E/E' and NT-proBNP with renal function in patients with essential hypertension. PLoS One 2013;8:e54513.

44. Nardi E, Cottone S, Mulè G, et al. Influence of chronic renal insufficiency on left ventricular diastolic function in hypertensives without left ventricular hypertrophy. J Nephrol 2007;20:320–8.

45. Verdecchia P, Schillaci G, Guerrieri M, et al. Prevalence and determinants of left ventricular filling abnormalities in an unselected hypertensive population. Eur Heart J 1990;11:679–91.

46. de Simone G, Kitzman DW, Chinali M, et al. Left ventricular concentric geometry is associated with impaired relaxation in hypertension: the Hypergen study. Eur Heart J 2005;26:1039–45.

47. Zanchetti A, Cuspidi C, Comarella L, et al. Left ventricular diastolic dysfunction in elderly hypertensives: results of the APROS-diadys study. J Hypertens 2007;25: 2158–67.

48. Sciarretta S, Paneni F, Ciavarella GM, et al. Evaluation of systolic properties in hypertensive patients with different degrees of diastolic dysfunction and normal ejection fraction. Am J Hypertens 2009;22:437–43.

49. Ballo P, Nistri S, Cameli M, et al. Association of left ventricular longitudinal and circumferential systolic dysfunction with diastolic function in hypertension: a nonlinear analysis focused on the interplay with left ventricular geometry. J Card Fail 2014;20:110–20.

50. Kalam K, Otahal P, Marwick TH. Prognostic implications of global LV dysfunction: a systematic review and meta-analysis of global longitudinal strain and ejection fraction. Heart 2014;100:1673–80.
51. Shah AM, Claggett B, Sweitzer NK, et al. Prognostic importance of impaired systolic function in heart failure with preserved ejection fraction and the impact of spironolactone. Circulation 2015;132:402–14.
52. Shah SJ, Aistrup GL, Gupta DK, et al. Ultrastructural and cellular basis for the development of abnormal myocardial mechanics during the transition from hypertension to heart failure. Am J Physiol Heart Circ Physiol 2014;306:H88–100.
53. Galderisi M. Diagnosis and management of left ventricular diastolic dysfunction in the hypertensive patient. Am J Hypertens 2011;24:507–17.
54. Schillaci G, Pasqualini L, Verdecchia P, et al. Prognostic significance of left ventricular diastolic dysfunction in essential hypertension. J Am Coll Cardiol 2002;39:2005–11.
55. Wang M, Yip GW, Wang AY, et al. Tissue Doppler imaging provides incremental prognostic value in patients with systemic hypertension and left ventricular hypertrophy. J Hypertens 2005;23:183–91.
56. Sharp AS, Tapp RJ, Thom SA, et al. Tissue Doppler E/E' ratio is a powerful predictor of primary cardiac events in a hypertensive population: an ASCOT substudy. Eur Heart J 2010;31:747–52.
57. Wachtell K, Palmieri V, Gerdts E, et al. Prognostic significance of left ventricular diastolic dysfunction in patients with left ventricular hypertrophy and systemic hypertension (the LIFE Study). Am J Cardiol 2010;106:999–1005.
58. Peterson GE, de Backer T, Contreras G, et al. Relationship of left ventricular hypertrophy and diastolic function with cardiovascular and renal outcomes in African Americans with hypertensive chronic kidney disease. Hypertension 2013;62:518–25.
59. Terpstra WF, May JF, Smit AJ, et al. Long-term effects of amlodipine and lisinopril on left ventricular mass and diastolic function in elderly, previously untreated hypertensive patients: the ELVERA trial. J Hypertens 2001;19:303–9.
60. Muller-Brunotte R, Kahan T, Malmqvist K, et al. Tissue velocity echocardiography shows early improvement in diastolic function with irbesartan and atenolol therapy in patients with hypertensive left ventricular hypertrophy. Results from the Swedish irbesartan left ventricular hypertrophy investigation vs atenolol (SILVHIA). Am J Hypertens 2006;19:927–36.
61. Solomon SD, Verma A, Desai A, et al. Effect of intensive versus standard blood pressure lowering on diastolic function in patients with uncontrolled hypertension and diastolic dysfunction. Hypertension 2010;55:241–8.
62. Tapp RJ, Sharp A, Stanton AV, et al. Differential effects of antihypertensive treatment on left ventricular diastolic function: an ASCOT (Anglo-Scandinavian Cardiac Outcomes Trial) substudy. J Am Coll Cardiol 2010;55:1875–81.
63. Ikonomidis I, Mazarakis A, Papadopoulos C, et al. Weight loss after bariatric surgery improves aortic elastic properties and left ventricular function in individuals with morbid obesity: a 3-year follow-up study. J Hypertens 2007;25:439–47.
64. Carluccio E, Biagioli P, Alunni G, et al. Effect of revascularizing viable myocardium on left ventricular diastolic function in patients with ischaemic cardiomyopathy. Eur Heart J 2009;30:1501–9.

Heart Failure and Hypertension

Importance of Prevention

Marc A. Pfeffer, MD, PhD

KEYWORDS

- Heart failure • Randomized clinical trials • Antihypertensive agents • Prevention

KEY POINTS

- Elevated blood pressure has the greatest population attributable risk for the development of heart failure.
- The mortality rates following the clinical recognition of heart failure is increased multifold.
- The treatment of hypertension with antihypertensive agents is particularly effective in preventing heart failure, which makes it the most effective therapy for heart failure.

Cumulative successes from randomized controlled clinical trials (RCTs) over the last 30 years in the treatment of patients with symptomatic heart failure with pharmacologic therapies as well as electrophysiological devices such as cardiac resynchronization therapy and autonomic implantable cardiac defibrillators have resulted in tangible improvements in prognosis.[1,2] These advancements are manifested by both an older age at which the first hospitalization for management of heart failure occurs as well as a lower rate of death following this initial hospitalization.[3] However, the RCTs that generated the evidence for these interventions that have favorably altered clinical practice, to date, have been entirely limited to the segment of the heart failure population with reduced ejection fraction (HFrEF). Those with symptomatic heart failure with a left ventricular ejection fraction (LVEF) that is only mildly impaired or even within the range considered normal (previously termed diastolic heart failure), now designated as heart failure with preserved ejection fraction (HFpEF), manifest the same signs and symptoms and have a similarly impaired quality of life.[4] These patients with HFpEF have only relatively recently been the focus of interventional clinical outcome RCTs. At present, none of the handful of RCTs targeting patients with HFpEF that were large enough to ascertain whether clinical outcomes can be altered has provided sufficiently robust evidence for an improvement in the prognosis for these patients.

Division of Cardiology, Department of Medicine, Brigham and Women's Hospital, Harvard Medical School, 75 Francis Street, Boston, MA 02115, USA
E-mail address: mpfeffer@rics.bwh.harvard.edu

Med Clin N Am 101 (2017) 19–28
http://dx.doi.org/10.1016/j.mcna.2016.08.012
0025-7125/17/© 2016 Elsevier Inc. All rights reserved.

Once heart failure becomes manifested by signs and symptoms, the subsequent risk of death is generally increased by a factor of 5- to 10-fold compared with similar cohorts that do not develop clinical heart failure. This major detrimental impact of heart failure on lifespan can be readily demonstrated within epidemiologic cohorts as well as with RCTs. In broad representative community populations such as the Framingham Heart Study and Atherosclerosis Risk In Communities (ARIC), the mortality following clinical heart failure has been between 40% to 50% within 5 years of the initial diagnosis.[5,6] This multifold heightened risk for death following the clinical recognition of heart failure regardless of LVEF has been recapitulated within RCTs. For example, in clinical trials that excluded those with heart failure or conducted analyses of those without a prior history of this syndrome, the development of the signs and symptoms of heart failure had a clear multifold detrimental impact on longevity. In the Heart Outcomes Protection Evaluation (HOPE), which excluded those with heart failure as well as reduced ejection fraction, those manifesting heart failure had a much higher mortality than the remainder of the population even after adjusting for other pertinent differences (**Fig. 1**).[7] Similarly, in Cholesterol And Recurrent Events (CARE), an early statin trial in patients with coronary artery disease, 28% of the 243 patients who developed heart failure died in 3.5 years compared with 7% mortality within 5 years of the remaining 3617 patients.[8] In the Aliskiren Trial in Type 2 Diabetes Using Cardio-Renal Endpoints (ALTITUDE), hospitalization for heart failure was the most common initially nonfatal major cardiovascular event compared with myocardial infarction and stroke, and was associated with the near sixfold increased risk of death compared with those in the study who did not have an initial nonfatal event.[9]

The adverse impact of heart failure goes beyond shortened life span, as frequent exacerbations of signs and symptoms requiring hospitalization are a hallmark of the severe morbidity of this clinical syndrome. With therapeutic advancements, especially for heart failure with reduced ejection fraction, and with the shift in the population demographics with a larger number of those aged 65 years and older living with heart failure, the burden of this frequent disorder both individually and to society with increased health care utilization expenses, has continued to increase. Indeed, heart failure remains the leading cause for hospitalization in the Medicare population.[10,11] That the prevalence of heart failure continues to expand can be considered a reflection on the advances in treatments. However, the important observation of an older age at

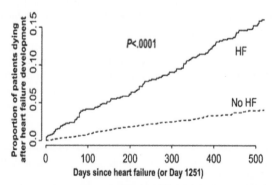

Fig. 1. Comparison of mortality rates between those who did and did not develop heart failure in the HOPE trial. (*From* Arnold JM, Yusuf S, Young J, et al. Prevention of heart failure in patients in the Heart Outcomes Prevention Evaluation (HOPE) Study. Circulation 2003;107:1285; with permission.)

which the initial hospitalization for heart failure occurs from unselected nationwide data, is in many respects even more important.[3] This key observation cannot be attributed to the many treatment advances for those with symptomatic heart failure; rather it provides clear evidence and a tribute to the effectiveness of preventive measures.

Heart failure should indeed be considered as a preventable disease. The critical importance of prevention was vividly underscored by the American College of Cardiology/American Heart Association (ACC/AHA) Staging Classification (A,B,C,D) of Heart Failure introduced in 2003.[12] That the first 2 of the 4 stages (A and B) designate individuals in the general population, those that do not even have heart failure is a major affirmation by the guideline writers of the critical importance for prevention. In fact, most in Stage A, by far the largest segment of adults in the community (those without symptomatic heart failure or overt structural heart disease), will never develop the clinical syndrome (**Fig. 2**). The emphasis on multiple prudent nonpharmacologic lifestyles choices underscores wise options to promote healthy aging, not just avoiding heart failure. Without any downside, abstinence from smoking lowers cancer as well as general cardiovascular risks. Because sensible lifestyle measures such as avoidance of smoking, maintaining a moderate level of physical activity, and prudent dietary selections are all associated with the benefits of lower cardiovascular risks without any overt negative consequences, they are uniformly promoted in primary (as well as secondary) prevention guidelines.[13,14]

Maintaining a reasonable level of physical activity has multiple virtues such as associated weight control and lowering risk for diabetes. Physical inactivity is considered an important modifiable risk factor for coronary heart disease.[15] A clear and statistically robust inverse association between activity levels above sedentary and risk of developing heart failure has also been consistently reported.[16] Indeed, a recent

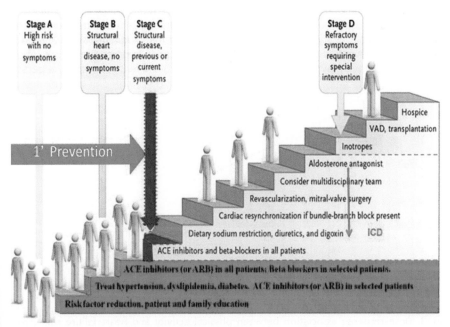

Fig. 2. Stages of heart failure and treatment options for systolic heart failure. (*Adapted from* Jessup M, Brozena S. Heart failure. N Engl J Med 2003;348:2013.)

meta-analysis of over 350,000 participants in prospective cohort studies showed a progressive lowering in the hazard ratio for developing heart failure as a function of physical activity levels (**Fig. 3**).[17] In the Framingham Heart Study, this protective association between physical activity was observed for the risk of both preserved and reduced ejection fraction heart failure.[18]

As a consequence of the increasing incidence of obesity and related diabetes along with great strides in acute coronary care management leading to more survivors of myocardial infarction, the at-risk reservoir for heart failure continues to expand. Hypertension is, however, the leading treatable predisposing risk factor for the development of symptomatic heart failure. This inauspicious distinction is a function of both the wide prevalence of elevated arterial pressure in aging adults and the magnitude of the adverse impact higher blood pressure has for the manifestation of heart failure.[19] The lifetime risk of developing heart failure represents another quantitative expression of the importance of elevated blood pressure and these other contributors. It is estimated that 1 in 5 adults will develop heart failure and that this number is approximately 1 in 3 or 4 for those with a blood pressure greater than 160 mm Hg. Consider a 60-year-old man with a blood pressure less than 140 mm Hg having a lifetime risk of 17.4% rising to 29% for those with a blood pressure of 160 mm Hg or greater. Similarly, the lifetime risk of a 60-year-old woman with a blood pressure less than 140 mm Hg goes from 14.4% to 27% for those with a blood pressure of 160 mm Hg.[19] These numbers would be hollow and would have little impact were it not for the ability to meaningfully and substantially lower this risk with antihypertensive agents.

Focusing on nonmutually exclusive contributors to the development of heart failure should not be considered as a contest, as there are no winners, but rather as collective opportunities to lower one's chance of living a fuller life without the morbidity and premature mortality associated with heart failure and other major cardiovascular conditions. Conceptually, if the risk factor is modifiable, then the higher the attributable risk, the greater the potential is to avoid or prevent. As a more global risk assessment is made for each individual, physicians and their patients have a broader perspective combining multiple lifestyle and when appropriate pharmacologic therapies to reduce the hazards of adverse cardiovascular events. The decision to prescribe chronic pharmacologic therapy to lower risks for future cardiovascular events exposes the person

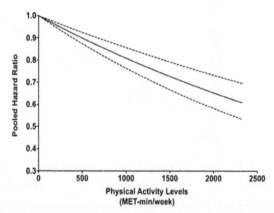

Fig. 3. Dose–response association between physical activity and heart failure risk. (*From* Pandey A, Garg S, Khunger M, et al. Dose-response relationship between physical activity and risk of heart failure: a meta-analysis. Circulation 2015;132:1792; with permission.)

to the potential for adverse drug effects as well as medical expenses and inconveniences. Physicians and patients need convincing data regarding both the potential benefits and the undesirable aspects of therapy to make informed decisions. This is especially pertinent when treating asymptomatic individuals in whom motivation is essential to sustain long-term therapy.

Effective primary prevention requires a more global assessment of risk profile rather than addressing 1 aspect of the multifactorial process. In addition to recommendations for lifestyle changes for appropriate individuals, pharmacologic therapies can have highly important favorable impacts on risks.[13,14] When viewed as multiple opportunities rather than single approaches, statins and antihypertensive therapies are probably the most important pharmacologic cornerstones for prevention. Statins are obviously administered to reduce risk for atherosclerotic events such as vascular death, myocardial infarction, and stroke. A meta-analysis of over 170,000 patients in well conducted RCTs provide some of the strongest data regarding the efficacy and safety of these agents.[20] Although used to reduce atherosclerotic events, it should be appreciated that favorable outcomes for heart failure have also been demonstrated. Indeed, in the first major clinical outcome trial of a statin, the Scandinavian Simvastatin Survival Study (4S), which demonstrated a survival benefit of a statin in a high-risk, high-cholesterol population, also showed that fewer people randomized to simvastatin developed heart failure.[21] Even more recent studies concentrating on the intensity of lipid-lowering therapy provide clear evidence of lower rates of hospitalization for heart failure with the use of higher doses of statins (**Fig. 4**).[22]

Perhaps the most impressive heritage of RCTs to generate data for clinical decision making in cardiovascular medicine concerns the use of antihypertensive medications to prevent morbidity and prolong survival in subjects with elevated arterial pressure. The initial and now truly historic first 2 randomized clinical outcome trials in cardiovascular medicine, the Veterans Cooperative Studies, clearly showed that the use of pharmacologic agents to lower blood pressure resulted in reduced rates of heart failure, stroke, abdominal aortic aneurysm, and premature cardiovascular death.[23,24] These early pioneering trials from the late 1960s and early 1970s demonstrating the benefits

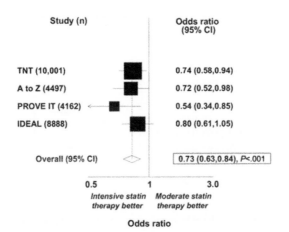

Fig. 4. Differential reduction in heart failure with higher doses of statins. (*From* Scirica BM, Morrow DA, Cannon CP, et al. Intensive statin therapy and the risk of hospitalization for heart failure after an acute coronary syndrome in the PROVE IT-TIMI 22 study. J Am Coll Cardiol 2006;47:2329; with permission.)

of chronic antihypertensive therapies were repeatedly confirmed and extended in much larger populations of subjects with less severe hypertension.[25] As such, chronic pharmacologic treatment of elevated blood pressure is a cornerstone for prevention of cardiovascular diseases.

Because the epidemiology of blood pressure and risk does not have a discrete threshold, multiple studies have been done addressing the level of blood pressure where the benefits of pharmacologic treatment outweighed the adverse effects of therapy. Elevated systolic pressure was subsequently found to be a more appropriate target in adults for initiating pharmacologic therapy for therapy.[26,27] In the Systolic Hypertension in the Elderly Program (SHEP), the primary outcome of fatal and nonfatal stroke was reduced by 36% with the use of stepped care antihypertensive agents (chlorthalidone, atenolol, reserpine) compared with placebo. It is noteworthy that heart failure was also reduced by an even greater degree, 54% in the active therapy group.[27] In a meta-analysis demonstrating that major reductions in cardiovascular death, stroke, and heart failure were all readily achieved compared with placebo, the largest benefit observed with antihypertensive therapy was in the prevention of heart failure (**Fig. 5**).[28] Similarly, in the more recent Hypertension in the Very Elderly Trial (HYVET), and perhaps the last placebo-controlled trial in hypertension, patients age 80 year or older with a systolic pressure 160 mm Hg or more were enrolled. The primary endpoint of fatal or nonfatal stroke was marginally reduced by 30% in the active therapy group ($P = .06$). However, there was a more marked 64% reduction in the rate of heart failure ($P<.001$) in the group assigned to antihypertensive agents (indapamide followed by perindodril) compared with placebo.[29]

The importance of antihypertensive therapy is so well documented and ingrained that many of the recent studies compare antihypertensive agents to each other rather than to placebo. In the largest of these efforts, the Antihypertensive and Lipid Lowering to Prevent Heart Attack Trial (ALLHAT), chlorthalidone, a diuretic, was found to be superior to either the angiotensin converting enzyme (ACE) inhibitor linsinopril or the calcium channel blocker amlodipine, with respect to the development of heart failure.[30] It is important to note that an arm of this study comparing the alpha blocker doxazosin to chlorthalidone was stopped prematurely when concerning higher rates of congestive heart failure (LVEF not determined) were observed in the doxazosin

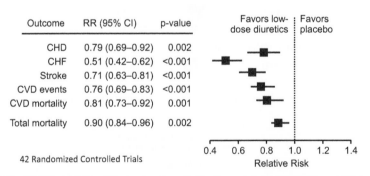

Fig. 5. Risk reductions with antihypertensive medications versus placebo for multiple cardiovascular outcomes. (*Adapted from* Psaty BM, Lumley T, Furberg CD, et al. Health outcomes associated with various antihypertensive therapies used as first-line agents: a network meta-analysis. JAMA 2003;289:2541.)

group.[31] Other comparative studies have suggested additional differences between antihypertensive agents, with fewer strokes with the use of the angiotensin receptor blocker losartan compared with a beta blocker atenolol in Losartan Intervention For Endpoint (LIFE), with no difference in the development of heart failure in the 2 active therapy arms.[32] However, in general, most experts emphasize the importance of blood pressure reduction rather than the specific pharmacologic agent utilized.[33] In practical terms, because most patients with hypertension require more than 1 agent to adequately control their elevated blood pressure, the question of 1 drug versus another becomes secondary to the importance of obtaining and sustaining adequate control of elevated blood pressure.

With the importance of initiating antihypertensive agents to control blood pressure in those with hypertension so firmly established, a more recent focus of major RCTs was on the determining the desired target level of blood pressure to strive to achieve with antihypertensive drugs. This practical question of the target pressure level is a critical issue, since increased intensity translates to more drugs and higher doses that are not without adverse consequences. Improved clinical outcomes would be the only justification for this approach, and reliable data from RCTs on the benefits and risks are needed to base these recommendations. Fortunately, this important aspect of clinical care issue was addressed in the Action to Control Cardiovascular Risk in Diabetes (ACCORD) and the Systolic Blood Pressure Intervention Trial (SPRINT). Both trials randomized large numbers of high-risk cardiovascular patients with (ACCORD) or without diabetes (SPRINT), and compared cardiovascular event rates in those allocated to a target systolic blood pressure of either less 120 mm Hg

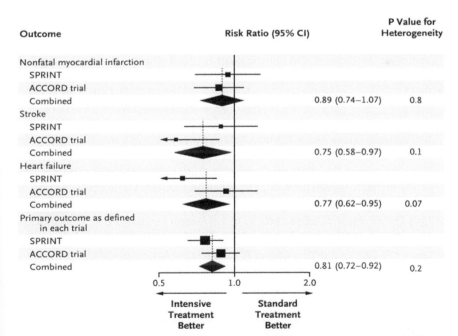

Fig. 6. Combined outcome data from ACCORD and SPRINT showing important reductions in heart failure and stroke with the target blood pressure of 120 mm Hg systolic compared with less than 140 mm Hg. (*From* Perkovic V, Rodgers A. Redefining blood-pressure targets–SPRINT starts the marathon. N Engl J Med 2015;373:2177; with permission.)

(intensive) or 140 mm Hg (standard).[34,35] In ACCORD, there was not a clear clinical benefit demonstrated with the more intensive strategy.[34] However, in larger SPRINT of high cardiovascular risk populations (excluding patients with diabetes), the improvements in prognosis with higher-intensity antihypertensive therapy were so profound that the trial stopped prematurely for efficacy.[35] An accompanying editorial provides an important perspective, indicating that the collective results of these 2 major recent trials support the lower blood pressure goals.[36] Indeed, the most blood pressure-sensitive endpoints of heart failure and stroke were reduced when the outcomes of the 2 trials were combined (**Fig. 6**).

The treatment of hypertension has many profound favorable outcomes and is a key factor for the prevention of heart failure. Moreover, prevention should be considered the most effective therapy for heart failure (both reduced and preserved ejection fraction). However, treating an asymptomatic individual with pharmacologic agents to prevent a possible future adverse cardiovascular event requires motivation (belief in the data). The translation of the results of SPRINT into clinical practice means recommending more pills, which requires a degree of trust between the caregivers and patients. Few physicians will anticipate hearing "Thank you doctor for the additional pill to lower my risk." The motivation must come from legacy RCTs.

REFERENCES

1. Yancy CW, Jessup M, Bozkurt B, et al. 2016 ACC/AHA/HFSA focused update on new pharmacological therapy for heart failure: an update of the 2013 ACCF/AHA guideline for the management of heart failure: a report of the American College of Cardiology/American Heart Association Task Force on clinical practice guidelines and the Heart Failure Society of America. J Am Coll Cardiol 2016;68: 1476–88.

2. Ponikowski P, Voors AA, Anker SD, et al. 2016 ESC guidelines for the diagnosis and treatment of acute and chronic heart failure: the task force for the diagnosis and treatment of acute and chronic heart failure of the European Society of Cardiology (ESC). Developed with the special contribution of the Heart Failure Association (HFA) of the ESC. Eur J Heart Fail 2016;18(8):891–975.

3. Jhund PS, Macintyre K, Simpson CR, et al. Long-term trends in first hospitalization for heart failure and subsequent survival between 1986 and 2003: a population study of 5.1 million people. Circulation 2009;119:515–23.

4. Lewis EF, Lamas GA, O'Meara E, et al. Characterization of health-related quality of life in heart failure patients with preserved versus low ejection fraction in CHARM. Eur J Heart Fail 2007;9:83–91.

5. Levy D, Kenchaiah S, Larson MG, et al. Long-term trends in the incidence of and survival with heart failure. N Engl J Med 2002;347:1397–402.

6. Loehr LR, Rosamond WD, Chang PP, et al. Heart failure incidence and survival (from the Atherosclerosis Risk in Communities study). Am J Cardiol 2008;101: 1016–22.

7. Arnold JM, Yusuf S, Young J, et al. Prevention of heart failure in patients in the Heart Outcomes Prevention Evaluation (HOPE) study. Circulation 2003;107: 1284–90.

8. Lewis EF, Moyé LA, Rouleau JL, et al. Predictors of late development of heart failure in stable survivors of myocardial infarction: the CARE study. J Am Coll Cardiol 2003;42:1446–53.

9. Jhund PS, McMurray JJ, Chaturvedi N, et al. Mortality following a cardiovascular or renal event in patients with type 2 diabetes in the ALTITUDE trial. Eur Heart J 2015;36:2463–9.

10. Ziaeian B, Fonarow GC. Epidemiology and aetiology of heart failure. Nat Rev Cardiol 2016;13:368–78.

11. Roger VL. Epidemiology of heart failure. Circ Res 2013;113:646–59.

12. Jessup M, Brozena S. Heart failure. N Engl J Med 2003;348:2007–18.

13. Goff DC Jr, Lloyd-Jones DM, Bennett G, et al. 2013 ACC/AHA guideline on the assessment of cardiovascular risk: a report of the American College of Cardiology/American Heart Association Task Force on practice guidelines. J Am Coll Cardiol 2014;63:2935–59.

14. Piepoli MF, Hoes AW, Agewall S, et al. European guidelines on cardiovascular disease prevention in clinical practice: The sixth joint task force of the european society of cardiology and other societies on cardiovascular disease prevention in clinical practise (constituted by representatives of 10 societies and by invited experts). Developed with the special contribution of the european association for cardiovascular prevention & rehabilitation (EACPR). Eur Heart J 2016;37: 2315–81.

15. Eckel RH, Jakicic JM, Ard JD, et al. 2013 AHA/ACC guideline on lifestyle management to reduce cardiovascular risk: a report of the American College of Cardiology/American Heart Association Task Force on Practice Guidelines. Circulation 2014;129:S76–99.

16. Andersen K, Mariosa D, Adami HO, et al. Dose-response relationship of total and leisure time physical activity to risk of heart failure: a prospective cohort study. Circ Heart Fail 2014;7:701–8.

17. Pandey A, Garg S, Khunger M, et al. Dose-response relationship between physical activity and risk of heart failure: a meta-analysis. Circulation 2015;132: 1786–94.

18. Kraigher-Krainer E, Lyass A, Massaro JM, et al. Association of physical activity and heart failure with preserved vs. reduced ejection fraction in the elderly: the Framingham Heart Study. Eur J Heart Fail 2013;15:742–6.

19. Lloyd-Jones DM, Larson MG, Leip EP, et al. Lifetime risk for developing congestive heart failure: the Framingham Heart Study. Circulation 2002;106:3068–72.

20. Baigent C, Blackwell L, Embersen J, et al. Efficacy and safety of more intensive lowering of LDL cholesterol: a meta-analysis of data from170,000 participants in 26 randomised trials. Lancet 2010;376:1670–81.

21. Kjekshus J, Pedersen TR, Olsson AG, et al. The effects of simvastatin on the incidence of heart failure in patients with coronary heart disease. J Card Fail 1997;3: 249–54.

22. Scirica BM, Morrow DA, Cannon CP, et al. Intensive statin therapy and the risk of hospitalization for heart failure after an acute coronary syndrome in the PROVE IT-TIMI 22 study. J Am Coll Cardiol 2006;47:2326–31.

23. Veterans Administration Cooperative Study Group on Antihypertensive Agents. Effects of treatment on morbidity in hypertension. Results in patients with diastolic blood pressures averaging 115 through 129 mm Hg. JAMA 1967;202:1028–34.

24. Veterans Administration Cooperative Study Group on Antihypertensive Agents. Effects of treatment on morbidity in hypertension: II. Results in patients with diastolic blood pressure averaging 90 through 114 mmHg. JAMA 1970;213: 1143–52.

25. Pfeffer MA, McMurray JJV. Lessons in uncertainty and humility - Clinical trials involving hypertension. N Eng J Med 2016; Nov (in press).

26. Staessen JA, Fagard R, Thijs L, et al. Randomised double-blind comparison of placebo and active treatment for older patients with isolated systolic hypertension. The Systolic Hypertension in Europe (Syst-Eur) Trial Investigators. Lancet 1997;350:757–64.

27. Prevention of stroke by antihypertensive drug treatment in older persons with isolated systolic hypertension. Final results of the Systolic Hypertension in the Elderly Program (SHEP). SHEP Cooperative Research Group. JAMA 1991;265: 3255–64.

28. Psaty BM, Lumley T, Furberg CD, et al. Health outcomes associated with various antihypertensive therapies used as first-line agents: a network meta-analysis. JAMA 2003;289:2534–44.

29. Beckett NS, Peters R, Fletcher AE, et al. Treatment of hypertension in patients 80 years of age or older. N Engl J Med 2008;358:1887–98.

30. ALLHAT Officers and Coordinators for the ALLHAT Collaborative Research Group, The Antihypertensiveand Lipid-Lowering Treatment to Prevent Heart Attack Trial. Major outcomes in high-risk hypertensive patients randomized to angiotensin-converting enzyme inhibitor or calcium channel blocker vs diuretic: the Antihypertensive and Lipid-Lowering Treatment to Prevent Heart Attack Trial (ALLHAT). JAMA 2002;288:2981–97.

31. ALLHAT Collaborative Research Group. Major cardiovascular events in hypertensive patients randomized to doxazosin vs chlorthalidone: the Antihypertensive and Lipid-Lowering Treatment to Prevent Heart Attack Trial (ALLHAT). JAMA 2000;283:1967–75.

32. Dahlof B, Devereux RB, Kjeldsen SE, et al. Cardiovascular morbidity and mortality in the Losartan Intervention For Endpoint reduction in hypertension study (LIFE): a randomised trial against atenolol. Lancet 2002;359:995–1003.

33. Turnbull F. Effects of different blood-pressure-lowering regimens on major cardiovascular events: results of prospectively-designed overviews of randomised trials. Lancet 2003;362:1527–35.

34. Cushman WC, Evans GW, Byington RP, et al. Effects of intensive blood-pressure control in type 2 diabetes mellitus. N Engl J Med 2010;362:1575–85.

35. Wright JT Jr, Williamson JD, Whelton PK, et al. A randomized trial of intensive versus standard blood-pressure control. N Engl J Med 2015;373:2103–16.

36. Perkovic V, Rodgers A. Redefining blood-pressure targets–SPRINT starts the marathon. N Engl J Med 2015;373:2175–8.

Hypertension, Left Ventricular Hypertrophy, and Myocardial Ischemia

Tony Stanton, MBChB, PhD, FCSANZ, FESC, FRCP, FRACP[a],
Francis G. Dunn, MBChB, FRCP[b],*

KEYWORDS

- Hypertension • Ischemia • Perfusion • Mechanisms • Management

KEY POINTS

- Myocardial ischemia contributes in a major way to the morbidity and mortality associated with hypertension and hypertensive heart disease (HHD).
- There are a variety of mechanisms that contribute to the production of myocardial ischemia in hypertension. Although coronary artery disease (CAD) may be an important associated factor in the production of ischemia, it is not a prerequisite and many patients with hypertension have ischemia with normal coronary arteries.
- Management of such patients should include a search for myocardial ischemia and, if present, a tailored approach to treatment that encompasses both risk factors management and selection of medications that can effectively control arterial pressure and prevent or lessen myocardial ischemia.

INTRODUCTION AND OVERVIEW

The devastating effects of hypertension on the heart prior to the introduction of antihypertensive therapy are inclined to be forgotten. Patients graphically describe a feeling of drowning as pulmonary edema takes hold. One of the authors (FD) remembers being a young physician treating such patients. One of the most dramatic benefits of antihypertensive therapy has been the reduction in morbidity and mortality from HHD. This considerable benefit is comparable with the reduction in stroke and in renal failure using similarly well-selected antihypertensive therapy.

Hypertension, dyslipidemia, glucose intolerance, cigarette smoking, and left ventricular hypertrophy (LVH) are the main, independent modifiable risk factors for cardiovascular disease.[1] In addition, hypertension is a pathophysiologic template for

Disclosure Statement: We have no commercial, financial, or funding sources relevant to this article.
[a] Nambour Hospital, School of Medicine, University of Queensland, Medical Suites, Level 2, Nambour, Queensland 4556, Australia; [b] University of Glasgow, Glasgow G12 8QQ, Scotland
* Corresponding author. Stobhill Hospital, Glasgow G21 3UW, Scotland.
E-mail address: fgdunn@sky.com

Med Clin N Am 101 (2017) 29–41
http://dx.doi.org/10.1016/j.mcna.2016.08.003
0025-7125/17/© 2016 Elsevier Inc. All rights reserved.

medical.theclinics.com

myocardial ischemia and there is secure epidemiologic evidence demonstrating its importance as a risk factor for angina, myocardial fibrosis, myocardial infarction, and sudden death.[1,2] Furthermore, this relationship strengthens progressively as the arterial pressure rises and when LVH coexists as identified by Electrocardiography (ECG) or echocardiography.[2] An excess of 40% of the attributable risk for these manifestations of ischemia is due to hypertension.

It is worth dwelling in particular on sudden death. Men with hypertension and LVH have a 6-fold to 8-fold, and women 3-fold, increased risk of sudden cardiac death presumably due to ventricular arrhythmias. Despite major ongoing research, this problem remains a most elusive condition to predict and, therefore, to prevent. Myocardial ischemia is a potent stimulus for ventricular tachydysrhythmias and hypertension provides a perfect medium for these catastrophic events, which are increased further in the presence of LVH.

The development of CAD in patients with hypertension is a complex interaction of direct hemodynamic effects, genetic predisposition, endothelial dysfunction, oxidative stress, and humoral factors. Although associated obstructive CAD is a key factor in this kaleidoscope, other factors are involved as a consequence of hypertension and LVH. Understanding the background pathophysiology to myocardial ischemia allows therapy to be targeted more effectively with subsequent reduction in these clinical sequelae (**Fig. 1**).

PATHOPHYSIOLOGY OF MYOCARDIAL ISCHEMIA IN HYPERTENSIVE HEART DISEASE

HHD is the heart's response to sustained arterial hypertension. It is initially a functionally adaptive process in response to increased left ventricular (LV) afterload. The hallmarks of this process are the development of LVH, myocardial ischemia, diastolic dysfunction, myocardial fibrosis, apoptosis, cardiomyocyte growth, endothelial dysfunction, and increased arterial stiffness.[3] These factors combine to produce a maladaptive feedback loop (**Fig. 2**). The most easily identifiable phenotypic expression of HHD is LV remodeling, which ultimately leads to LVH.

Types of Left Ventricular Remodeling

Cardiac remodeling is defined as "alterations in size, geometry, shape, composition and function of the heart resulting from cardiac load or injury."[4] There are 3 recognized types of remodeling[5]: concentric, eccentric, and post–myocardial infarction, which has particular relevance to this article. A mixed picture occurs as the infarcted myocardium becomes stretched, leading to an increase in LV cavity size, with subsequent increased pressure on the noninfarcted myocardium to maintain stroke volume.

In hypertension, the development of LVH occurs as the heart remodels in the presence of increased LV load. This sustained rise in blood pressure (BP) produces increased LV wall stress. This is compensated for physiologically with the changes in wall thickness and radius.

As BP increases there is increased LV wall stress, compensated for by thickening of the LV wall (concentric remodeling).[6] Thus, the increased LV wall stress is a major determinant of myocardial oxygen demand and myocardial ischemia is a hallmark of this process.

FACTORS PREDISPOSING TO LEFT VENTRICULAR HYPERTROPHY
Nonhemodynamic Factors

Hypertension provides a sustained hemodynamic load on the LV, which remodels in an attempt to normalize wall stress and regulate myocardial oxygen consumption.

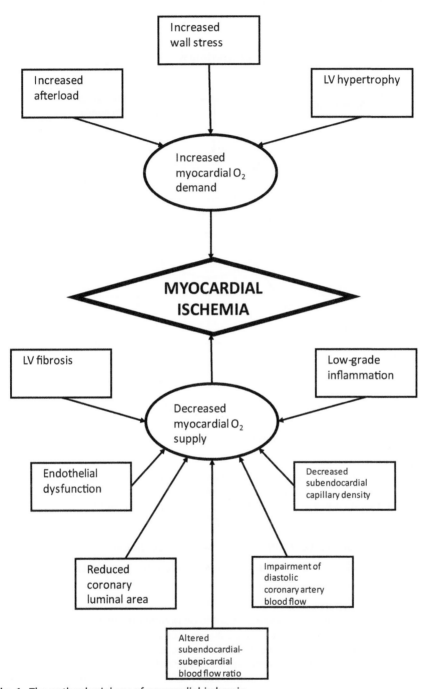

Fig. 1. The pathophysiology of myocardial ischemia.

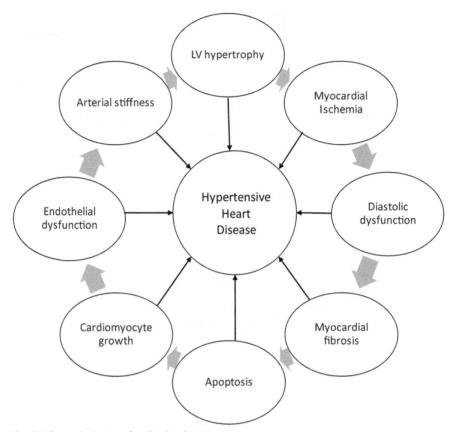

Fig. 2. The maladaptive feedback of HHD.

There are numerous nonhemodynamic factors, however, which influence the development of LVH, including gender, ethnicity, genetics, diabetes, obesity, and dietary salt intake. Although intensive advice and support are often supplied to hypertensive patients, lifestyle intervention is not usually effective.[7]

Hemodynamic Factors: Ventricular and Systemic Maladaptation

The typical maladaptive changes seen in myocardial architecture include the following.

Cardiomyocyte hypertrophy

Traditionally, cardiomyocytes were thought to be postmitotic, with the heart unable to regenerate cardiomyocytes after cell death (eg, postmyocardial infarction). Contemporary evidence suggests, however, that cardiac cells, both cardiomyocytes and interstitial cells, are continually replaced by newer cell populations. It is likely, therefore, that LVH results from a combination of both extracellular fibrosis and hypertrophy.[8]

Concentric remodeling is classically due to the addition of new sarcomeres in parallel, causing an increase in cardiomyocyte width whereas in eccentric hypertrophy the addition of sarcomeres in series increases cardiomyocyte length.[9] The exact molecular mechanism by which this difference in response occurs is not yet elucidated.

Myocardial fibrosis

Pressure overload and humoral stimuli, such as catecholamines, local components of the renin-angiotensin system, endothelins, and certain growth factors, have all been shown to promote myocardial fibrosis as evidenced by increased interstitial and perivascular collagen deposition.[10] Hypertension is a potent stimulus for fibrosis, with 1 postmortem study showing that the volume fraction of fibrosis in hypertensive hearts was 31.1% compared with 6.5% in nonhypertensive controls.[11]

Seminal work by Frohlich[12] demonstrated that fibrosis was also a part of the normal aging process, which can then be accelerated by hypertension. Experimental work demonstrated a progressive increase in collagen deposition was linked to evolving myocardial ischemia, evident as reduced LV and right ventricular coronary blood flow and flow reserve.

Fibrosis is, however, a dynamic process as shown by the ability of medications that inhibit the renin-angiotensin system to substantially reduce it.[13] The antifibrotic effects of mineralocorticoid receptor antagonists, such as spironolactone, have also been shown in hypertension.[14] The development, and thus the prevention, of myocardial fibrosis is important given this is a critical factor in the development of diastolic dysfunction and eventual cardiac failure.[15]

Arterial stiffness

The vasculature undergoes similar changes to the myocardium in response to hypertension. Direct pressure overload, humoral stimulation, angiotensin II, endothelins, and nitric oxide all contribute to excessive collagen deposition in the vessels walls.[16] Vascular smooth muscle mass and tone are increased with overall stiffening of large vessels. Raised pulse pressure, the major hemodynamic consequence of increased aortic pulse wave velocity, has been shown to be a potent risk marker in hypertensive patients independent of BP.[17]

Endothelial dysfunction

Among hypertensive patients, 60% exhibit impaired small artery vasodilatation in vitro.[18] Critical to this process is the impaired synthesis of nitric oxide from the amino acid L-arginine by the coronary endothelium. There is an increase in reactive oxygen species (oxidative stress), which scavenge available nitric oxide leading to the impaired vasodilatation of vascular smooth muscle cells and end-organ ischemia. Endothelial dysfunction can be improved in hypertension by administration of L-arginine.[19]

Inflammation

Inflammation, most commonly measured using plasma C-reactive protein (CRP) levels, has been linked to hypertension, the development of LVH, and subsequent cardiovascular morbidity and mortality.[20] The anti-inflammatory action of statins is one of the putative methods by which they promote LV mass regression, although a recent randomized study of rosuvastatin failed to show a reduction in LV mass despite a reduction in CRP levels in hypertensive individuals.[21] Conversely, angiotensin II receptor blockers have been shown to reduce microscopic evidence of fibrosis, CRP, markers of inflammation (high-sensitivity–tumor necrosis factor α and interleukin-6), vasoconstriction, and, ultimately, cardiac fibrosis in hypertension.[22,23]

Apoptosis

Apoptosis is programmed cell death most often by a biological stimulus. Hypertension is a common, progressive cause of cardiomyocyte apoptosis, especially in LVH. Increased angiotensin II is often the causative stimulus.[24] It is thought that apoptosis plays a pivotal role in the transition from preserved ventricular function to cardiac failure. Inhibition of angiotensin II, using the angiotensin II receptor blocker losartan, has been shown to attenuate cardiac apoptosis, independent of the effect on BP, in both animal and human studies.[24,25]

MYOCARDIAL ISCHEMIA
Hypertension and Myocardial Ischemia with Associated Coronary Artery Disease

Hypertension is an established risk factor for atherosclerotic CAD and cerebrovascular disease.[26] The development of CAD in patients with hypertension is a complex interaction of direct hemodynamic effects, genetic predisposition, endothelial dysfunction, oxidative stress, and humoral factors, such as angiotensin II and catecholamines (discussion of which is beyond the scope of this review).

Hypertension and Myocardial Ischemia Without Coronary Artery Disease

Myocardial ischemia is a hallmark of HHD even in the absence of CAD. There is evidence of reduced coronary flow reserve (CFR) and subendocardial and microvascular ischemia[27] at all levels of hypertension (**Box 1**).[3]

As LV mass increases, there is increased oxygen demand. Cardiomyocytes hypertrophy to compensate for this. There is no corresponding increase, however, in capillary numbers with a resultant mismatch between capillary and myocyte numbers (reduced relative capillary density). Thus, as oxygen demand increases, perfusion is unable to compensate accordingly. Pathophysiologically, there is a reduction in CFR (the ratio of hyperemic to baseline myocardial blood flow) and an increase in minimal coronary vascular resistance.[28] This phenomenon is termed, *coronary microvascular dysfunction*. Commonly, this causes no problems at rest during resting condition with decompensation occurring when the myocardium is placed under stress (eg, exercise or pharmacologic agents). This explains the high prevalence of myocardial ischemia seen in hypertensive patients with nonobstructive CAD[29] and the subsequent elevated risk of major adverse cardiac events and all-cause mortality.[30]

Coronary microvascular dysfunction is assessed indirectly given the absence of a technique to visualize the microcirculation in vivo. Although invasive techniques exist that allow the assessment of CFR using intracoronary Doppler guide wires, this technique is rarely used in HHD. Detailed assessment of the subendocardium, which is particularly vulnerable to ischemia in HHD, can, however, be undertaken noninvasively.[31]

Box 1
Factors in hypertensive heart disease resulting in ischemia

- Ventricular fibrosis with associated extraventricular ischemia
- Coronary arteriolar constriction due to fibrosis.
- Endothelial dysfunction of coronary resistance vessels
- Reduced coronary luminal area in relation to increased LV mass
- Increased LV wall tension
- Altered subendocardial-subepicardial blood flow ratio
- Impairment of diastolic coronary artery blood flow
- Decreased subendocardial capillary density
- Inflammatory responses

DETECTION OF MYOCARDIAL ISCHEMIA IN HYPERTENSION

Because hypertension can produce myocardial ischemia, clinical assessment is required to assess this. A thorough history with direct questioning on possible symptoms of ischemia is required with an assessment of cardiovascular risk factors. Other precipitants for ischemia, such as atrial fibrillation, aortic stenosis, hypertrophic cardiomyopathy, anemia, and thyrotoxicosis, should be sought as should clinical evidence of atherosclerotic disease.

Electrocardiography

ST and T-wave repolarization changes (LV strain pattern) on a resting ECG are known markers of adverse prognosis.[32] Measurement of myocardial strain and CFR using echocardiography have shown that this pattern is due to subendocardial microcirculatory and reduced CFR.[33] Increased QRS duration and QT prolongation have also been linked to all-cause and cardiovascular death in hypertensive patients.[34] Again, myocardial ischemia is thought to be one of the main factors in the origin of these changes.

Previously unsuspected myocardial infarction or ischemic changes may also be seen as well as more subtle abnormalities, such as left atrial abnormality. The importance of left atrial abnormality as both an early sign of LV involvement and hemodynamic changes was demonstrated 50 years ago[35] and is as relevant today with the ongoing interest in diastolic dysfunction and in atrial fibrillation in patients with hypertension. Atrial fibrillation can precipitate myocardial ischemia in this already vulnerable group of patients.

Silent ischemia is also common in hypertensive patients and can be detected by ambulatory monitoring.[36] This manifests as ST-segment depression without accompanying chest discomfort. It has a prevalence of 20% to 26% in hypertensive patients[37] and is triggered by variations in BP, heart rate, and circadian rhythm.[38] Silent ischemia brings an accompanying increase in cardiovascular risk.[39]

Echocardiography

Echocardiography is able to detect changes early in HHD.[40] One of these is integrated backscatter, which is a measure of myocardial collagen content. There are some limitations to this technique, although changes have been documented in hypertensive LVH.[41]

CFR can be assessed using transthoracic Doppler echocardiography by placing a pulsed-wave Doppler sample placed on the color signal of the left anterior descending artery. CFR is defined as the ratio between hyperemic and basal peak diastolic coronary flow velocities and has been shown to be reduced in patients with hypertension.[42] The main drawback is that the variability is thought to be in the region of 10%.[43]

Myocardial contrast echocardiography uses gas-filled microbubbles (3–5 μm in diameter), which can pass through the coronary microcirculation. Application of high-energy ultrasound causes bubble destruction and the rate of replenishment within the myocardium is a measure of microcirculatory perfusion. Reduced vasodilation capacity of the microcirculation has been shown in patients with hypertension.[44]

Myocardial deformation imaging (strain and strain rate) can detect abnormalities in subendocardial perfusion and function. The myocardial deformation response to stress is illustrative of the interaction of LV geometry and myocardial ischemia.[45] The detrimental effects of LVH and ischemia are incremental and predictive of mortality over long-term follow-up.[46] These parameters are sensitive markers of interstitial fibrosis and subendocardial function.[47,48]

Cardiac MRI

Stress perfusion cardiac MRI, using gadolinium-based contrast media, allows the examination of ventricular mass and function, stress and rest perfusion, and viability. Perfusion images are obtained using adenosine stress. A contrast washout period is then allowed prior to the measurement of perfusion at rest. Finally, late gadolinium enhancement images are obtained.[49]

Although most commonly used in the setting of CAD, the technique has been applied in HHD. In a series of more than 100 patients with mild to moderate hypertension, normal coronary arteries, preserved ventricular function, and symptoms of ischemia, reduced myocardial perfusion both at baseline and on stress was found compared with healthy controls. These changes were independent of LV mass or LVH.[50] Other investigators have shown a significant correlation between delayed contrast enhancement and ST-segment depression during exercise stress testing in hypertensive patients with normal coronary arteries.[51]

Nuclear Imaging

PET has demonstrated that patients with hypertension and LVH have transmurally blunted CFR in response to stress, most likely a consequence of microvascular dysfunction.[52] Endothelial dysfunction has also been identified in hypertensive patients using this technique.[53]

Computed Tomography

Advances in computational fluid dynamics permit the accurate assessment of fractional flow reserve using computed tomography scanning, which is highly comparable to invasively measured fractional flow reserve.[54] From this CFR can be calculated. Although this technique shows promise in the evaluation of microvascular functional assessment out with CAD, further studies are required.

MANAGEMENT ISSUES

HHD is a potent risk for the development of cardiac failure, atrial fibrillation, and sudden death. The myocardial ischemia seen in HHD often a mediator of these complications (**Fig. 3**).

Myocardial Ischemia Due to Coronary Artery Disease

Hypertension is a major independent risk factor of CAD. For every rise in systolic BP of 20 mm Hg (or rise of diastolic BP by 10 mm Hg), there is a doubling of risk of CAD mortality and subsequent adequate treatment has shown concomitant reductions in risk. In those with coexistent CAD, a lower BP target of less than 130/80 mm Hg is advocated if there is known CAD or cerebrovascular disease. β-Blockers are the first choice agent given that they are also efficacious in the management of angina, through their effect on reducing myocardial oxygen demand. If there is a history of previous MI, LV dysfunction, diabetes, or chronic kidney disease, then the addition of an angiotensin-converting enzyme inhibitor or angiotensin II receptor blocker is indicated.[26] Treatment of hypertension in these patients must be associated with optimization of lifestyle and addressing all other cardiovascular risk factors.

The current evidence base in regard to the presence of myocardial ischemia in patients with hypertension mandates a focused approach to therapy. Currently there are several agents that act through balancing the myocardial oxygen supply/demand relationship. The point has not yet been reached of having optimal medication for his condition but there is much to recommend in drugs that combine a BP lowering effect with

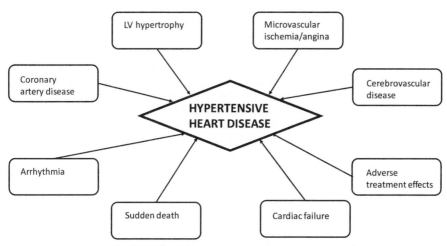

Fig. 3. The spectrum of risk conferred by HHD on cardiovascular morbidity and mortality.

an anti-ischemic effect. β-Blockers and calcium antagonists have a proved track record in this regard. β-Blockers lower the major determinates of oxygen consumption and the calcium antagonists improve myocardial flow through vasodilation.

Myocardial Ischemia Without Coronary Artery Disease

Microvascular dysfunction seen in HHD results in a high prevalence of myocardial ischemia. Up to 50% of all patients undergoing invasive coronary angiography for the investigation of chest pain turn out to have nonobstructed coronary arteries.[55] Despite this, there remains a high risk of subsequent major adverse cardiac events and all-cause mortality.[30] The dihydropyridine–calcium channel blocker benidipine seems to stimulate nitric oxide production in hypertensive rats and thereby reduce the effect of hypertension on vascular remodeling and CFR.[56] Amlodipine (but not nifedipine or diltiazem) reversed perivascular fibrosis and prevented myocardial ischemia in nitric oxide–deficient rats.[56] In humans, treatment with felodipine reduced asymptomatic ischemic episodes compared with a thiazide diuretic despite a similar reduction in BP and double product.[57]

The weight of evidence for improvement in endothelial function, reduction in oxidative stress, and beneficial vascular remodeling favors calcium channel blockers and angiotensin-converting enzyme inhibitors as first-line therapy for hypertension with associated myocardial ischemia and normal coronary arteries.[58] β-Blockers may have a role if there are ongoing anginal symptoms. Aldosterone antagonists also have a role in BP reduction and in reducing myocardial fibrosis, which can contribute to ischemia.

The value of the late sodium current inhibitor, ranolazine, which had shown promise in earlier studies,[59] has recently been called into question in a randomized, double-blind, placebo-controlled trial.[60]

Sudden Death

Management to prevent sudden death should address all the elements contributing to its risk in HHD. Therefore, the comments pertaining to management of ischemia, heart failure, reducing fibrosis, and LVH are all relevant in this regard. There remains no effective screening tool to predict sudden death in this population.

SUMMARY AND FUTURE CHALLENGES

Hypertension and HHD remain silent killers. Structural pathologic changes have been shown to occur early in the disease with a concomitant elevation of risk. End-organ dysfunction, such as LVH and ischemia, are high-risk markers and merit urgent treatment. Advances in cardiac imaging have allowed greater understanding of the molecular, humoral, and structural changes seen in HHD. Despite this, there still are few effective therapies that specifically target these mechanisms. Myocardial ischemia is a significant driver of patient symptoms, hospital presentations, and cardiovascular morbidity and mortality. Proved treatments for myocardial ischemia in the absence of CAD are lacking and BP reduction, treatment of heart failure, and regression of LVH remain the focus.

Sir Thomas Lewis in his classic monograph, *Diseases of the Heart*, stated, "in patients with hypertension, the chief consideration in individual prognosis is the state of the heart."[61] No effective medication was available then. Today there is a plethora of agents, yet this ominous prognostic picture continues and to a significant degree as a result of myocardial ischemia. Despite considerable progress in this area, the tenure of Lewis's statement remains as valid today as it did almost 100 years ago.

REFERENCES

1. Kannel WB. Some lessons in cardiovascular epidemiology from Framingham. Am J Cardiol 1976;37(2):269–82.
2. Kannel WB. Left ventricular hypertrophy as a risk factor: the Framingham experience. J Hypertens Suppl 1991;9(2):S3–8 [discussion: S8–9].
3. Díez J, Frohlich ED. A translational approach to hypertensive heart disease. Hypertension 2010;55(1):1–8.
4. Cohn JN, Ferrari R, Sharpe N. Cardiac remodeling–concepts and clinical implications: a consensus paper from an international forum on cardiac remodeling. Behalf of an International Forum on Cardiac Remodeling. J Am Coll Cardiol 2000;35(3):569–82.
5. Opie LH, Commerford PJ, Gersh BJ, et al. Controversies in ventricular remodelling. Lancet 2006;367(9507):356–67.
6. Grossman W, Jones D, McLaurin LP. Wall stress and patterns of hypertrophy in the human left ventricle. J Clin Invest 1975;56(1):56–64.
7. Reid CM, Maher T, Jennings GL, Heart Project Steering Committee. Substituting lifestyle management for pharmacological control of blood pressure: a pilot study in Australian general practice. Blood Press 2000;9(5):267–74.
8. Du Y, Plante E, Janicki JS, et al. Temporal evaluation of cardiac myocyte hypertrophy and hyperplasia in male rats secondary to chronic volume overload. Am J Pathol 2010;177(3):1155–63.
9. Frohlich ED, Susic D. Pressure overload. Heart Fail Clin 2012;8(1):21–32.
10. Querejeta R, Varo N, Lopez B, et al. Serum carboxy-terminal propeptide of procollagen type I is a marker of myocardial fibrosis in hypertensive heart disease. Circulation 2000;101(14):1729–35.
11. Rossi MA. Pathologic fibrosis and connective tissue matrix in left ventricular hypertrophy due to chronic arterial hypertension in humans. J Hypertens 1998; 16(7):1031–41.
12. Frohlich ED. Risk mechanisms in hypertensive heart disease. Hypertension 1999; 34(2):782–9.
13. Diez J, Querejeta R, Lopez B, et al. Losartan-dependent regression of myocardial fibrosis is associated with reduction of left ventricular chamber stiffness in hypertensive patients. Circulation 2002;105(21):2512–7.

14. Brilla CG, Matsubara LS, Weber KT. Antifibrotic effects of spironolactone in preventing myocardial fibrosis in systemic arterial hypertension. Am J Cardiol 1993; 71(3):12A–6A.
15. Kuwahara F, Kai H, Tokuda K, et al. Transforming growth factor-beta function blocking prevents myocardial fibrosis and diastolic dysfunction in pressure-overloaded rats. Circulation 2002;106(1):130–5.
16. Dzau VJ. Significance of the vascular renin-angiotensin pathway. Hypertension 1986;8(7):553–9.
17. Blacher J, Asmar R, Djane S, et al. Aortic pulse wave velocity as a marker of cardiovascular risk in hypertensive patients. Hypertension 1999;33(5):1111–7.
18. Park JB, Schiffrin EL. Small artery remodeling is the most prevalent (earliest?) form of target organ damage in mild essential hypertension. J Hypertens 2001; 19(5):921–30.
19. Lekakis JP, Papathanassiou S, Papaioannou TG, et al. Oral L-arginine improves endothelial function in patients with hypertension. Int J Cardiol 2002;86(2–3):317–23.
20. Iwashima Y, Horio T, Kamide K, et al. C-reactive protein, left ventricular mass index, and risk of cardiovascular disease in essential hypertension. Hypertens Res 2007;30(12):1177–85.
21. Folkeringa RJ, de Vos C, Pinto YM, et al. No effect of rosuvastatin on left ventricular hypertrophy in patients with hypertension: a prospective randomised open-label study with blinded endpoint assessment. Int J Cardiol 2010;145(1):156–8.
22. Fliser D, Buchholz K, Haller H, EUropean Trial on Olmesartan and Pravastatin in Inflammation and Atherosclerosis (EUTOPIA) Investigators. Antiinflammatory effects of angiotensin II subtype 1 receptor blockade in hypertensive patients with microinflammation. Circulation 2004;110(9):1103–7.
23. Shibasaki Y, Nishiue T, Masaki H, et al. Impact of the angiotensin II receptor antagonist, losartan, on myocardial fibrosis in patients with end-stage renal disease: assessment by ultrasonic integrated backscatter and biochemical markers. Hypertens Res 2005;28(10):787–95.
24. Gonzalez A, Lopez B, Ravassa S, et al. Stimulation of cardiac apoptosis in essential hypertension: potential role of angiotensin II. Hypertension 2002;39(1):75–80.
25. Diep QN, El Mabrouk M, Yue P, et al. Effect of AT(1) receptor blockade on cardiac apoptosis in angiotensin II-induced hypertension. Am J Physiol Heart Circ Physiol 2002;282(5):H1635–41.
26. Rosendorff C, Lackland DT, Allison M, et al. Treatment of hypertension in patients with coronary artery disease: a scientific statement from the American Heart Association, American College of Cardiology, and American Society of Hypertension. Hypertension 2015;65(6):1372–407.
27. Laine H, Raitakari OT, Niinikoski H, et al. Early impairment of coronary flow reserve in young men with borderline hypertension. J Am Coll Cardiol 1998; 32(1):147–53.
28. Bache RJ. Effects of hypertrophy on the coronary circulation. Prog Cardiovasc Dis 1988;30(6):403–40.
29. Sara JD, Widmer RJ, Matsuzawa Y, et al. Prevalence of coronary microvascular dysfunction among patients with chest pain and nonobstructive coronary artery disease. JACC Cardiovasc Interv 2015;8(11):1445–53.
30. Jespersen L, Hvelplund A, Abildstrom SZ, et al. Stable angina pectoris with no obstructive coronary artery disease is associated with increased risks of major adverse cardiovascular events. Eur Heart J 2012;33(6):734–44.
31. Stanton T, Marwick TH. Assessment of subendocardial structure and function. JACC Cardiovasc Imaging 2010;3(8):867–75.

32. Okin PM, Oikarinen L, Viitasalo M, et al. Prognostic value of changes in the electrocardiographic strain pattern during antihypertensive treatment: the Losartan Intervention for End-Point Reduction in Hypertension Study (LIFE). Circulation 2009;119(14):1883–91.
33. Arita Y, Hirata K, Wada N, et al. Altered coronary flow velocity reserve and left ventricular wall motion dynamics: a phenomenon in hypertensive patients with ECG strain. Echocardiography 2013;30(6):634–43.
34. Oikarinen L, Nieminen MS, Viitasalo M, et al. QRS duration and QT interval predict mortality in hypertensive patients with left ventricular hypertrophy: the Losartan Intervention for Endpoint Reduction in Hypertension Study. Hypertension 2004; 43(5):1029–34.
35. Tarazi RC, Miller A, Frohlich ED, et al. Electrocardiographic changes reflecting left atrial abnormality in hypertension. Circulation 1966;34(5):818–22.
36. Pringle SD, Dunn FG, Tweddel AC, et al. Symptomatic and silent myocardial ischaemia in hypertensive patients with left ventricular hypertrophy. Br Heart J 1992;67(5):377–82.
37. Uen S, Un I, Fimmers R, et al. Myocardial ischemia during everyday life in patients with arterial hypertension: prevalence, risk factors, triggering mechanism and circadian variability. Blood Press Monit 2006;11(4):173–82.
38. Xanthos T, Ekmektzoglou KA, Papadimitriou L. Reviewing myocardial silent ischemia: specific patient subgroups. Int J Cardiol 2008;124(2):139–48.
39. Boon D, Piek JJ, van Montfrans GA. Silent ischaemia and hypertension. J Hypertens 2000;18(10):1355–64.
40. Dunn FG, Chandraratna P, deCarvalho JG, et al. Pathophysiologic assessment of hypertensive heart disease with echocardiography. Am J Cardiol 1977;39(6): 789–95.
41. Lucarini AR, Talarico L, Di Bello V, et al. Increased myocardial ultrasonic reflectivity is associated with extreme hypertensive left ventricular hypertrophy: a tissue characterization study in humans. Am J Hypertens 1998;11(12):1442–9.
42. Mahfouz RA. Relation of coronary flow reserve and diastolic function to fractional pulse pressure in hypertensive patients. Echocardiography 2013;30(9):1084–90.
43. Rigo F, Richieri M, Pasanisi E, et al. Usefulness of coronary flow reserve over regional wall motion when added to dual-imaging dipyridamole echocardiography. Am J Cardiol 2003;91(3):269–73.
44. Di Bello V, Pedrinelli R, Giorgi D, et al. Coronary microcirculation in essential hypertension: a quantitative myocardial contrast echocardiographic approach. Eur J Echocardiogr 2002;3(2):117–27.
45. Stanton T, Ingul CB, Hare JL, et al. Interaction of left ventricular geometry and myocardial ischemia in the response of myocardial deformation to stress. Am J Cardiol 2009;104(7):897–903.
46. Stanton T, Ingul CB, Hare JL, et al. Association of myocardial deformation with mortality independent of myocardial ischemia and left ventricular hypertrophy. JACC Cardiovasc Imaging 2009;2(7):793–801.
47. Park TH, Nagueh SF, Khoury DS, et al. Impact of myocardial structure and function postinfarction on diastolic strain measurements: implications for assessment of myocardial viability. Am J Physiol Heart Circ Physiol 2006;290(2):H724–31.
48. Hashimoto I, Li X, Hejmadi Bhat A, et al. Myocardial strain rate is a superior method for evaluation of left ventricular subendocardial function compared with tissue Doppler imaging. J Am Coll Cardiol 2003;42(9):1574–83.
49. Costa MA, Shoemaker S, Futamatsu H, et al. Quantitative magnetic resonance perfusion imaging detects anatomic and physiologic coronary artery disease

as measured by coronary angiography and fractional flow reserve. J Am Coll Cardiol 2007;50(6):514–22.

50. Kawecka-Jaszcz K, Czarnecka D, Olszanecka A, et al. Myocardial perfusion in hypertensive patients with normal coronary angiograms. J Hypertens 2008; 26(8):1686–94.

51. Andersen K, Hennersdorf M, Cohnen M, et al. Myocardial delayed contrast enhancement in patients with arterial hypertension: initial results of cardiac MRI. Eur J Radiol 2009;71(1):75–81.

52. Rimoldi O, Rosen SD, Camici PG. The blunting of coronary flow reserve in hypertension with left ventricular hypertrophy is transmural and correlates with systolic blood pressure. J Hypertens 2014;32(12):2465–71 [discussion: 2471].

53. Alexanderson E, Jacome R, Jimenez-Santos M, et al. Evaluation of the endothelial function in hypertensive patients with 13N-ammonia PET. J Nucl Cardiol 2012; 19(5):979–86.

54. Norgaard BL, Leipsic J, Gaur S, et al. Diagnostic performance of noninvasive fractional flow reserve derived from coronary computed tomography angiography in suspected coronary artery disease: the NXT trial (analysis of coronary blood flow using CT angiography: next steps). J Am Coll Cardiol 2014;63(12):1145–55.

55. Patel MR, Peterson ED, Dai D, et al. Low diagnostic yield of elective coronary angiography. N Engl J Med 2010;362(10):886–95.

56. Kobayashi N, Kobayashi K, Hara K, et al. Benidipine stimulates nitric oxide synthase and improves coronary circulation in hypertensive rats. Am J Hypertens 1999;12(5):483–91.

57. de Oliveira CF, Nathan LP, Metze K, et al. Effect of Ca2+ channel blockers on arterial hypertension and heart ischaemic lesions induced by chronic blockade of nitric oxide in the rat. Eur J Pharmacol 1999;373(2–3):195–200.

58. Trenkwalder P, Dobrindt R, Aulehner R, et al. Antihypertensive treatment with felodipine but not with a diuretic reduces episodes of myocardial ischaemia in elderly patients with hypertension. Eur Heart J 1994;15(12):1673–80.

59. Tagliamonte E, Rigo F, Cirillo T, et al. Effects of ranolazine on noninvasive coronary flow reserve in patients with myocardial ischemia but without obstructive coronary artery disease. Echocardiography 2015;32(3):516–21.

60. Bairey Merz CN, Handberg EM, Shufelt CL, et al. A randomized, placebo-controlled trial of late Na current inhibition (ranolazine) in coronary microvascular dysfunction (CMD): impact on angina and myocardial perfusion reserve. Eur Heart J 2016;37(19):1504–13.

61. Lewis T. Diseases of the heart. London: Macmillan; 1933.

The Hypertensive Myocardium

From Microscopic Lesions to Clinical Complications and Outcomes

María U. Moreno, PhD[a,d], Rocío Eiros, MD[b],
Juan J. Gavira, MD, PhD[b,d], Catalina Gallego, MD[a,c],
Arantxa González, PhD[a,d], Susana Ravassa, PhD[a,d],
Begoña López, PhD[a,d], Javier Beaumont, PhD[a,d],
Gorka San José, PhD[a,d], Javier Díez, MD, PhD[a,b,d],*

KEYWORDS

- Arterial hypertension • Hypertensive heart disease • Left ventricular hypertrophy
- Cardiomyocyte hypertrophy • Cardiomyocyte apoptosis • Myocardial fibrosis
- Microcirculation abnormalities

KEY POINTS

- The chronic hemodynamic load imposed by hypertension on the left ventricle leads to lesions in the cardiomyocyte and noncardiomyocyte components of the myocardium that results in its structural remodeling.
- Myocardial remodeling provides structural support for the alterations of cardiac function, perfusion, and electrical activity that adversely influence the clinical evolution of hypertensive heart disease.
- Managing hypertensive heart disease must focus on detecting, reducing, and reversing left ventricular hypertrophy as well as the detection and repair of the microscopic lesions responsible for myocardial remodeling.

Continued

Funding Sources: Ministry of Economy and Competitiveness, Spain (Instituto de Salud Carlos III grants RD12/0042/0009 and PI15/01909), and the European Commission FP7 Programme, Belgium (MEDIA project grant HEALTH-2010-261409, and FIBRO-TARGETS project grant FP7-HEALTH-2013-602904).
Disclosure Statement: The authors have nothing to disclose.
[a] Program of Cardiovascular Diseases, Center of Applied Medical Research, University of Navarra, Edificio CIMA, Av. Pío XII, 55, Pamplona 31008, Spain; [b] Department of Cardiology and Cardiac Surgery, University Clinic, University of Navarra, Av. Pío XII, 36, Pamplona 31008, Spain; [c] Programa de Cardiología Clínica, Clínica CardioVID, Universidad Pontificia Bolivariana, Calle 78B 75-21, Medellín, Colombia; [d] IdiSNA, Navarra Institute for Health Resarch, Pamplona, Spain
* Corresponding author. Programa de Enfermedades Cardiovasculares, Edificio CIMA, Av. Pío XII, 55, Pamplona 31008, Spain.
E-mail address: jadimar@unav.es

Med Clin N Am 101 (2017) 43–52
http://dx.doi.org/10.1016/j.mcna.2016.08.002
0025-7125/17/© 2016 Elsevier Inc. All rights reserved.

Continued

- The reduction of the burden currently associated with hypertensive heart disease can be targeted using personalized treatment.
- The noninvasive, biomarker-mediated identification of homogeneous subsets of patients with hypertensive heart disease is essential to provide personalized treatment.

INTRODUCTION

The heart is very sensitive to physiologic stimuli or pathologic states, and even slight perturbations may lead to severe cardiac changes, eventually with detrimental outcomes. For instance, in conditions of pressure overload owing to systemic hypertension, the left ventricle undergoes extensive growth, leading to left ventricular hypertrophy (LVH), which is the anatomic hallmark of hypertensive heart disease (HHD). From the point of view of cardiac function, HHD is characterized by an initial process that helps the heart to maintain cardiac output despite the increased afterload imposed by systemic hypertension.[1] However, long-term exposure to biomechanical stress associated with the hemodynamic load imposed by hypertension, eventually leads to an impaired inotropic/lusitropic function that, in many cases, progresses to LV dysfunction and heart failure (HF).[1] This maladaptive change is likely owing to alterations in the histologic composition of the myocardium that result in its structural remodeling (**Fig. 1**).[2]

Myocardial remodeling is a complex process driven by the responses of the cardiomyocytic and the noncardiomyocytic components of the heart to dynamic mechanical, neurohumoral, inflammatory, and oxidative stimuli.[3,4] Because of the interrelationships of these responses, they are likely to recognize common mediators. For instance, it has been reported recently that myocardin-related transcription factor-A mediates both

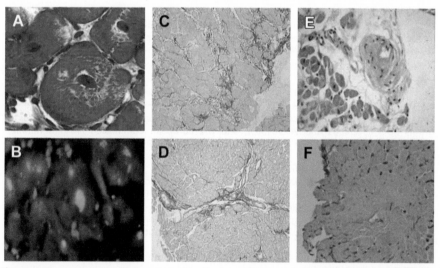

Fig. 1. Main microscopic lesions found in the hypertensive myocardium: (*A*) cardiomyocyte hypertrophy (Masson's trichrome staining, 100×), (*B*) cardiomyocyte apoptosis (TUNEL, 100×), (*C*) interstitial fibrosis (picro-sirius red staining, 20×), (*D*) perivascular fibrosis (picro-sirius red staining, 20×), (*E*) reduced lumen:wall ratio of an intramyocardial artery (Masson's trichrome staining, 20×), and (*F*) capillary rarefaction (von Willebrand staining, 20×).

mechanical stretch-induced and neurohumoral stimulation-induced gene and hyper-trophic responses in cardiomyocytes.[5] Furthermore, myocardin-related transcription factor-A plays a critical role in promoting conversion of cardiac fibroblasts to myofibro-blasts in response to mechanical and humoral factors by activating a fibrotic gene program.[6]

Owing to myocardial remodeling, pathologic LVH is an independent cardiovascular risk factor that is related to cardiovascular complications in hypertensive patients. Considered as a categorical variable, LVH significantly increases the risk of coronary artery disease, HF frequently with preserved ejection fraction (HFpEF), stroke, cardiac arrhythmia, and sudden death.[7] In addition, it has been shown that the cardiovascular risk decreases significantly in hypertensive patients in whom LVH regresses with anti-hypertensive treatment compared with patients in whom LVH persists and de novo development of LVH despite similar hemodynamic effectiveness of the treatment.[8] This article reviews the major pathologic components of myocardial remodeling in HHD, highlighting their main mechanisms and their impact on cardiac function and pa-tient's clinical outcome.

CARDIOMYOCYTE LESIONS

The response of the cardiomyocyte to pressure overload must not be considered sim-ply an adaptive compensation, but as a detrimental consequence.[9]

Hypertrophy

Hypertrophic growth of cardiomyocytes is the primary mechanism by which the heart reduces stress on the LV wall imposed by pressure overload. It entails stimulation of intracellular signaling cascades that activate gene expression and promotes protein synthesis, protein stability, or both, with consequent increases in protein content and in the size and organization of force-generating units (sarcomeres) that, in turn, leads to increased size of individual cardiomyocytes with resulting augmentation in LV mass and thus LVH.[10] The mechanisms whereby mechanical stretch of cardiomyo-cytes is transduced across the cell membrane are unclear. They probably involve stretch-sensitive ion channels, a Na^+/H^+ exchanger, integrins and integrin-interacting molecules, and other internal and membrane-bound stretch sensors in a complex network that links the extracellular matrix, the cytoskeleton, the sarcomere, calcium (Ca^{2+})-handling proteins, and the nucleus.[11]

The changes in genetic expression characteristic of the cardiomyocyte hypertrophic response involve isogenic shifts, which result in reexpression of a fetal gene program, as well as repression of postdevelopmental genes (**Box 1**).[12] The long-held views are that, in response to pressure overload, these morphologic and genetic changes serve to restore cardiac muscle economy and counteract myocardial dysfunction. However, evidence indicates that a blunting of cardiomyocyte hypertrophy and attenuation of the fetal gene reexpression does not necessarily result in immediate LV dysfunction or HF despite the pressure overload. Therefore, a paradigm shift occurs, in the sense that genetic reprograming associated with cardiomyocyte hypertrophy may no longer be considered as an adaptive process.[13] In fact, a detailed analysis of the genetic changes that accompany cardiomyocyte hypertrophy leads us to the conclusion that they translate into derangements in energy metabolism, contractile cycle and excitation–contraction coupling, cytoskeleton and membrane properties. These changes determine mechanical dysfunction which, in turn, provides the basis for car-diomyocyte malfunction, which is associated with LVH and predisposes the ventricle to diastolic and/or systolic dysfunction.[14]

Box 1
Changes of gene expression during cardiomyocyte hypertrophy

Genes whose expression is reactivated

β-Myosin heavy chain

Embryonic myosin light chain in ventricles

IVS3A form of calcium channel

α3-Subunit of Na^+, K^+-ATPase

Switch from fatty acid oxidation to glycolysis genes

Lactate dehydrogenase M subunits

B subunit of creatine kinase

Ventricular expression of atrial natriuretic factor

Genes directing cardiomyocyte lengthening

Genes whose expression is blunted

Calcium ATPase of sarcoplasmic reticulum (SERCA2)

β_1-Adrenergic receptors

M_2-Muscarinic receptors

Early transient K^+ current, I_{to}

Myoglobin

N2BA titin isoform

Death

Cardiomyocyte apoptosis is abnormally stimulated in patients with HHD with HF.[15] Cardiomyocyte apoptosis has been proposed to occur as a result of an imbalance between the factors that induce or block apoptosis. Thus, in arterial hypertension inducers of cardiomyocyte apoptosis (eg, mechanical stretching and angiotensin II) predominate over suppressors (eg, agonists of the gp130/LIFR survival pathway).[16] Apoptosis of cardiomyocytes may contribute to the development of LV dysfunction/ failure of the hypertensive myocardium through 3 different pathways. First, an association of increased cardiomyocyte apoptosis with diminished cardiomyocyte number has been found in hypertensive patients,[16] suggesting that apoptosis may serve as 1 mechanism involved in the loss of contractile mass and function in hypertensive patients. Second, some mechanisms that are activated during the apoptotic process may also interfere with the function of viable cardiomyocytes before death.[17] In fact, caspase-3 cleaves cardiac myofibrillar proteins, resulting in an impaired force/Ca^{2+} relationship and myofibrillar ATPase activity. In addition, the release of cytochrome C from mitochondria during apoptosis may impair oxidative phosphorylation and ATP production, thus leading to energetic compromise and functional impairment. Third, in addition to contributing to histologic remodeling of the myocardium, cardiomyocyte apoptosis may also contribute to geometric remodeling of the LV chamber. In fact, severe cardiomyocyte apoptosis may lead to side-to-side slippage of cells, mural thinning, and chamber dilatation. Thus, wall restructuring secondary to severe cardiomyocyte apoptosis may create an irreversible state of the myocardium, conditioning progressive dilatation, and the continuous deterioration of LV hemodynamics and performance with time.[18]

Although apoptosis is a hallmark of HHD, it is important to point out that in the response to any given cardiac injury various modalities of cell death, including apoptosis, necrosis, and autophagy, are stimulated, because they are interconnected by common cellular pathways at multiple points.[19] For instance, autophagy is activated during hypertensive LVH, serving to maintain cellular homeostasis.[20] Excessive autophagy eliminates, however, essential cellular elements and possibly provokes cardiomyocyte death, which contributes to myocardial remodeling.

NONCARDIOMYOCYTE LESIONS

Studies performed over the past 2 decades have evidenced that beyond cardiomyocytic lesions, changes in myocardial extracellular matrix and microvasculature are part of the structural remodeling of the myocardium that ultimately develops in HHD and have a profound detrimental impact on the overall cardiac function.

Myocardial Fibrosis

Myocardial fibrosis, secondary to an exaggerated accumulation of collagen types I and III fibers within the interstitium and surrounding intramural coronary arteries and arterioles, is one of the key features of hypertensive myocardial remodeling. The excess of myocardial collagen present in hypertensive LVH is suggested to result from the combination of several alterations[21]: (i) increased procollagen synthesis by fibroblasts and phenotypically transformed fibroblastlike cells or myofibroblasts, (ii) increased extracellular conversion of procollagen into microfibril-forming collagen by specific proteinases, (iii) increased spontaneous microfibril assembly to form fibrils, (iv) enhanced lysyl oxidase–mediated cross-linking of fibrils to form fibers; and (v) unchanged or decreased fiber degradation by matrix metalloproteinases (MMPs).

Fibrosis might contribute to the pathophysiologic changes of HHD through different pathways. First, a linkage between fibrosis and LV dysfunction may be established.[22] Initially, the accumulation of collagen fibers compromises the rate of relaxation, diastolic suction, and passive stiffness, thereby contributing to impaired diastolic function. Continued accumulation of collagen fibers, accompanied by changes in their spatial orientation, further impairs diastolic filling. These changes further compromise cardiomyocyte contraction and myocardial force development thus impairing systolic performance. Second, impaired coronary flow reserve associated with LVH might be related to several factors, including perivascular fibrosis.[23] In fact, the amount of perivascular collagen has been correlated inversely with coronary flow reserve in patients with LVH.[24] Third, increased deposition of fibrotic tissue, which occurs in association with hypertension and LVH, results in diffusion problems in a situation in which oxygen and nutritional demands are increased.[25] Fourth, interstitial fibrosis may also contribute to ventricular arrhythmias in hypertension.[26] Thus, hypertensive patients with dysrhythmias exhibit higher values of LV mass and myocardial collagen than patients without arrhythmias, despite the finding that the ejection fraction and the frequency of coronary vessels with significant stenosis may be similar in the 2 groups of patients. Fibrosis induces conduction abnormalities thereby promoting local reentry arrhythmias. Finally, whereas the key role of ectopic foci in pulmonary veins, which may trigger atrial fibrillation, has been recognized, atrial fibrosis has been identified as the main mechanism for atrial fibrillation.[27] This suggests that atrial fibrosis in hypertensive patients (namely those with chronic HF) may promote more widespread changes in the myocardial collagen matrix.

Of interest, the alterations in the quality and quantity of the myocardial collagen matrix also may influence adversely the clinical outcome in patients with HHD, namely in those with HF. For instance, it has been shown that whereas increased collagen type I cross-linking is associated per se with HF hospitalization in patients with HHD and HF,[28] the coincidence of increased collagen type I cross-linking with severe collagen type I deposition is associated with HF hospitalization and mortality (cardiovascular and all cause).[29]

Microvascular Alterations

The hypertensive myocardium is characterized by different structural alterations in the small intramyocardial vessels.[30] Hyperplasia or hypertrophy and altered vascular smooth muscle cellular alignment may promote encroachment of the tunica media into the lumen, thereby causing both increased medial thickness/lumen ratio or reduced maximal cross-sectional area of intramyocardial arteries. In contrast, vascular density in LVH becomes relatively decreased. This seems to result from capillary rarefaction or inadequate vascular growth in response to increasing muscle mass. These microcirculatory alterations, together with perivascular fibrosis contribute to decreased coronary flow reserve of patients with HHD.[31] Interestingly, associations have been found between decreased coronary flow reserve and LV systolic and diastolic dysfunction in HHD during stress maneuvers.[32–34]

In 1 report, the role of coronary microvascular endothelial inflammation associated with systemic conditions (eg, hypertension, obesity, and diabetes mellitus) was highlighted in patients with HFpEF.[35] Coronary microvascular endothelial inflammation would decrease the bioavailability of nitric oxide and cyclic guanosine monophosphate content, resulting in decreasing cardiomyocyte protein kinase G activity. Thus, low protein kinase G activity may promote cardiomyocyte hypertrophy, hypophosphorylation of the cytoskeletal protein titin, stimulation of cardiac fibroblastic differentiation into myofibroblasts with high fibrogenic activity, and increased myocardial stiffness. This sequence of events suggests that coronary microvascular endothelial inflammation may be responsible for myocardial remodeling in HFpEF. This was recently supported by the demonstration that HFpEF was associated with microvascular endothelial activation[36] and a reduction of coronary flow reserve.[37]

CLINICAL IMPLICATIONS

Although current management of HHD remains focused on controlling blood pressure and reducing the increased LV mass,[38] the impact of currently available antihypertensive agents on myocardial remodeling may not be optimal (**Table 1**). Therefore, additional strategies aimed at noninvasive biochemical[39] or imaging[40] diagnosis and therapeutic repair[41] of the microscopic changes responsible for hypertensive myocardial remodeling are needed.

The problem of myocardial fibrosis may help to understand this approach. The degree of lysyl oxidase-mediated cross-linking between collagen type I fibrils determines the stiffness of the collagen type I fiber and its resistance to proteolysis by MMP-1 or interstitial collagenase, resulting in diminished cleavage of a small carboxy-terminal telopeptide of the fiber (CITP).[42] Thus, a low serum CITP:MMP-1 ratio has been associated independently with increased myocardial collagen type I cross-linking in patients with HHD and HF.[28] In support, a low serum CITP:MMP-1 ratio was associated with hospitalization for HF in these patients.[28]

Interestingly, in patients of hypertensive HF, administration of torasemide (in addition to standard HF therapy) was associated with reduced myocardial expression of active lysyl oxidase, the degree of collagen type I cross-linking, and collagen type I deposition.[43,44] Additionally, treatment with torasemide was accompanied by normalization of LV stiffness and improved function in 80% of the patients.[43] None of these

Table 1
Clinical evidence-based hemodynamic and cardiac effects of antihypertensive agents

Pharmacologic Class	Decrease of Blood Pressure	Reduction of LV Mass	Repair of Remodeling Lesions[a]
Diuretics	Yes	Mild	Proven for torasemide[44]
β-Blockers	Yes	Mild to moderate	Apparently not
α-Blockers	Yes	Mild	Unknown
Calcium antagonists	Yes	Moderate	Apparently not
Angiotensin-converting enzyme inhibitors	Yes	Marked	Proven for lisinopril[46]
Angiotensin receptor blockers	Yes	Marked	Proven for losartan[47]
Aldosterone antagonists	Yes	Mild-moderate	Proven for spironolactone[48]
Direct renin inhibitors	Yes	Marked	Unknown
Angiotensin receptor blocker and neprylisin inhibitor	Yes	Unknown	Unknown

Abbreviation: LV, left ventricular.
[a] Refers to some of the lesions (namely, fibrosis).

beneficial effects were observed in furosemide-treated HF patients.[43,44] Whether HF patients with a low serum CITP:MMP-1 ratio would benefit more from the antifibrotic properties of torasemide than the remaining HF patients is a hypothesis that remains to be studied further. Interestingly, in 1 open-label randomized trial performed in patients with HF receiving standard therapy, addition of torasemide was associated with a lower rate of hospitalization for HF than the addition of furosemide.[45]

SUMMARY

The histologic alterations that develop in both the myocardial parenchyma and the microvasculature of the hypertensive left ventricle provide structural support for the

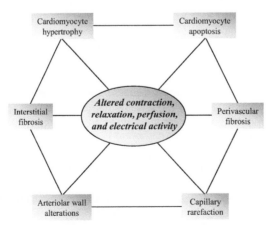

Fig. 2. Mosaic of interactions among the microscopic lesions found in the hypertensive myocardium that result in alterations in left ventricular function, ischemia (namely, in conditions of stress), and propensity to arrhythmias.

alterations of cardiac function, perfusion, and electrical activity that adversely influ-ence the clinical evolution of patients with HHD (**Fig. 2**). Therefore, a major unmet need in HHD therapy is the ability to identify homogeneous subsets of patients whose underlying histologic lesions are driven by specific mechanisms that can be solely tar-geted using personalized treatment. From this perspective, to detect noninvasively and to repair effectively, the structural myocardial remodeling must be considered as part of the overall clinical management in patients with HHD. In doing so, adverse outcomes associated with HHD could be prevented more effectively.

REFERENCES

1. Lazzeroni D, Rimoldi O, Camici PG. From left ventricular hypertrophy to dysfunc-tion and failure. Circ J 2016;80:555–64.
2. Díez J, González A, López B, et al. Mechanisms of disease: pathologic structural remodeling is more than adaptive hypertrophy in hypertensive heart disease. Nat Clin Pract Cardiovasc Med 2005;2:209–16.
3. Díez J. Towards a new paradigm about hypertensive heart disease. Med Clin North Am 2009;93:637–45.
4. McMaster WG, Kirabo A, Madhur MS, et al. Inflammation, immunity, and hyper-tensive end-organ damage. Circ Res 2015;116:1022–33.
5. Kuwahara K, Kinoshita H, Kuwabara Y, et al. MRTF-A is a common mediator of mechanical stress- and neurohumoral stimulation-induced cardiac hypertrophic signaling leading to activation of BNP gene expression. Mol Cell Biol 2010;30: 4134–48.
6. Small EM, Thatcher JE, Sutherland LB, et al. Myocardin-related transcription factor-A controls myofibroblast activation and fibrosis in response to myocardial infarction. Circ Res 2010;107:294–304.
7. Cramariuc D, Gerdts E. Epidemiology of left ventricular hypertrophy in hyperten-sion: implications for the clinic. Expert Rev Cardiovasc Ther 2016;17:1–12.
8. Devereux RB, Wachtell K, Gerdts E, et al. Prognostic significance of left ventric-ular mass change during treatment of hypertension. JAMA 2004;292:2350–6.
9. Frohlich ED, González A, Díez J. Hypertensive left ventricular hypertrophy risk: beyond adaptive cardiomyocytic hypertrophy. J Hypertens 2011;29:17–26.
10. Sugden PH, Clerk A. Cellular mechanisms of cardiac hypertrophy. J Mol Med (Berl) 1998;76:725–46.
11. Clerk A, Cullingford TE, Fuller SJ, et al. Signaling pathways mediating cardiac myocyte gene expression in physiological and stress responses. J Cell Physiol 2007;212:311–22.
12. Kuwahara K, Nishikimi T, Nakao K. Transcriptional regulation of the fetal cardiac gene program. J Pharmacol Sci 2012;119:198–203.
13. Meijs MF, de Windt LJ, de Jonge N, et al. Left ventricular hypertrophy: a shift in paradigm. Curr Med Chem 2007;14:157–71.
14. Dhalla NS, Saini-Chohan HK, Rodriguez-Leyva D, et al. Subcellular remodelling may induce cardiac dysfunction in congestive heart failure. Cardiovasc Res 2009;81:429–38.
15. González A, Ravassa S, López B, et al. Apoptosis in hypertensive heart disease: a clinical approach. Curr Opin Cardiol 2006;21:288–94.
16. Fortuño MA, Ravassa S, Fortuño A, et al. Cardiomyocyte apoptotic cell death in arterial hypertension. Mechanisms and potential management. Hypertension 2001;38:1406–12.

17. Narula J, Arbustini E, Chandrashekhar Y, et al. Apoptosis and the systolic dysfunction in congestive heart failure. Story of apoptosis interruptus and zombie myocytes. Cardiol Clin 2001;19:113–26.

18. Chandrashekhar Y. Role of apoptosis in ventricular remodeling. Curr Heart Fail Rep 2005;2:18–22.

19. Whelan RS, Kaplinskiy V, Kitsis RN. Cell death in the pathogenesis of heart disease: mechanisms and significance. Annu Rev Physiol 2010;72:19–44.

20. Wang ZV, Rothermel BA, Hill JA. Autophagy in hypertensive heart disease. J Biol Chem 2010;285:8509–14.

21. Berk BC, Fujiwara K, Lehoux S. ECM remodeling in hypertensive heart disease. J Clin Invest 2007;117:568–75.

22. Brower GL, Gardner JD, Forman MF, et al. The relationship between myocardial extracellular matrix remodeling and ventricular function. Eur J Cardiothorac Surg 2006;30:604–10.

23. Schwartzkopff B, Motz W, Frenzel H, et al. Structural and functional alterations of the intramyocardial coronary arterioles in patients with arterial hypertension. Circulation 1993;88:993–1003.

24. Dai Z, Aoki T, Fukumoto Y, et al. Coronary perivascular fibrosis is associated with impairment of coronary blood flow in patients with non-ischemic heart failure. J Cardiol 2012;60:416–21.

25. Frohlich ED. Fibrosis and ischemia: the real risks in hypertensive heart disease. Am J Hypertens 2001;14:194S–9S.

26. McLenachan JM, Dargie JH. Ventricular arrhythmias in hypertensive left ventricular hypertrophy. Relation to coronary artery disease, left ventricular dysfunction, and myocardial fibrosis. Am J Hypertens 1990;3:735–40.

27. Boldt A, Wetzel U, Lauschke J, et al. Fibrosis in left atrial tissue of patients with atrial fibrillation with and without underlying mitral valve disease. Heart 2004; 90:400–5.

28. López B, Ravassa S, González A, et al. Myocardial collagen cross-linking is associated with heart failure hospitalization in patients with hypertensive heart failure. J Am Coll Cardiol 2016;67:251–60.

29. González Miqueo A, López N, Ravassa S, et al. Combining collagen type I-related biomarkers identifies a malignant phenotype of myocardial fibrosis in hypertensive heart failure. Eur J Heart Fail 2016;18:394–5 (abstract).

30. Feihl F, Liaudet L, Levy BI, et al. Hypertension and microvascular remodelling. Cardiovasc Res 2008;78:274–85.

31. Kelm M, Strauer BE. Coronary flow reserve measurements in hypertension. Med Clin North Am 2004;88:99–113.

32. Galderisi M, Cicala S, Caso P, et al. Coronary flow reserve and myocardial diastolic dysfunction in arterial hypertension. Am J Cardiol 2002;90:860–4.

33. Kozàkovà M, Ferrannini E, Palombo C. Relation between left ventricular midwall function and coronary vasodilator capacity in arterial hypertension. Hypertension 2003;42:528–33.

34. Ikonomidis I, Tzortzis S, Paraskevaidis I, et al. Association of abnormal coronary microcirculatory function with impaired response of longitudinal left ventricular function during adenosine stress echocardiography in untreated hypertensive patients. Eur Heart J Cardiovasc Imaging 2012;13:1030–40.

35. Paulus WJ, Tschöpe C. A novel paradigm for heart failure with preserved ejection fraction: comorbidities drive myocardial dysfunction and remodeling through coronary microvascular endothelial inflammation. J Am Coll Cardiol 2013;62:263–7.

36. Franssen C, Chen S, Unger A, et al. Myocardial microvascular inflammatory endothelial activation in heart failure with preserved ejection fraction. JACC Heart Fail 2016;4:312–24.
37. Kato S, Saito N, Kirigaya H, et al. Impairment of coronary flow reserve evaluated by phase contrast cine-magnetic resonance imaging in patients with heart failure with preserved ejection fraction. J Am Heart Assoc 2016;5:e002649.
38. Schiattarella GG, Hill JA. Inhibition of hypertrophy is a good therapeutic strategy in ventricular pressure overload. Circulation 2015;131:1435–47.
39. González A, López B, Ravassa S, et al. Biochemical markers of myocardial remodelling in hypertensive heart disease. Cardiovasc Res 2009;81:509–18.
40. Hoey ET, Pakala V, Teoh JK, et al. The role of imaging in hypertensive heart disease. Int J Angiol 2014;23:85–92.
41. González A, Ravassa S, Beaumont J, et al. New targets to treat the structural remodeling of the myocardium. J Am Coll Cardiol 2011;58:1833–43.
42. Visse R, Nagase H. Matrix metalloproteinases and tissue inhibitors of metalloproteinases: structure, function, and biochemistry. Circ Res 2003;92:827–39.
43. López B, Querejeta R, González A, et al. Impact of treatment on myocardial lysyl oxidase expression and collagen cross-linking in patients with heart failure. Hypertension 2009;53:236–42.
44. López B, Querejeta R, González A, et al. Effects of loop diuretics on myocardial fibrosis and collagen type I turnover in chronic heart failure. J Am Coll Cardiol 2004;43:2028–35.
45. Murray MD, Deer MM, Ferguson JA, et al. Open-label randomized trial of torsemide compared with furosemide therapy for patients with heart failure. Am J Med 2001;111:513–20.
46. Brilla CG, Funck RC, Rupp H. Lisinopril-mediated regression of myocardial fibrosis in patients with hypertensive heart disease. Circulation 2000;102(12): 1388–93.
47. Diez J, Querejeta R, Lopez B, et al. Losartan-dependent regression of myocardial fibrosis is associated with reduction of left ventricular chamber stiffness in hypertensive patients. Circulation 2002;105(21):2512–7.
48. Izawa H, Murohara T, Nagata K, et al. Mineralocorticoid receptor antagonism ameliorates left ventricular diastolic dysfunction and myocardial fibrosis in mildly symptomatic patients with idiopathic dilated cardiomyopathy: a pilot study. Circulation 2005;112(19):2940–5.

Hypertension in Patients with Cardiac Transplantation

Amanda L. Bennett, MD[a],*, Hector O. Ventura, MD[b]

KEYWORDS

• Hypertension • Calcineurin inhibitors • Cardiac transplantation

KEY POINTS

- The physiology of the development of hypertension (HTN) after cardiac transplantation is explored.
- The importance of calcineurin inhibitors on the development of HTN after cardiac transplantation is discussed.
- The management of patients with HTN after cardiac transplantation is outlined.

INTRODUCTION

Despite the clinical success and improvement in survival of cardiac transplantation in the last 20 years, many patients develop chronic problems such as cardiac allograft vasculopathy and hypertension (HTN). The incidence of HTN after cardiac transplantation varies from 50% to 80% of recipients.[1] Development of HTN after cardiac transplantation is multifactorial. In the complex biosystem created by transplantation, patients are susceptible to multiple mechanisms for HTN. The unique physiology created by the cardiac allograft places these patients at risk for continued complications from cardiovascular disease and long-term mortality. Among these mechanisms are the use of immunosuppressive therapy (calcineurin inhibitors [CI] and glucocorticoids), surgical denervation, development of restrictive physiology, ventricular vascular uncoupling, and fluid sensitivity. This review describes the state of current literature pertaining to the pathophysiology and treatment of HTN in patients after cardiac transplantation.

[a] Department of Internal Medicine, Ochsner Clinic Foundation, 1514 Jefferson Highway, New Orleans, LA 70121, USA; [b] Department of Cardiomyopathy & Heart Transplantation, John Ochsner Heart and Vascular Institute, 1514 Jefferson Highway, New Orleans, LA 70121, USA
* Corresponding author.
E-mail address: amanda.bennett@ochsner.org

Med Clin N Am 101 (2017) 53–64
http://dx.doi.org/10.1016/j.mcna.2016.08.011
0025-7125/17/© 2016 Elsevier Inc. All rights reserved.

MECHANISMS OF HYPERTENSION AFTER CARDIAC TRANSPLANTATION
Predisposing Factors of the Recipient

Traditional risk factors of the recipient before cardiac transplantation, such as HTN, smoking, hypercholesterolemia, and pretransplant body weight do not have any correlation with the development of posttransplant HTN.[2] However, HTN as part of the pretransplant metabolic syndrome or its development within the first 3 months posttransplant, is associated with a greater risk of mortality and long-term renal dysfunction.[3]

Calcineurin Inhibitor–Mediated Effects

Although the use of CIs have greatly improved the success and survival of cardiac transplant recipients, these agents have several adverse effects, the most common being HTN and nephrotoxicity.[4,5] The development of posttransplant HTN and its possible underlying mechanisms has been studied most closely with relation to the use of cyclosporine.[6,7] It has been shown that patients receiving cyclosporine develop new-onset HTN requiring pharmacologic treatment in 82% of cases compared with 64% of those treated with tacrolimus.[8] Although in the new era of tacrolimus-based immunosuppression the incidence of HTN is less, it still represents a significant problem in the management of these patients. HTN has been shown to correlate with the use of cyclosporine for autoimmune diseases as well as for immunosuppression after other solid organ transplants.[9] We will discuss some of the mechanisms by which CIs, more specifically cyclosporine, can cause an increase in blood pressure in patients with cardiac transplantation.

Inhibition of peripheral vasodilation

CIs have a direct effect on free and intramuscular calcium ion concentrations through the involvement of the calcium-calmodulin–dependent phosphatase mechanism.[10] Increased calcium within the vascular smooth muscle leads to constriction and arterial HTN. Attenuation of this mechanism decreases the production of nitric oxide (NO), effectively leading to an inhibition of vasodilatation.[11]

Increased vasoconstrictor production

HTN, in cyclosporine-treated cardiac transplant recipients, is associated with reductions in cardiac output, increased vasoconstrictor sensitivity,[12] decreased prostaglandin levels, and increased thromboxane A2 synthesis.[13] Decreased prostaglandin synthesis leads to vasoconstriction of the afferent arterioles, which activates activation of the renin–angiotensin–aldosterone system (RAAS). This effect can be reversed within the renal vasculature through the use of thromboxane A2 antagonists, but such reversal does not demonstrate effects on systemic HTN.[14] Endothelin-1 is thought to contribute to stimulation of proinflammatory cytokines, tissue damage, and fibrosis seen in patients after transplantation.[15] Although the levels of endothelin-1 are independent of degree of HTN, it is thought that cyclosporine may have a role in increasing the endothelin receptors in the renal microvessels, which in turn produces vasoconstriction and renal-modulated HTN.[16,17]

Left ventricular remodeling and left ventricular hypertrophy

Calcineurin activates the genes that are associated with the development of left ventricular hypertrophy by dephosphorylating nuclear factor of activated T cells (specifically NFATc3); however, the use of CIs is not proven to prevent the development of left ventricular hypertrophy in animal models.[18] Similarly, after cardiac transplantation, patients with HTN, obesity, and CI-based immunosuppression demonstrate an increased in left ventricular mass and left ventricular hypertrophy, which may have long-term consequences for the function of the allograft. Increases in left ventricular mass associated with cyclosporine use are greater than with the use of other immune-modulating therapies.[19]

Nephrotoxicity
A dose-dependent increase in blood urea nitrogen, serum creatinine, hyperkalemia, metabolic acidosis, and chronic interstitial nephritis with irreversible renal toxicity is associated with CI use.[20,21] Reductions in the glomerular filtration rate are a direct result of decreased renal blood flow caused by CIs.[22] Although the mechanisms for renal injury from the use of CIs are not well-understood, histologically proven evidence of renal–vascular damage suggests direct nephrotoxic effects, leading to the loss of renal function and resultant HTN.[6]

Activation of the renin–angiotensin–aldosterone system
It has been shown that CIs stimulate the RAAS leading to an increase in angiotensin II levels and corresponding renal vasoconstriction and the development of HTN.[23,24] However, Bellet and colleagues[25] demonstrated that there is no difference in plasma renin levels between cardiac transplant patients receiving azathioprine and prednisone compared with patients receiving CI-based immunosuppressive therapy. Moreover, it has been shown that treatment with RAAS blocking agents such as captopril or lisinopril do not prevent CI-induced reductions in the renal blood flow, effectively negating the activation of angiotensin II as the underlying mechanism for the development of HTN and renal toxicity.[8,26]

Increased sodium sensitivity
The WNK/SPAK kinase pathway is a major factor in the blood pressure homeostasis through the regulation of the sodium and potassium reabsorption pathway within the nephron.[27] Encoding for the serine threonine kinase expressed in distal nephron, the WNK4 gene is responsible for the nephron's ability to switch between volume retention via RAAS and aldosterone-mediated potassium wasting.[28] Via regulation of the sodium chloride cotransporter found in the distal nephron, WNK4 expression conveys sensitivity to thiazide-type diuretics.[29] CIs such as cyclosporine and tacrolimus have direct metabolic side effects on the WNK4 system.[30] Activation of this renal sodium chloride cotransporter within the nephron contributes to HTN.[31]

Posttransplant weight gain
HTN can be related to weight gain after transplantation.[32] When compared with tacrolimus, cyclosporine is associated with additional weight gain of 2.3 kg in the first year after solid organ transplantation; however, it should be noted that this difference was not significant 3 years after transplantation.[33]

Activation of the sympathetic nervous system
Cyclosporine initiation acutely activates sympathetic activity by increasing renal afferent signaling through neurogenic vasoconstriction and by induction of central modulation of glutaminergic neurotransmission.[34] Continued use of cyclosporine does not portent the same effects.[35] Recent studies in animals have demonstrated that this effect is mediated by Ca^2 calmodulin-dependent phosphatase calcineurin, leading to vasoconstriction and an increase in blood pressure.[36]

Glucocorticoid-Mediated Effects

Increased response to catecholamines
The use of corticosteroids in immunosuppression protocols is associated with numerous side effects. The incidence of steroid-related HTN is around 15%.[37]

Although renal sodium retention and intravascular volume overload contribute to HTN, especially early in the course of the use of corticosteroids, a nonrenal mechanism (increase in peripheral vascular resistance) is also involved in the development and maintenance of HTN.[37] The concept of nonrenal actions of corticosteroids in the development of HTN was shown by a study that demonstrated acute elevations in blood pressure as a response to deoxycorticosterone acetate in dogs and rats devoid of renal mass.[38] Several investigations suggest that glucocorticoids act on adrenergic receptors to potentiate the vascular actions of catecholamines and thus producing vasoconstriction.[39,40] Glucocorticoid use is also associated with an increase in aortic smooth muscle cell angiotensin II receptor IA messenger RNA by stimulating angiotensin II receptor IA promoter activity thereby activating RAAS and contributing to HTN.[41]

Nitric oxide–mediated effects

Another mechanism by which corticosteroids can produce HTN is through inhibition of the NO pathway. Dexamethasone has been shown to attenuate acetylcholine-mediated vasodilatory response.[42] In addition, glucocorticoids reduce endothelial NO synthase III messenger RNA by decreasing transcription and increasing degradation thereby inhibiting NO-mediated peripheral vascular dilatation.[43]

Restrictive–Constrictive Physiology

HTN after heart transplantation is associated with increased peripheral vascular resistance and normal cardiac output. Cardiac transplant recipients have normal right atrial and pulmonary capillary wedge pressures at rest; however, an increase in pulmonary capillary wedge pressure and abnormalities in right atrial filling waves can be noted during stress.[44,45] The presence of a hemodynamic pattern suggestive of a restrictive–constrictive physiology is common early after transplant, but the incidence decreases during the first year.[46] Patients with diastolic dysfunction have been shown to have impaired systolic function, but no differences in either mean arterial pressure or systemic vascular resistance between patients with or without constrictive–restrictive physiology have been detected.[47] It is unclear whether one or the aggregate of cardiac denervation, myocardial pathology, HTN, volume overload, and pericardial disease explains these hemodynamic observations. The presence of abnormal left ventricular end-diastolic pressure, ejection fraction, and left ventricular end-diastolic pressure-to-volume ratio is found to accompany the development of HTN.[48] Additionally, it has been shown that there is no relationship between markers of rejection such as fibrosis or inflammation on endomyocardial biopsy and the mild-to-moderate hemodynamic abnormalities seen in cardiac transplant patients in the immediate post-transplant period.[48,49]

Despite that, the abnormal hemodynamics may explain the early development of HTN; it has been shown that hemodynamics parameters and exercise capacity return to normal within 1 year of transplantation.[50] Progressive exercise capacity improvement is often accompanied by reduction of the reflex-induced HTN and systemic vascular resistance in this population[51]; however, requirements for antihypertensive medications do not show a corresponding decrease as time passes from the initial transplant.

Ventricular Vascular Uncoupling

Ventricular and vascular uncoupling in cardiac transplant recipients is multifactorial and may be owing to a combination of stiffness of the recipient peripheral vasculature and the development of HTN, as well as a direct effect of cyclosporine in the peripheral vasculature. The denervated donor heart is faced with acute and high vascular impedance after transplantation, which produces a potential mismatch between the donor heart and the recipient vasculature.[52] In any case, the presence of ventricular vascular uncoupling may cause deleterious long-term changes in the ventricular function of the cardiac allograft. Over time, mismatch and uncoupling may ultimately affect the function of the transplanted heart as it does in the nontransplanted heart and contribute to the development of HTN.[53]

Denervation and Deregulation of Parasympathetic Regulation

Transection of the autonomic fibers during heart transplantation results sympathetic and vagal denervation causing delayed and blunted heart rate (HR) response to exercise as well as an increased resting HR.[54] Posttransplant, the ventricular tissues have normal beta-adrenergic receptor affinity and density but reduced catecholamine and alpha-tubulin contents, consistent with intrinsic sympathetic cardiac nervous system remodeling.[55] Despite evidence of sympathetic remodeling, parasympathetic remodeling and control of donor HR is absent in the majority of patients up to 96 months after transplantation.[56]

Tachycardia is closely associated with increased blood pressure in normal populations as well as insulin resistance and heart failure.[57] A typical posttransplant resting HR is between 90 and 110 beats per minute.[58] An inappropriately high resting HR has been demonstrated to be an adverse prognostic sign in long-term survivors of cardiac transplantation.[59] Prolonged and uncontrolled tachycardia may lead to a tachycardia-mediated cardiomyopathy and increases the risk of sudden cardiac death.[60]

MANAGEMENT OF HYPERTENSION AFTER CARDIAC TRANSPLANTATION
Modulation of Immunosuppression

One the first goals in the management of HTN after cardiac transplantation is to modulate immunosuppression therapy to a minimally tolerated dose.[4] Recently, withdrawal of corticosteroids has been proposed; however, studies and reports vary on the time course for reduction or taper of steroid use. Rapid discontinuation of steroids is not only associated with increased acute rejection, but also with decreased in adverse effects of these agents, including HTN.[61] It has been shown that corticosteroid withdrawal is associated with reduced mortality and decreased cardiovascular event risk through either early (<3 months posttransplant) or late (3–12 months posttransplant) withdrawal that is attributable to the modulations in other risk factors such as hyperglycemia, hyperlipidemia, and HTN.[62,63]

Reduction of oral doses of CI is associated with a dose-dependent reduction in blood pressure.[64] New evidence suggests that the transition from CI-based regimens to belatacept-based therapy has identified improvements in cardiovascular risk profile and blood pressure management; however, this agent is not widely in use at this time.[65] Mammalian target of rapamycin inhibitors or mycophenolic acid derivatives are an alternative to the use of CIs or used in CI minimization strategies. Although these agents are not associated with the development of HTN, their efficacy and safety profiles must be taken into account before initiation.[66]

Importance of Diurnal Variation

The circadian rhythm of blood pressure is disturbed after cardiac transplantation.[67] Posttransplant, patients no longer experience nocturnal blood pressure decreases seen in nontransplanted patients and are consequently exposed to an overall greater 24-hour hypertensive burden.[68] Appropriate antihypertensive therapy has the potential to bring about significant benefits in the heart transplant recipient because of the greater exposure and multitude of metabolic processes disturbed by the necessity of immunosuppressive therapy in these patients.[69] Optimal blood pressure management may be achieved by giving larger doses of antihypertensive agents at bedtime. Targeting treatment for the specific time of the day that blood pressure is typically highest may also be effective.

Clinical Trials

A multicenter, randomized trial investigating the short-term effectiveness of the calcium antagonist diltiazem versus the angiotensin-converting enzyme inhibitor lisinopril has been performed in the postcardiac transplant population.[70] The study included 116 patients with HTN after cardiac transplantation (blood pressure 140/90 mm Hg on separate visits) despite dietary sodium restriction. Fifty-five patients were randomized to sustained-release diltiazem up to 360 mg/d and, of these patients, 21 (38%) were responders achieving a diastolic blood pressure of less than 90 mm Hg, 23 (42%) were nonresponders, and 11 (20%) were withdrawn from the study. Sixtyone patients were randomized to lisinopril up to 40 mg/d, and of this group, 28 patients (46%) were responders, 22 (36%) were nonresponders, and 11 (18%) were withdrawn from the study. Systolic and diastolic blood pressure decreased significantly with both drugs in the responder group. The most common side effect observed with diltiazem was peripheral edema, whereas hyperkalemia and hypotension were more common with lisinopril. A total of 35 adverse effects were reported with both drugs; these side effects were minor and resolved with the discontinuation of the agent. The authors concluded that both agents are safe but only achieve blood pressure control as monotherapy in fewer than 50% of cardiac transplant recipients with cyclosporine-induced HTN. This study highlights the importance of multiple antihypertensive agents to achieve blood pressure control in cardiac transplant recipients.

Choice of Antihypertensive Therapy

Adjuvant therapy
The treatment of posttransplant HTN is often difficult despite the use of multiple drug regimens. Initial efforts to administer the lowest possible doses of CIs and steroids are imperative and may dictate the choice of further therapy. It is also important to avoid the use of nonsteroidal antiinflammatory medications in patients with HTN after cardiac transplantation owing to the risk of further impairment in renal function associated with the use of these agents.

Calcium channel blockers
Calcium antagonists (calcium channel blockers) and angiotensin-converting enzyme inhibitors are the first-line agents in the treatment of HTN after cardiac transplantation. Diltiazem has been shown not only an antihypertensive effect and a decrease in mortality, but also significant decreases in oral doses of cyclosporine required to reach therapeutic serum levels.[71] It has been shown that creatinine clearance was better preserved in patients receiving nifedipine, indicating a possible protective effect of this calcium channel antagonist in the kidney. Other nondihydropyridine calcium channel blockers such as amlodipine can be also used.

Angiotensin-converting enzyme inhibitors and angiotensin receptor blockers
Angiotensin-converting enzyme inhibitors and angiotensin receptor blockers have been shown to regulate blood pressure in patients after cardiac transplantation. In addition, they prevent cardiac allograft remodeling.[72] The blockade of the

renin–angiotensin system attenuates the glucocorticoid-mediated increase in blood pressure and[73] alleviates the fibrosis in the kidneys owing to CIs.[74]

Diuretics
Diuretics are used to control increase in fluid overload after cardiac transplantation. Cardiac transplant recipients demonstrate abnormal responses to volume expansion with an affinity for salt and water retention that is present despite a normal cardiac index.[75] CIs induce sodium retention; diuretics counteract this effect.[29] Meticulous attention to dietary sodium intake is important. Care should be taken in the use of these medications because the diuretic benefit may come at the cost of decreased renal function or an increase in serum creatinine, which may alter the pharmacodynamics of CI dosing.[4]

Vasoactive agents
For HTN that is present in the chronic renal failure population and potentially in those transplant recipients with CN-induced renal damage, alpha blockade with medications such as prazosin may be a viable treatment option.[76] Alpha-adrenergic antagonists can lower blood pressure by reducing peripheral vascular resistances and may decrease levels of triglycerides and cholesterol.[77]

To affect vascular resistance, many treatment options are available. The direct vasodilator minoxidil may be added in severe cases of HTN, but should be paired with the use of diuretics and beta-blockers to prevent edema and tachycardia.[78] Central alpha-agonists such as clonidine are also commonly used for refractory HTN and have shown to have no impact on the glomerular filtration rate or renal plasma flow, which may improve renal function in the posttransplant setting.[79] Supplementation of fatty acids (3–4 g/d) with high concentrations of eicosanoic and docosanoic acids has been shown to reduce peripheral vascular resistance and subsequent HTN and may be particularly beneficial in CI-induced HTN.[80,81]

Direct renin inhibitors
In animal models, the direct renin inhibitor aliskiren has shown protective effects against tacrolimus-induced nephrotoxicity and may be able to counteract nephrotic syndrome associated with immunosuppressant use.[82] However, there is currently little to no experience using this medication in transplant therapy. Current studies are underway to evaluate the safety and interaction profile of direct renin inhibitors and CIs.

SUMMARY

HTN is a common complication among post cardiac transplant recipients affecting more than 95% of patients.[83] Increased blood pressure poses a significant cardiovascular morbidity and mortality in these patients; it should be identified quickly and needs to be managed appropriately. Understanding the pathophysiology and contributing factors to this disease in these complex and unique patients is the key to appropriate treatment selection.

Editor's comment by Edward D. Frohlich, MD, MACP, FACP

HTN in patients who required a cardiac transplantation is a frequently encountered management problem. These 2 major problems require clinical management by extraordinary clinicians with the broad specialty experience of well-trained specialists, the patience and management experience of knowledgeable physicians with the commitment of a committed primary care physician, and the desire requires prompt answers. This is the not infrequent problem of the postcardiac transplantation patient who presents with never-before-known and -treated HTN.

This dilemma was faced by well-trained and experienced internists, including an experienced chief of an active cardiac transplantation having a large and highly regarded training program frequently confronted with many major questions. Thus, the question arose as to the treatment of the cardiac transplanted patient with never-before-encountered HTN.

Dr Bennett was first confronted with this situation after a careful search of the existing literature failed to satisfy this straightforward question. Thus, the questions were, which were the potential underlying mechanisms (left ventricular remodeling, nephrotoxicity, activation of the renin-angiotensin systems, sodium sensitivity, neurogenic mechanisms, and problems with any of the prescribed medications including with immunosuppressive therapy)? And, what might have been the experience of others with this question confronted at any large teaching hospital with a long experience with cardiac transplanted patients? After a thorough search of the literature and discussion with chief of the unit, Dr Ventura, she presented her written conclusion, which seemed a straightforward response to me.

After reading about their thinking presented herein, I thought that the way their problem was confronted was best expressed in their answer, which provided a stimulating and most provoking discussion for this monograph.

REFERENCES

1. Textor SC, Taler SJ, Canzanello VJ, et al. Posttransplantation hypertension related to calcineurin inhibitors. Liver Transpl 2000;6(5):521–30.
2. Olivari MT, Antolick A, Ring S. Arterial hypertension in heart transplant recipients treated with triple drug immunosuppressive therapy. J Heart Transplant 1989;8: 34–9.
3. Martínez-Dolz L, Sánchez-Lázaro IJ, Almenar-Bonet L, et al. Metabolic syndrome in heart transplantation: impact on survival and renal function. Transpl Int 2013; 26(9):910–8.
4. Ventura HO, Mehra MR, Stapleton DD, et al. Cyclosporine-induced hypertension in cardiac transplantation. Med Clin North Am 1997;81(6):1347–57.
5. Aparicio LS, Alfie J, Barochiner J, et al. Hypertension: the neglected complication of transplantation. ISRN Hypertension 2013:165937.
6. Hosenpud JD, Novick RJ, Bennet LE, et al. The Registry of the International Society for heart and lung transplantation: thirteenth official report 1996. J Heart Lung Transplant 1996;15:655–74.
7. Starling RC, Cody RJ. Cardiac transplant hypertension. Am J Cardiol 1990;65: 106–11.
8. Canzanello VJ, Textor SC, Taler SJ, et al. Late hypertension after liver transplantation: a comparison of cyclosporine and tacrolimus (FK 506). Liver Transpl Surg 1998;4(4):328–34.
9. Bennett WM, Porter G. Cyclosporine-associated hypertension. Am J Med 1988; 85:131–3.
10. Luke RG, Curtis JJ. Biology and treatment of transplant hypertension. In: Laragh JH, Brenner BM, editors. Hypertension: pathophysiology, diagnosis and management. 2nd edition. New York: Raven Press; 1995. p. 2471–81.
11. Sanders M, Victor RG. Hypertension after cardiac transplantation: pathophysiology and management. Curr Opin Nephrol Hypertens 1995;4:443–51.
12. Ventura HO, Lavie CJ, Messerli FH, et al. Cardiovascular adaptation to cyclosporine-induced hypertension. J Hum Hypertens 1994;8:233–7.

13. Coffman IM, Carr DR, Yarger WF, et al. Evidence that renal prostaglandins and thromboxane production is stimulated in chronic cyclosporine nephrotoxicity. Transplantation 1987;43:282–5.

14. Garr MD, Paller MS. Cyclosporine augments renal but not systemic vascular reactivity. Am J Physiol 1990;258:211–7.

15. Cauduro RL, Costa C, Lhulier F, et al. Endothelin-1 plasma levels and hypertension in cyclosporine-treated renal transplant patients. Clin Transplant 2005;19(4): 470–4.

16. Forslund T, Hannonen P, Reitamo S, et al. Hypertension in cyclosporine A-treated patients is independent of circulating endothelin levels. J Intern Med 1995; 238(1):71–5.

17. Cavarape A, Endlich K, Feletto F, et al. Contribution of endothelin receptors in renal microvessels in acute cyclosporine-mediated vasoconstriction in rats. Kidney Int 1998;53(4):963–9.

18. Molkentin JD, Lu JR, Antos CL, et al. A calcineurin-dependent transcriptional pathway for cardiac hypertrophy. Cell 1998;93:215–28.

19. Ventura HO, Johnson MR, Grusk B, et al. Cardiac adaptation to obesity and hypertension after heart transplantation. J Am Coll Cardiol 1992;19:55–9.

20. Kahan BD. Cyclosporine nephrotoxicity: pathogenesis, prophylaxis, therapy, and prognosis. Am J Kidney Dis 1986;8:323–31.

21. Murray BM, Paller MS, Ferris TF. Effect of cyclosporine administration on renal hemodynamics in conscious rats. Kidney Int 1985;28:767–74.

22. Porter GA, Bennett WM, Sheps SG. Cyclosporine-associated hypertension. National High Blood Pressure Education Program. Arch Intern Med 1990;150:280–3.

23. Karabesheh S, Verma DR, Jain M, et al. Clinical and hemodynamic effects of renin-angiotensin system blockade in cardiac transplant recipients. Am J Cardiol 2011;108(12):1836–9.

24. Bantle JP, Nath KA, Sutherland DE, et al. Effects of cyclosporine on the renin-angiotensin-aldosterone system and potassium excretion in renal transplant recipients. Arch Intern Med 1985;145(3):505–8.

25. Bellet M, Cabrol C, Sessano P, et al. Systemic hypertension after cardiac transplantation: effect of cyclosporine on the renin-angiotensin-aldosterone system. Am J Cardiol 1985;56:927–31.

26. Schaaf MR, Hene RJ, Floor M, et al. Hypertension after renal transplantation: calcium channel or converting enzyme blockade? Hypertension 1995;25:77–81.

27. Hoorn EJ, Nelson JH, McCormick JA, et al. The WNK kinase network regulating sodium, potassium, and blood pressure. J Am Soc Nephrol 2011;22(4):605–14.

28. Peng JB, Warnock DG. WNK4-mediated regulation of renal ion transport proteins. Am J Physiol Renal Physiol 2007;293(4):F961–73.

29. Subramanya AR, Yang CL, McCormick JA, et al. WNK kinases regulate sodium chloride and potassium transport by the aldosterone-sensitive distal nephron. Kidney Int 2006;70(4):630–4.

30. Melnikov S, Mayan H, Uchida S, et al. Cyclosporine metabolic side effects: association with the WNK4 system. Eur J Clin Invest 2011;41(10):1113–20.

31. Hoorn EJ, Walsh SB, McCormick JA, et al. The calcineurin inhibitor tacrolimus activates the renal sodium chloride cotransporter to cause hypertension. Nat Med 2011;17(10):1304–9.

32. Stogsdill G, Gonzales D, Hays N, et al. Post-liver transplant weight gain and its effect on cardiovascular disease risk factors. FASEB J 2011;25:971.39.

33. Canzanello VJ, Schwartz L, Taler SJ, et al. Evolution of cardiovascular risk after liver transplantation: a comparison of cyclosporine A and tacrolimus (FK506). Liver Transpl Surg 1997;3(1):1–9.

34. Victor RG, Thomas GD, Marban E, et al. Presynaptic modulation of cortical synaptic activity by calcineurin. Proc Natl Acad Sci U S A 1995;92(14):6269–73.

35. Klein IH, Abrahams AC, van Ede T, et al. Differential effects of acute and sustained cyclosporine and tacrolimus on sympathetic nerve activity. J Hypertens 2010;28(9):1928–34.

36. Lyson T, Ermel LD, Belshaw PJ, et al. Cyclosporine- and FK506-induced sympathetic activation correlates with calcineurin-mediated inhibition of T-cell signaling. Circ Res 1993;73(3):596–602.

37. Veenstra DL, Best JH, Hornberger J, et al. Incidence and long-term cost of steroid-related side effects after renal transplantation. Am J Kidney Dis 1999; 33(5):829–39.

38. Langford HG, Snavely JR. Effect of DCA on development of renoprival hypertension. Am J Physiol 1959;196:449–50.

39. Yard AC, Kadowitz PJ. Studies on the mechanism of hydrocortisone potentiation of vasoconstrictor responses to epinephrine in the anesthetized animal. Eur J Pharmacol 1972;20:1–9.

40. Besse JC, Bass AD. Potentiation by hydrocortisone of responses to catecholamines in vascular smooth muscle. J Pharmacol Exp Ther 1966;154:224–38.

41. Uno S, Guo DF, Nakajima M, et al. Glucocorticoid induction of rat angiotensin II type 1A receptor gene promoter. Biochem Biophys Res Commun 1994;204: 210–5.

42. Wallerath T, Witte K, Schafer SC, et al. Down-regulation of the expression of endothelial NO synthase is likely to contribute to glucocorticoid-mediated hypertension. Proc Natl Acad Sci U S A 1999;96:13357–62.

43. Whitworth JA, Schyvens CG, Zhang Y, et al. The nitric oxide system in glucocorticoid-induced hypertension. J Hypertens 2002;20:1035–43.

44. Humen DP, McKenzie FN, Kostuk WJ. Restricted myocardial compliance one year following cardiac transplantation. J Heart Transplant 1984;3:341–5.

45. Cotts WG, Oren RM. Function of the transplanted heart: unique physiology and therapeutic implications. Am J Med Sci 1997;314(3):164–72.

46. Tallaj JA, Kirklin JK, Brown RN, et al. Post-heart transplant diastolic dysfunction is a risk factor for mortality. J Am Coll Cardiol 2007;50(11):1064–9.

47. Valantine HA, Appelton CP, Hatle LK, et al. A hemodynamic and Doppler echocardiographic study of ventricular function in long-term cardiac allograft recipients: etiology and prognosis of restrictive-constrictive physiology. Circulation 1989;79:66–75.

48. Murali S, Uretsky BF, Reddy S, et al. Hemodynamic abnormalities following cardiac transplantation: relationship to hypertension and survival. Am Heart J 1989;118:334–41.

49. Greenbert ML, Uretsky BF, Reddy S, et al. Long-term hemodynamic follow-up of cardiac transplant patients treated with cyclosporine and prednisone. Circulation 1985;71(3):487–94.

50. Rudas L, Pflugfelder PW, Kostuk WJ. Hemodynamic observations following orthotopic cardiac transplantation: evolution of rest hemodynamics in the first year. Acta Physiol Hung 1992;79(1):57–64.

51. Crisafulli A, Tocco F, Milia R, et al. Progressive improvement in hemodynamic response to muscle metaboreflex in heart transplant recipients. J Appl Physiol (1985) 2013;114(3):421–7.

52. Patel ND, Weiss ES, Nwakanma LU, et al. Cardiac transplantation and surgery for heart failure impact of donor-to-recipient weight ratio on survival after heart transplantation: analysis of the United Network for organ sharing database. Circulation 2008;118:S83–8.
53. Borlaug BA, Kass DA. Ventricular-vascular interaction in heart failure. Heart Fail Clin 2008;4(1):23–36.
54. Ambrosi P, Kreitmann B, Habib G. Does heart rate predict allograft vasculopathy in heart transplant recipients? Int J Cardiol 2010;145:256–7.
55. Murphy DA, Thompson GW, Ardell JL, et al. The heart reinnervates after transplantation. Ann Thorac Surg 2000;69(6):1769–81.
56. Arrowood JA, Minisi AJ, Goudreau E, et al. Absence of parasympathetic control of heart rate after human orthotopic cardiac transplantation. Circulation 1997;96:3492–8.
57. Palatini P, Casiglia E, Pauletto P, et al. Relationship of tachycardia with high blood pressure and metabolic abnormalities: a study with mixture analysis in three populations. Hypertension 1997;30:1267–73.
58. Kobashigawa JK. Physiology of the transplanted heart. In: Norma DJ, Turka LA, editors. Primer on transplantation. 2nd edition. Thorofare (NJ): American Society of Transplant Physicians; 2001. p. 358–62.
59. Scott CD, McComb JM, Dark JH. Heart rate and late mortality in cardiac transplant recipients. Eur Heart J 1993;14:530–3.
60. Nerheim P, Birger-Botkin S, Piracha L, et al. Heart failure and sudden death in patients with tachycardia-induced cardiomyopathy and recurrent tachycardia. Circulation 2004;110:247–52.
61. Matas AJ. Steroid elimination-who, when, how? Transplant Proc 2008;40(10 supplement):S52–6.
62. Arnol M, de Mattos AM, Chung JS, et al. Late steroid withdrawal and cardiovascular events in kidney transplant recipients. Transplantation 2008;86(12):1844–8.
63. Jaber JJ, Feustel PJ, Elbahloul O, et al. Early steroid withdrawal therapy in renal transplant recipients: a steroid-free sirolimus and CellCept-based calcineurin inhibitor-minimization protocol. Clin Transplant 2007;21(1):101–9.
64. Ekberg H, Grinyo J, Nashan B, et al. Cyclosporine sparing with mycophenolate mofetil, daclizumab and corticosteroids in renal allograft recipients: the CAESAR study. Am J Transplant 2007;7(3):560–70.
65. Artz MA, Boots JMM, Ligtenberg G, et al. Conversion from cyclosporine to tacrolimus improves quality-of-life indices, renal graft function and cardiovascular risk profile. Am J Transplant 2004;4(6):937–45.
66. Gonzalez-Vilchez F, Vazquez de Prada JA, Paniagua MJ, et al. Use of mTOR inhibitors in chronic heart transplant recipients with renal failure: calcineurin-inhibitors conversion or minimization? Int J Cardiol 2014;171(1):15–23.
67. Reeves RA, Shapiro AP, Thompson ME, et al. Loss of nocturnal decline in blood pressure after cardiac transplantation. Circulation 1986;73:401–8.
68. Wenting GJ, vd Meiracker AH, Simoons ML, et al. Circadian variation of heart rate but not of blood pressure after heart transplantation. Transplant Proc 1987;19:2554–5.
69. Lindenfeld J, Page RL 2nd, Zolty R, et al. Drug therapy in the heart transplant recipient part III: common medical problems. Circulation 2005;111:113–7.
70. Brozena SC, Johnson MR, Ventura H, et al. Effectiveness and safety of diltiazem or lisinopril in treatment of hypertension after heart transplantation Results of a prospective, randomized multicenter trial. J Am Coll Cardiol 1996;27(7):1707–12.

71. Schroeder JS, Gao SZ, Alderman EL, et al. A preliminary study of diltiazem in the prevention of coronary artery disease in heart-transplant recipients. N Engl J Med 1993;328:164–70.
72. Suwelack B, Gerhardt U, Hausberg M, et al. Comparison of quinapril versus atenolol: effects on blood pressure and cardiac mass after renal transplantation. Am J Cardiol 2000;86(5):583–5.
73. Suzuki H, Handa M, Kondo K, et al. Role of renin-angiotensin system in glucocorticoid hypertension in rats. Am J Physiol 1982;243:E48–51.
74. Heinze G, Mitterbauer C, Regele H, et al. Angiotensin converting enzyme inhibitor or angiotensin II type 1 receptor antagonist therapy is associated with prolonged patient and graft survival after renal transplantation. J Am Soc Nephrol 2006; 17(3):889–99.
75. Corcos T, Tamburino C, Leger P. Early and late hemodynamic evaluation after cardiac transplantation: a study of 28 cases. J Am Coll Cardiol 1988;11:264–9.
76. Curtis JR, Bateman FJA. Use of prazosin in management of hypertension in patients with chronic renal failure and in renal transplant recipients. Br Med J 1975; 4(5994):432–4.
77. Nash DT. Alpha-adrenergic blockers: mechanism of action, blood pressure control, and effects of lipoprotein metabolism. Clin Cardiol 1990;13:764.
78. Kleiner JP, Ball JH, Nelson WP, et al. The outpatient treatment of refractory hypertension with minoxidil. South Med J 1977;70:814–7.
79. Green S, Zawada ET Jr, Muakkassa W, et al. Effect of clonidine therapy on renal hemodynamics in renal transplant hypertension. Arch Intern Med 1984;144(6): 1205–8.
80. Skulas-Ray AC, Kris-Etherton PM, Harris WS, et al. Effects of marine-derived omega-3 fatty acids on systemic hemodynamics at rest and during stress: a dose–response study. Ann Behav Med 2012;44(3):301–8.
81. Ventura HO, Milani RV, Smart FW, et al. Cyclosporine induced hypertension: efficacy of omega-3 fatty acids in patients following cardiac transplantation. Circulation 1993;88:II281–285.
82. Al-Harbi NO, Imam F, Al-Harbi MM, et al. Treatment with aliskiren ameliorates tacrolimus-induced nephrotoxicity in rats. J Renin Angiotensin Aldosterone Syst 2015;16:1329–36.
83. Taylor DO, Edwards LB, Mohacsi PJ, et al. The registry of the International Society for Heart and Lung Transplantation: twentieth official adult heart transplant report—2003. J Heart Lung Transplant 2003;22:616–24.

Renal Arterial Disease and Hypertension

Stephen C. Textor, MD

KEYWORDS

- Renovascular • Renal artery stenosis • Hypertension • Angiotensin • Kidney
- Ischemic nephropathy

KEY POINTS

- Renal artery disease produces a spectrum of progressive clinical manifestations ranging from minor degrees of hypertension to circulatory congestion and kidney failure.
- Moderate reductions in renal blood flow do not induce tissue hypoxia or damage, making medical therapy for renovascular hypertension feasible for many patients.
- Several prospective trials indicate that optimized medical therapy using agents that block the renin-angiotensin system should be the initial management.
- Evidence of progressive disease and/or treatment failure should allow recognition of high-risk subsets that benefit from renal revascularization.
- Severe reductions in kidney blood flow ultimately activate inflammatory pathways that do not reverse with restoring blood flow alone.

Renovascular hypertension has been recognized for more than 80 years, since seminal experimental studies showed that progressive occlusion of the renal vessels produces an increase in systemic arterial pressure. These data established a central role of the kidney in blood pressure regulation and provided one of the most widely studied models of angiotensin-dependent hypertension.[1] This condition can occur at levels of renal pressure greater than those that impair kidney function, although progressive reduction in renal blood flow leads to additional disturbances, including impaired volume control, circulatory congestion, and ultimately irreversible kidney injury. Hence, occlusive renovascular disease (RVD) comprises a spectrum of disorders ranging from incidental, minor disease to incipient occlusion with tissue ischemia, as shown in **Fig. 1**.

EPIDEMIOLOGY

The dominant cause (at least 85%) of RVD in Western countries is atherosclerotic renal artery stenosis (ARAS). This condition often develops as part of systemic atherosclerotic disease affecting multiple vascular beds, including coronary, cerebral, and

Disclosures: Nothing to disclose.
Division of Nephrology and Hypertension, Mayo Clinic, 200 1st Street, Rochester, MN 55905, USA
E-mail address: textor.stephen@mayo.edu

Med Clin N Am 101 (2017) 65–79
http://dx.doi.org/10.1016/j.mcna.2016.08.010
0025-7125/17/© 2016 Elsevier Inc. All rights reserved.

Manifestations of Renovascular Disease

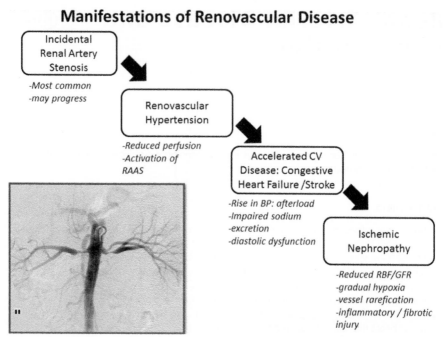

Incidental
Renal Artery
Stenosis

-*Most common*
-*may progress*

Renovascular
Hypertension

-*Reduced perfusion*
-*Activation of*
RAAS

Accelerated CV
Disease: Congestive
Heart Failure /Stroke

-*Rise in BP: afterload*
-*Impaired sodium*
-*excretion*
-*diastolic dysfunction*

Ischemic
Nephropathy

-*Reduced RBF/GFR*
-*gradual hypoxia*
-*vessel rarefication*
-*inflammatory / fibrotic*
injury

Fig. 1. Progressively more severe clinical manifestations associated with occlusive RVD. Minor degrees of lumen obstruction manifest as incidental lesions of minimal hemodynamic importance. As obstruction leads to reduced pressures and flow beyond the lesion, renovascular hypertension and acceleration of cardiovascular events ensue, particularly when associated with impaired sodium excretion. Ultimately, severe and long-standing RVD activates injury pathways within the kidney parenchyma that may no longer depend primarily on hemodynamic effects of stenosis and respond only partially to restoring vessel patency. BP, blood pressure; CV, cardiovascular; GFR, glomerular filtration rate; RAAS, renin-angiotensin-aldosterone system; RBF, renal blood flow.

peripheral vessels. Community-based studies suggest that up to 6.8% of individuals older than 65 years have ARAS with more than 60% occlusion.[2] Screening studies indicate an increasing prevalence of detectable ARAS in hypertensive subjects, from 3% (ages 50–59 years) to 25% (ages >70 years).[3] Clinically significant atherosclerotic RVD often is manifest by worsening or accelerating blood pressure increases in older individuals with preexisting hypertension.

Any flow-limiting vascular lesion within the renal circulation can produce renovascular hypertension (RVH). This can arise from a variety of fibromuscular dysplasias (FMDs), such as medial fibroplasia, which typically presents the appearance of a string-of-beads, or focal narrowing in the midportion of the renal artery[4] (**Fig. 2**). Some form of FMD may be detected incidentally in up to 3% of normotensive men or women presenting as potential kidney donors.[5] Those who progress to develop renovascular hypertension are predominantly women, some of whom are smokers. This gender predominance suggests that hormonal factors modulate the progression of this disorder and its clinical phenotype. Other disorders that produce RVH include renal trauma, arterial occlusion from dissection or thrombosis, and embolic occlusion of the renal artery (**Box 1**). Particularly in Asia, inflammatory vascular disorders such as Takayasu arteritis commonly affect the renal circulation. An emerging iatrogenic form of RVD includes occlusion of

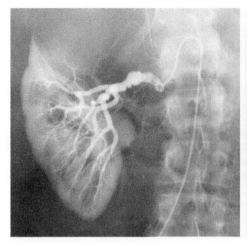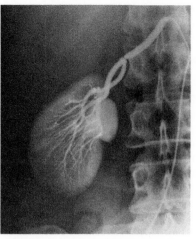

Fig. 2. Examples of fibromuscular RVD. (*Left*) Angiogram with a string-of-beads appearance typical of medial fibroplasia. Indentation of the vessel wall represents a series of internal webs that reduce distal perfusion and trigger RVH. Such lesions can respond to intra-arterial balloon angioplasty (percutaneous transluminal renal angioplasty). (*Right*) angiogram showing a focal stenosis causing severe hypertension. Recent classification schemes distinguish mainly between multifocal disease (*left*) and focal disease (*right*).

Box 1
Renal arterial lesions that produce the syndrome of renovascular hypertension

Unilateral disease (analogous to 1-clip–2-kidney hypertension)

Unilateral ARAS

Unilateral FMD
  Medial fibroplasia
  Perimedial fibroplasia
  Intimal fibroplasia
  Medial hyperplasia

Renal artery aneurysm

Arterial embolus

Arteriovenous fistula (congenital/traumatic)

Segmental arterial occlusion (posttraumatic)

Extrinsic compression of renal artery; for example, pheochromocytoma

Renal compression; for example, metastatic tumor

Bilateral disease or solitary functioning kidney (analogous to 1-clip–1-kidney model)

Stenosis to a solitary functioning kidney

Bilateral renal arterial stenosis

Aortic coarctation

Systemic vasculitis (eg, Takayasu, polyarteritis)

Atheroembolic disease

Vascular occlusion caused by endovascular aortic stent graft the renal arteries from endovascular aortic stent grafts, for which landing zones may migrate or be deliberately placed across the origins of the renal arteries.[6]

PATHOPHYSIOLOGY

RVH is triggered initially by activation of the renin-angiotensin-aldosterone system (RAAS). Studies over several decades have identified multiple actions of angiotensin II (Ang II), including its role as a direct vasoconstrictor, stimulation of adrenal release of aldosterone, and induction of sodium retention. Ang II recruits additional pressor mechanisms, such as sympathetic adrenergic pathways, vascular remodeling, and modification of prostaglandin-dependent vasodilatation.[7] Blockade of the renin-angiotensin system or genetic knockout of angiotensin I (AT-1) receptors prevents the development of experimental RVH.[8] After some time, secondary vasoconstrictor pathways can become dominant, with the result that pharmacologic RAAS blockade and/or renal revascularization may no longer completely reverse RVH.

Two major models of RVH have been proposed, depending on the functional role of the remaining kidney (the nonstenotic or contralateral kidney).[9] When the contralateral kidney is normal, it responds to increasing systemic pressure with suppression of its own renin release and enhanced pressure natriuresis. This 2-kidney–1-clip condition is characterized by unilateral release of renin into the renal veins, increased levels of plasma renin activity, and arterial pressure that demonstrably depends on the pressor effects of Ang II. The second model has been designated 1-kidney–1-clip RVD, in which either a functional contralateral kidney is not present or is not capable of ongoing pressure natriuresis. As a result, the increase in systemic pressure no longer is offset by increased sodium excretion, leading to volume expansion and secondary reduction in renin release from the stenotic kidney. These events lead to lower values for circulating plasma renin activity, loss of renal vein renin lateralization, and loss of detectable angiotensin dependence of systemic hypertension, unless or until diuresis and volume contraction are accomplished. In reality, the contralateral kidney in 2-kidney–1-clip renovascular hypertension is rarely normal, possibly as a result of tissue injury from direct effects of angiotensin II and/or other pathways. As a result, impaired contralateral kidney function impairs sodium excretion in many patients with long-standing RVH. Hence, clinical laboratory manifestations in human patients vary widely between the extremes predicted by 1-kidney and 2-kidney experimental models.

Remarkably, studies using blood oxygen level–dependent (BOLD) magnetic resonance (MR) indicate that reductions in blood flow (up to 35%–40%) can occur without demonstrable tissue hypoxia or evident long-term kidney fibrosis.[10] This is partly caused by the overperfusion of the kidney cortex as part of its filtration function, consistent with the observation that less than 10% of oxygen is required to fulfil the energy requirements of the kidney.[11] By contrast, the medulla normally is supplied by postglomerular arterioles with lower blood flow and has greater oxygen extraction because of energy-dependent active solute transport.[12] Thus, the kidney normally has a large cortical-medullary oxygen gradient with areas of markedly reduced oxygen tension in deep medullary areas. Moderate reductions in blood flow therefore exert only minor effects on oxygen delivery to the cortex and the reductions in glomerular filtration that result also reduce the net solute transport and thereby reduce oxygen requirements in medullary regions. An important corollary of these observations is that medical therapy for renovascular hypertension, albeit commonly reducing blood flow to the poststenotic kidney, can be tolerated, sometimes for many years, without inducing parenchymal kidney damage.

However, renal tolerance to reduced blood flow has limits. More severe and prolonged reductions in blood flow eventually threaten both tissue oxygenation and viability of the poststenotic kidney.[13] Studies of both experimental and human RVD indicate that cortical hypoxia is eventually associated with activation of inflammatory pathways,[14] as shown in **Fig. 3**. These pathways are characterized by abundant renal vein levels of proinflammatory cytokines, (such as tumor necrosis factor alpha and monocyte chemoattractant protein-1) in addition to the appearance of T lymphocytes and macrophages within the tissue parenchyma.[15,16] Inflammatory changes associated with severe ischemia lead to obliteration of tubules with failure to regenerate intact epithelial surfaces, with resulting atubular glomeruli.[17] At some point, these processes become refractory to restoring vessel patency with revascularization, despite restoring renal blood flow and reversal of tissue hypoxia.[18] This transition from simply a hemodynamic reduction in blood flow triggering RVH to an inflammatory, profibrotic state complicates the clinical decisions regarding optimal timing for renal revascularization.

DIAGNOSIS: CLINICAL MANIFESTATIONS

RVH and ischemic nephropathy are diagnosed primarily by recognition of a clinical syndrome defined by progressive or severe hypertension with/without unexplained chronic kidney disease (CKD). Occlusive RVD produces a range of manifestations generally related to the severity of vascular occlusion, as shown in **Fig. 1**. Many

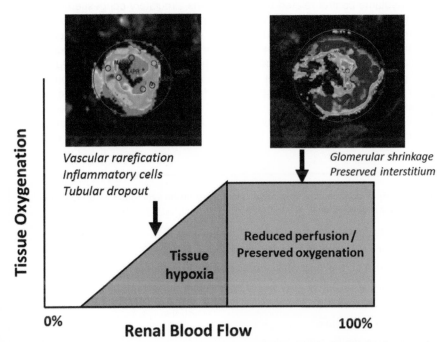

Fig. 3. Tissue oxygenation as measured by BOLD MR remains stable during moderate reductions in renal blood flow in atherosclerotic RVD. At some level, severe and prolonged blood flow reductions lead to overt tissue hypoxia associated with rarefication of small vessels, activation of inflammatory pathways, and interstitial fibrosis. Eventually, restoration of large vessel patency no longer reverses this process.

incidental lesions are now identified during imaging procedures for other indications, including computed tomography (CT) and/or MR angiography. It should be emphasized that hemodynamic effects of lumen occlusion, such as changes in either translesional pressure or flow, are barely detectable until lumen occlusion reaches a critical level (in the vicinity of 70% to 80% lumen occlusion).[19] Studies in humans subjected to stepwise partial balloon obstruction of the renal artery indicate that gradients of at least 10% to 20% reductions in postobstruction pressures are required to detect measurable renin release.[20] An important corollary is that failure to identify a pressure gradient across such a vascular lesion makes it unlikely that renal revascularization will have clinical benefit.

Clinical characteristics of atherosclerotic RVH include rapid changes in arterial pressure, often in patients with preexisting hypertension (**Box 2**). The average age of recent interventional reports for RVH is more than 70 years. Arterial pressure increases with age in Western societies, so most of these individuals have preexisting hypertension already treated with antihypertensive drugs. Recognizing progression and increasing antihypertensive drug requirements should raise the question of a superimposed secondary process such as atherosclerotic RVH. Compared with essential hypertension, patients with RVH have more evident activation of the renin-angiotensin system and increased sympathetic nerve activation, sometimes associated with wide pressure fluctuations and variability. Target organ manifestations, including vascular injury, left ventricular hypertrophy, and renal dysfunction, are more common with RVH compared with age-matched patients with essential hypertension of similar levels.[21]

Occlusive RVD and RVH can accelerate manifestations of other vascular diseases. Impaired volume control related to RVD worsens circulatory congestion associated with left ventricular dysfunction. When RVD triggers additional increases in arterial pressure, the resulting left ventricular outflow resistance can precipitate congestive heart failure, sometimes named flash pulmonary edema,[22,23] which is a recognizable clinical syndrome that is often associated with rapid worsening of renal function as arterial pressure is reduced and/or diuresis is achieved. Observational series report higher rates of mortality and rehospitalization for patients with combined congestive heart failure and RVD.[24,25]

Ultimately, progressive atherosclerotic RVD leads to loss of kidney function in the affected kidney. Prospective trials, including angioplasty and stenting for renal artery

---

Box 2
Clinical features of patients with renovascular hypertension syndromes associated with renovascular hypertension

1. Early or late onset hypertension (<30 years, >50 years)
2. Acceleration of treated essential hypertension
3. Deterioration of renal function in treated essential hypertension
4. Acute renal failure during treatment of hypertension
5. Flash pulmonary edema
6. Progressive renal failure
7. Refractory congestive cardiac failure

These syndromes should alert clinicians to the possible contribution of RVD. The last 3 are most common in patients with bilateral disease, many of whom are treated as essential hypertension until these characteristics appear (see text).

lesions (ASTRAL) and cardiovascular outcomes in renal atherosclerotic lesions (CORAL), indicate that 15% to 22% of patients with RVD progress to a renal end point over a follow-up period of between 3 and 4 years.[26] As a practical matter, establishing whether progressive CKD reflects underlying vascular disease should be a central concern for clinicians.

DIAGNOSIS: LABORATORY STUDIES

Current diagnostic studies and interpretation for RVD have been reviewed.[27] General values for hematologic and electrolyte levels are normal or consistent with the degree of glomerular filtration rate (GFR) reduction (level of CKD). Unexplained increases of serum creatinine levels merit further evaluation with at least ultrasonography duplex imaging. Urinalyses are typically bland, with few cellular elements and little proteinuria. The presence of significant albuminuria (or increase of urinary albumin/creatinine ratio) should raise concerns about other parenchymal renal disorders, including diabetic nephropathy.

Measurement of circulating plasma renin activity can be helpful, but is limited. As noted earlier, increased levels are consistent with RVH, although sodium retention, drug effects, and transitions to alternative pressor pathways sometimes leave these levels normal or low. The aldosterone/renin ratio typically is consistent with secondary aldosterone excess, and may account for hypokalemia observed either spontaneously or during diuretic therapy. Both hormonal and electrolyte levels are affected by many other factors, making their diagnostic value limited.

Measurement of renal vein renin levels was commonly performed during planning for surgical renal artery procedures when this was the primary therapy for RVH. Identification of overt lateralization to the poststenotic kidney along with suppression of renin release from the contralateral kidney has been associated with pressure reduction in more than 90% of patients.[27] Once again, the utility of this procedure is limited by variable conditions under which the measurements are made, which are often associated with external sodium chloride administration. Hence, failure to identify lateralization was associated with improved blood pressure in at least 50% of cases, rendering it of limited sensitivity and specificity. Repeat measurement after sodium depletion has been shown to unmask renal vein lateralization and identify RVH.[28] As a clinical measure, identifying a specific kidney as a pressor kidney with unilateral renin release is most useful when contemplating therapeutic nephrectomy for blood pressure control.

IMAGING STUDIES

Establishing the diagnosis of occlusive RVD intrinsically requires evidence of renal arterial obstruction. Hence, imaging studies are a sine qua non for this diagnosis. A detailed discussion of the relative benefits and characteristics of specific renovascular imaging methods is beyond the scope of this article. Before undertaking imaging procedures, some of which are expensive and potentially hazardous, clinicians would do well to establish exactly what the goals of the imaging study should be. Is the purpose simply to identify whether one or both kidneys have evident occlusive disease? Is it to establish the viability and functional characteristics of the poststenotic kidney? Is it to identify the specific location and severity of RVD for revascularization? Is it to identify translesional gradient information and/or response to revascularization? Perhaps most importantly, to what degree do the clinical conditions of the patient warrant consideration of acting on the imaging data, specifically regarding either renal revascularization or nephrectomy? Hence, the choice and pace of diagnostic imaging depend partly on the response to medical therapy and the clinical status of the patient. Duplex ultrasonography is often the first and least expensive study.

DIFFERENTIAL DIAGNOSIS

RVH remains one of the most common contributors to resistant hypertension. The differential diagnosis for resistant hypertension includes other secondary causes, including obstructive sleep apnea, primary renal diseases, and inappropriate aldosterone production/activity.[29] Most commonly, the question arises as to whether renal dysfunction represents parenchymal renal injury from hypertension (hypertensive nephrosclerosis), which is largely a diagnosis of exclusion, and it has been questioned whether nonmalignant forms of hypertension lead to renal failure.[30] Recent studies indicate that other factors, including specific genetic predisposition in African Americans, may determine the risk for renal dysfunction in such individuals. Some individuals have small vessel disease with or without thrombotic phenomena that mimics large vessel RVD, for which little can be done at present. In general, exclusion of RVD is an important step in the evaluation of otherwise unexplained renal dysfunction with or without hypertension.

Primary Medical and Antihypertensive Drug Therapy

Few conditions have undergone more radical paradigm shifts than the management of RVH. Although it remains a prototype for reversible causes of secondary hypertension, current practice has migrated to favor primary medical management as the mainstay of therapy. No doubt restoring vessel patency and perfusion pressures sometimes can decrease blood pressure to normal levels. This possibility is particularly applicable to younger individuals, such as women with renovascular hypertension from fibromuscular disease, whose hypertension sometimes regresses completely with technically successful renal artery angioplasty.[31] By contrast, older individuals with widespread atherosclerotic vascular disease and preexisting hypertension are likely to require ongoing medical antihypertensive therapy regardless of the success of revascularization.

Since the introduction of blockers of the renin-angiotensin system, medical therapy has achieved goal blood pressures more than 80% of the time, although multiple agents may be required[32] (**Fig. 4**). In such patients, pursuing expensive and invasive intervention is difficult to justify. Patients with RVH treated with angiotensin-converting enzyme (ACE)/angiotensin receptor blocker (ARB) therapy seem to have a long-term mortality benefit compared with those without such treatment.[33,34] Importantly, results from recent prospective, randomized trials fail to show substantial additional benefit from renal revascularization procedures for many patients who can be controlled with effective antihypertensive drug therapy.

Accordingly, management of RVH begins with optimizing medical therapy, which necessarily includes withholding tobacco use, introduction of statins, glucose control, and effective antihypertensive drug treatment, most often including either an ACE inhibitor or ARB.[34] If this approach achieves excellent blood pressure levels with stable renal function, no further action may be required, other than surveillance for disease progression.

However, atherosclerosis is intrinsically progressive, albeit at variable rates between individuals. Poststenotic perfusion pressures are lower than those in the aorta or prestenosis levels, thereby subjecting the kidney to reduced renal perfusion. As noted earlier, the kidney can tolerate moderate reductions in pressure without developing tissue hypoxia (as shown in **Fig. 3**) or structural renal injury,[35] sometimes for many years. However, at some point, overt tissue hypoxia does develop, along with inflammatory injury. Glomerular filtration at reduced renal perfusion pressure eventually depends on the postglomerular efferent arteriolar effects of angiotensin II. Hence

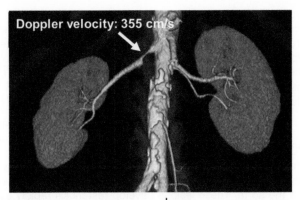

Medications: Lisinopril 40 mg | BP: 136 / 82 mm Hg
Amlodipine 5 mg | Creatinine 1.1 mg/dL
indapamide 1.25 mg | eGFR: 47 ml/min/1.73m2

Fig. 4. CT angiogram from a patient with unilateral atherosclerotic RVD manifest by high Doppler velocities and recently progressive hypertension. This condition was treated with drug therapy, including angiotensin-converting enzyme inhibition with satisfactory BP levels and GFR (serum creatinine, 1.1 mg/dL). Results of prospective, randomized trials indicate that little additional benefit is to be gained by further intervention (eg, renal revascularization) so long as this remains stable (see text). eGFR, estimated GFR.

blockade of the RAAS is particularly capable of reducing filtration pressure at critical levels of kidney perfusion. Progressive loss of GFR in such patients can sometimes recover substantially by withholding these ACE inhibitors and/or ARBs, as some investigators have advocated routinely.[36] Such a critical dependence signals near-critical levels of occlusive disease that may benefit from renal revascularization.

Revascularization for Renal Arterial Disease

Restoration of blood flow to the kidney beyond a stenotic lesion remains an obvious approach to improving renovascular hypertension and halting progressive vascular occlusive injury. A major shift from surgical reconstruction ensued in the 1990s in favor of endovascular stent procedures. Although some patients benefit enormously, revascularization procedures have both benefits and risks. In older patients with preexisting hypertension, the likelihood of a cure for hypertension is small. Although complications are not common, they can be catastrophic, including atheroembolic disease and aortic dissection. Knowing when the benefits of revascularization outweigh the risks is central to the challenges of managing RVD.

Angioplasty for Fibromuscular Disease

Most lesions of medial fibroplasia are located away from the renal artery ostium. Many of these have multiple webs within the vessel, which can be successfully traversed and opened by balloon angioplasty. Experience in the 1980s indicated more than 94% technical success rates. Some of these lesions (approximately 10%–15%) develop restenosis, for which repeat procedures have been used. Clinical benefit regarding blood pressure control has been reported in observational outcome studies in 65% to 75% of patients, although the rates of cure are less secure.[37] Cure of hypertension, defined as sustained blood pressure levels less than 140/90 mm Hg with no antihypertensive medications, may be obtained in 35% to 50% of patients. Predictors of cure (normal arterial pressures without medication beyond 6 months after angioplasty) include lower systolic blood pressures, younger age, and shorter duration of hypertension. Most patients with RVH and FMD are female and generally have less aortic disease and are at lower risk for major complications of angioplasty. Most clinicians favor early intervention for hypertensive patients with FMD with the hope of reduced antihypertensive medication requirements after successful angioplasty.

Angioplasty and Stenting for Atherosclerotic Renal Artery Stenosis

Angioplasty alone commonly fails to maintain patency for proximal or ostial atherosclerotic lesions, in part because of extensive recoil of the plaque extending into the main portion of the aorta. These lesions develop restenosis rapidly even after early success. Introduction of endovascular stents provides an indisputable advantage. An example of successful renal artery stenting is shown in **Fig. 5**. As technical success continues to improve, many reports suggest nearly 100% technical success in early vessel patency, although rates of restenosis continue to reach 14% to 25%.[38]

Several observational studies suggest that progression of renal failure attributed to ischemic nephropathy may be reduced by endovascular procedures. Harden and colleagues[39] presented reciprocal creatinine plots in 23 (of 32) patients, suggesting that the slope of loss of GFR could be favorably changed after renal artery stenting. It should be emphasized that 69% of patients improved or stabilized, indicating that 31% worsened, consistent with results from other series. Perhaps the most convincing group data in this regard derive from serial renal functional measurement in 33 patients with high-grade (>70%) stenosis to the entire affected renal mass (bilateral disease or stenosis to a solitary functioning kidney) with creatinine levels between 1.5 and 4.0 mg/dL. Follow-up over a mean of 20 months indicates that the slope of GFR loss converted from negative (-0.0079 dL/mg/mo) to positive (0.0043 dL/mg/mo).[40]

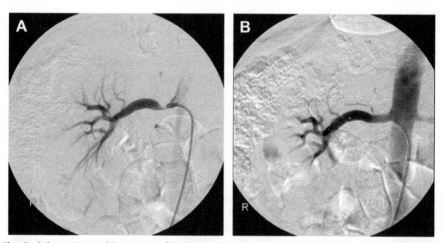

Fig. 5. (A) Angiographic image of high-grade stenosis manifest by new-onset accelerated hypertension more than 20 years after mantel radiation for malignancy. Drug therapy was associated with declining kidney function. (B) Endovascular stent placement in the proximal right renal artery achieved excellent recovery of lumen patency. This maneuver was followed with normalization of blood pressure and withdrawal of medications over 2 months.

These studies agree with other observations that long-term survival is reduced in bilateral disease and that the potential for renal dysfunction and accelerated cardiovascular disease risk is highest in such patients.[25,41]

Treatment Trials

Over the past 2 decades, several prospective randomized controlled trials have attempted to quantify a role for renal revascularization when added to medical therapy. Three early trials in renovascular hypertension from the 1990s addressed the added value of endovascular repair using percutaneous transluminal renal angioplasty (PTRA) without stenting compared with medical therapy for atherosclerotic RVH. Crossover rates for failure of medical therapy ranged from 22% to 44%, suggesting a role for PTRA in refractory hypertension, although the overall intention-to-treat analyses were negative.[42] There was greater blood pressure benefit after PTRA in patients with bilateral renal artery stenosis.

Recent prospective trials include stent placement and blood pressure and lipid-lowering for the prevention of progression of renal dysfunction caused by atherosclerotic ostial stenosis of the renal artery (STAR), ASTRAL, and CORAL as summarized in **Table 1**. In some cases, revascularization achieved slightly improved blood pressure levels and/or reduced drug requirements, but the differences have been minor. No definitive benefits regarding recovery of renal function, blood pressure control, or reduction of serious comorbid vascular events have been identified in any of these trials lasting 3 to 5 years.[43,44] These negative results have dampened the argument for early vascular intervention in atherosclerotic RVD.

The limitations of these trials have been substantial, particularly because many severe cases of rapidly progressive renal insufficiency, intractable hypertension, and/or episodic pulmonary edema have not been enrolled.[26,45] Hence, these trials underrepresent high-risk disease, as has been emphasized from registry[25,41] and observational reports.[46] These series identify high-risk subsets of patients with rapidly advancing disease and/or clinical problems related to fluid retention (pulmonary edema), acute kidney injury (AKI) during initiation of ACE/ARB therapy, or rapidly developing renal failure that benefit greatly from revascularization. An important role for clinicians remains to identify and intervene for such individuals.

MANAGEMENT STRATEGIES FOR RENOVASCULAR DISEASE

A clinical algorithm for managing RVH and ischemic nephropathy is presented in **Fig. 6**. In most cases, RVH manifests as progressive (or de-novo) hypertension with some decrement in kidney function. Reduction of cardiovascular risk is paramount and includes antihypertensive drug therapy to goal levels, along with removal of tobacco use, and likely initiation of statins and aspirin, particularly with atherosclerotic disease. Duplex imaging evaluates basic kidney structure, size, and whether occlusive disease is present, unilateral or bilateral. In most cases, drug therapy is sufficient to achieve blood pressure goals. If kidney function and blood pressure are stable on therapy, results of prospective, randomized trials suggest that little further is to be gained from revascularization, at least in follow-up intervals between 3 and 5 years. However, rates of progression and stability vary widely between individual patients. Important considerations include whether kidney function deteriorates in the presence of RAAS blockade and/or whether a high-risk syndrome develops, including circulatory congestion (pulmonary edema) and/or progressive renal insufficiency with failure to achieve blood pressure targets. In such cases, clinicians must carefully weigh the potential benefits and risks of restoring vessel

Table 1
Randomized clinical trials: PTRA with stenting versus medical therapy alone for renal function and/or cardiovascular outcomes with atherosclerotic RVD (ARVD)

Trials	N	Population	Inclusion Criteria	Exclusion Criteria	Outcomes
STAR (2009) 10 centers, f/up 2 y	Med Tx:76 PTRA: 64	Patients with impaired renal function, ostial ARVD detected by various imaging studies, and stable blood pressure on statin and aspirin	ARVD >50% Creatinine clearance <80 mL/min/1.73 m² Controlled blood pressure 1 mo before inclusion	Kidney <8 cm and, renal artery diameter <4 mm eCrCl <15 mL/min/1.73 m² DM with proteinuria (>3 g/dl), malignant hypertension	No difference in GFR decline (primary end point ≥20% change in clearance), but many did not undergo PTRA because of ARVD <50% on angiography Serious complication in the PTRA group Study was underpowered
ASTRAL (2009) 57 centers, f/up 5 y	Med Tx: 403 PTRA: 403	Patients with uncontrolled or refractory hypertension or unexplained renal dysfunction with unilateral or bilateral ARVD on statin and aspirin	ARVD substantial disease suitable for endovascular treatment and patient's doctor uncertain of clinical benefit from revascularization	High likelihood of PTRA in <6 mo Without ARVD, previous ARVD PTRA FMD	No difference in BP, renal function, mortality, CV events (primary end point: 20% reduction in the mean slope of the reciprocal of the serum creatinine level) Substantial risk in the PTRA group
CORAL (2013) 109 centers, f/up 5 y	Med Tx: 480 PTRA: 467	Hypertension; 2 or more antihypertensives or CKD stage ≥3 with ARVD with unilateral or bilateral disease on statin	SBP >155 mm Hg, at least 2 drugs ARVD >60% Subsequent changes included that the SBP >155 mm Hg for defining systolic hypertension was no longer specified as long as patient had CKD stage 3	FMD; creatinine >4.0 mg/dL; kidney length <7 cm; and use of >1 stent	No difference of death from CV or renal causes. Modest improvement of SBP in the stented group Total of 26 complications (5.5%)

Abbreviations: CV, cardiovascular; DM, diabetes mellitus; eCrCl, estimated creatinine clearance; f/up, follow-up; Med Tx, medical therapy; N, number of patients; SBP, systolic blood pressure.

Management of Renovascular Hypertension and Ischemic Nephropathy

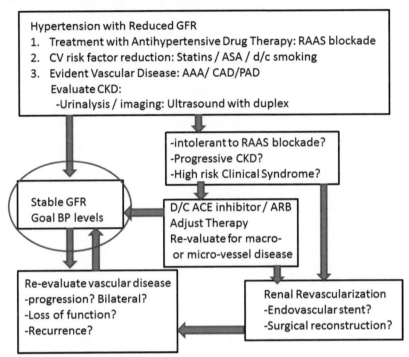

Fig. 6. Steps in the management of RVH and ischemic nephropathy. The foremost goals are to reduce morbidity associated with hypertension by reaching goal BP and to preserve kidney function. Should that not be achievable by medical therapy or should vascular disease progress, renal revascularization should be considered, either by endovascular or surgical intervention (see text).

patency and blood flow to the affected kidney at a point when renal function can be salvaged.

REFERENCES

1. Basso N, Terragno NA. History about the discovery of the renin-angiotensin system. Hypertension 2001;38:1246–9.
2. Hansen KJ, Edwards MS, Craven TE, et al. Prevalence of renovascular disease in the elderly: a population based study. J Vasc Surg 2002;36:443–51.
3. Coen G, Manni M, Giannoni MF, et al. Ischemic nephropathy in an elderly nephrologic and hypertensive population. Am J Nephrol 1998;18:221–7.
4. Meaney TF, Dustan HP, McCormack LJ. Natural history of renal arterial disease. Radiology 1968;91(5):881–7.
5. Lorenz EC, Vrtiska TJ, Lieske JC, et al. Prevalence of renal artery and kidney abnormalities by computed tomography among healthy adults. Clin J Am Soc Nephrol 2010;5:431–8.
6. Textor SC, Misra S, Oderich G. Percutaneous revascularization for ischemic nephropathy: the past, present and future. Kidney Int 2013;83(1):28–40.
7. Lerman LO, Nath KA, Rodriguez-Porcel M, et al. Increased oxidative stress in experimental renovascular hypertension. Hypertension 2001;37(2 Pt 2):541–6.

8. Cervenka L, Horacek V, Vaneckova I, et al. Essential role of AT1-A receptor in the development of 2K1C hypertension. Hypertension 2002;40:735–41.
9. Brunner HR, Kirshmann JD, Sealey JE, et al. Hypertension of renal origin: evidence for two different mechanisms. Science 1971;174:1344–6.
10. Gloviczki ML, Glockner JF, Lerman LO, et al. Preserved oxygenation despite reduced blood flow in poststenotic kidneys in human atherosclerotic renal artery stenosis. Hypertension 2010;55(4):961–6.
11. Epstein FH. Oxygen and renal metabolism. Kidney Int 1997;51:381–5.
12. Evans RG, Gardiner BS, Smith DW, et al. Intrarenal oxygenation: unique challenges and the biophysical basis of homeostasis. Am J Physiol Renal Physiol 2008;295(5):F1259–70.
13. Lerman LO, Chade AR. Angiogenesis in the kidney: a new therapeutic target? Curr Opin Nephrol Hypertens 2009;18:160–5.
14. Lerman LO, Textor SC. Gained in translation: protective paradigms for the poststenotic kidney. Hypertension 2015;65(5):976–82.
15. Gloviczki ML, Glockner JF, Crane JA, et al. BOLD magnetic resonance imaging identifies cortical hypoxia in severe renovascular disease. Hypertension 2011; 58(6):1066–72.
16. Gloviczki ML, Keddis MT, Garovic VD, et al. TGF expression and macrophage accumulation in atherosclerotic renal artery stenosis. Clin J Am Soc Nephrol 2013;8(4):546–53.
17. Lech M, Grobmayr R, Ryu M, et al. Macrophage phenotype controls long-term AKI outcomes–kidney regeneration versus atrophy. J Am Soc Nephrol 2014; 25(2):292–304.
18. Saad A, Herrmann SMS, Crane J, et al. Stent revascularization restores cortical blood flow and reverses tissue hypoxia in atherosclerotic renal artery stenosis but fails to reverse inflammatory pathways or glomerular filtration rate. Circ Cardiovasc Interv 2013;6(4):428–35.
19. Romero JC, Lerman LO. Novel noninvasive techniques for studying renal function in man. Semin Nephrol 2000;20:456–62.
20. De Bruyne B, Manoharan G, Pijls NHJ, et al. Assessment of renal artery stenosis severity by pressure gradient measurements. J Am Coll Cardiol 2006;48:1851–5.
21. Losito A, Fagugli RM, Zampi I, et al. Comparison of target organ damage in renovascular and essential hypertension. Am J Hypertens 1996;9:1062–7.
22. Messerli FH, Bangalore S, Makani H, et al. Flash pulmonary oedema and bilateral renal artery stenosis: the Pickering syndrome. Eur Heart J 2011;32(18):2231–7.
23. Gandhi SK, Powers JC, Nomeir AM, et al. The pathogenesis of acute pulmonary edema associated with hypertension. N Engl J Med 2001;344:17–22.
24. Kane GC, Xu N, Mistrik E, et al. Renal artery revascularization improves heart failure control in patients with atherosclerotic renal artery stenosis. Nephrol Dial Transplant 2010;25:813–20.
25. Ritchie J, Green D, Chrysochou C, et al. High-risk clinical presentations in atherosclerotic renovascular disease: prognosis and response to renal artery revascularization. Am J Kidney Dis 2014;63(2):186–97.
26. Herrmann SM, Saad A, Textor SC. Management of atherosclerotic renovascular disease after cardiovascular outcomes in renal atherosclerotic lesions (CORAL). Nephrol Dial Transplant 2015;30(3):366–75.
27. Herrmann SMS, Textor SC. Diagnostic criteria for renovascular disease: where are we now? Nephrol Dial Transplant 2012;27(7):2657–63.
28. Strong CG, Hunt JC, Sheps SG, et al. Renal venous renin activity: enhancement of sensitivity of lateralization by sodium depletion. Am J Cardiol 1971;27:602–11.

29. Calhoun DA, Jones D, Textor S, et al. Resistant hypertension: diagnosis, evaluation, and treatment: a scientific statement from the American Heart Association Professional Education Committee of the Council for High Blood Pressure Research. Circulation 2008;117(25):e510–26.
30. Freedman BI, Sedor JR. Hypertension-associated kidney disease–perhaps no more. J Am Soc Nephrol 2008;19(11):2047–51.
31. Olin JW, Sealove BA. Diagnosis, management, and future developments of fibromuscular dysplasia. J Vasc Surg 2011;53(3):826–36.
32. Canzanello VJ. Medical management of renovascular disease. In: Lerman LO, Textor SC, editors. Renal vascular disease. 1st edition. London: Springer; 2014. p. 305–16.
33. Hackam DG, Duong-Hua ML, Mamdani M, et al. Angiotensin inhibition in renovascular disease: a population-based cohort study. Am Heart J 2008;156: 549–55.
34. Chrysochou C, Foley RN, Young JF, et al. Dispelling the myth: the use of renin-angiotensin blockade in atheromatous renovascular disease. Nephrol Dial Transplant 2012;27(4):1403–9.
35. Textor SC, Lerman LO. Paradigm shifts in atherosclerotic renovascular disease: where are we now? J Am Soc Nephrol 2015;26:2074–80.
36. Onuigbo MAC. Is renoprotection with RAAS blockade a failed paradigm? Have we learnt any lessons so far? Int J Clin Pract 2010;64:1341–6.
37. Olin JW, Gornik HL, Bacharach JM, et al. Fibromuscular dysplasia: state of the science and critical unanswered questions: a scientific statement from the American Heart Association. Circulation 2014;129(9):1048–78.
38. Boateng FK, Greco BA. Renal artery stenosis: prevalence of, risk factors for and management of in-stent stenosis. Am J Kidney Dis 2013;61(1):147–60.
39. Harden PN, Macleod MJ, Rodger RS, et al. Effect of renal-artery stenting on progression of renovascular renal failure. Lancet 1997;349:1133–6.
40. Watson PS, Hadjipetrou P, Cox SV, et al. Effect of renal artery stenting on renal function and size in patients with atherosclerotic renovascular disease. Circulation 2001;102:1671–7.
41. Kalra PA, Chrysochou C, Green D, et al. The benefit of renal artery stenting in patients with atheromatous renovascular disease and advanced chronic kidney disease. Catheter Cardiovasc Interv 2010;75:1–10.
42. Balk E, Raman G, Chung M, et al. Effectiveness of management strategies for renal artery stenosis: a systematic review. Ann Intern Med 2006;145:901–12.
43. Cooper CJ, Murphy TP, Cutlip DE, et al. Stenting and medical therapy for atherosclerotic renal-artery stenosis. N Engl J Med 2014;370(1):13–22.
44. Wheatley K, Ives N, Gray R, et al, ASTRAL Investigators. Revascularization versus medical therapy for renal-artery stenosis. N Engl J Med 2009;361: 1953–62.
45. Textor SC, Misra S. Does renal artery stenting prevent clinical events? Clin J Am Soc Nephrol 2016;11(7):1125–7.
46. Textor SC. Attending rounds: a patient with accelerated hypertension and an atrophic kidney. Clin J Am Soc Nephrol 2014;9(6):1117–23.

The Pressure of Aging

Majd AlGhatrif, MD[a,b,1], Mingyi Wang, MD, PhD[a,1],
Olga V. Fedorova, PhD[a,1], Alexei Y. Bagrov, MD, PhD[a], Edward G. Lakatta, MD[a,*]

KEYWORDS

- Hemodynamics • Aging • Arterial wall remodeling
- Age-dependent salt-sensitive hypertension • Pulse wave velocity • Arterial fibrosis
- Angiotensin II • Marinobufagenin

KEY POINTS

- Although preclinical hemodynamic alterations observed early in life are not directly harmful, they form the basis for the deleterious hemodynamic effects observed with aging.
- The aortic biomechanics underlie the increase of salt sensitivity with advancing age, and a novel pro-fibrotic marker, an endogenous sodium pump ligand, marinobufagenin links aging, salt sensitivity, and arterial stiffness.
- A proinflammatory state in the arterial wall, with a pivotal role for angiotensin II (Ang II), is a key component of arterial aging.
- Pulsatile damage to the arterial wall and the proinflammatory state within the arterial wall interact in a vicious cycle, resulting in increasing arterial wall fibrosis.
- Therapies to prevent or delay Ang II signaling–related vascular changes that accompany aging to ultimately reduce the prevalence of hypertension should be aimed at breaking the vicious cycle at its early stages.

INTRODUCTION

Major hemodynamic alterations ensue with aging and are primarily attributable to central arterial stiffening[1]; these alterations become manifest in the ever-expanding epidemic of hypertension affecting 1 of every 3 Americans in general and a staggering rate of 7 of every 10 of those aged 65 years and older.[2] The burden of this epidemic is projected to increase with the aging of our population as the percentage of people aged 65 years and older increasing from 15% in 2014 to 22% in 2030.[3] This shift in demographics makes predominantly systolic hypertension, a challenging form of hypertension that becomes more prevalent with advancing age and that dominates the

[a] Laboratory of Cardiovascular Science, NIA, NIH, Baltimore, MD, USA; [b] Department of Medicine, Johns Hopkins Bayview Medical Center, Johns Hopkins School of Medicine, Baltimore, MD, USA
[1] Contributed equally.
* Corresponding author. Laboratory of Cardiovascular Science, Biomedical Research Center, 251 Bayview Boulevard, Suite 100, Room 09B116, Baltimore, MD 21224-6825.
E-mail address: LakattaE@grc.nia.nih.gov

Med Clin N Am 101 (2017) 81–101
http://dx.doi.org/10.1016/j.mcna.2016.08.006
0025-7125/17/Published by Elsevier Inc.

medical.theclinics.com

hypertension field.[4] All of these factors make hypertension a growing health burden with predicted hypertension-related health care costs reaching $389 billion in 2030.[5] Because aging is the major risk factor for predominantly systolic hypertension, the pivotal question to effectively address this hypertension epidemic is the following: What underlies arterial aging?

Evolutionary biologists proclaim that most of us are wired to be very healthy until around the end of childbearing age, because the main reason for our reality, they would say, is to perpetually insure the next generation of our species; after that, from an evolutionary perspective, there is no essential reason for us to be alive. However, we do remain alive longer well beyond our evolutionary life expectancy prescription because our environment has been enhanced by improved hygiene, better nutrition, better health care, and so forth. But, in outliving our Paleolithic gene set, disorder among molecules within our body progressively increases and functional declines accumulate with advancing age; beyond 40 years we become vulnerable to what are referred to as "degenerative chronic diseases of aging." Arterial aging and the associated alteration in hemodynamics are no exception.

The hypertension field has been struggling to better understand the complex relationship between arterial wall mechanical changes (ie, arterial wall stiffness) and hemodynamics (ie, arterial pressure alterations) and has been fixated on defining which factor is the culprit. The failure to reach an unequivocal answer is not surprising and is probably a reflection of the naivety of the question. In health homeostasis, a functional crosstalk between central and peripheral segments of the circulation is required for optimal operation. Once this homeostasis is broken, for any reason, a vicious cycle of minute alterations in central arterial mechanical and hemodynamics ensues and propagates, leading to the dramatic changes in arterial properties observed with aging. Thus, in this paradigm, it is close to impossible to detect the initial minute alteration and point to it as the culprit.

Given this extreme complexity, any efforts directed at treating or preventing the increase in blood pressure would be infertile without major efforts being committed to further explore the underpinning aging of the arterial wall. These efforts should be aimed at revealing early alterations, starting in young adulthood, before reaching the clinical threshold and developing stage/process-specific interventions rather than the one-size-fits-all approach that dominates hypertension. In the meantime, targeting elements of this vicious cycle, the master perpetuators of arterial aging, seems to be the most promising strategy to reduce the health burden of hypertension.

AGE-ASSOCIATED DYSFUNCTION OF CENTRAL ARTERIES AND HEMODYNAMIC ALTERATIONS

Epidemiologic studies have pursued the description of changes in arterial stiffness with aging and to answer the question of whether central arterial stiffness is a cause or an effect of elevated systolic and pulse blood pressure. One of the difficulties in addressing this issue relates to a degree of ambiguity and restrictions of the terms *blood pressure* and *arterial stiffness*. This question might be better articulated if we expand these terms and rename *arterial stiffness* as *arterial mechanical alterations* and *elevated blood pressure* as *hemodynamic alterations*; then, it becomes apparent that arterial mechanical properties and hemodynamics are inseparable and the question on what starts first, mechanical or hemodynamic alterations, seems to be somewhat naïve.

In the Beginning: Early Third Decade Arterial Mechanical Alterations and the Increase in Diastolic Blood Pressure

The initial evidence of age-associated arterial mechanical alterations is observed by the third decade of age with sharp declines in aortic strain, the difference between aortic systolic and diastolic diameter relative to the diastolic diameter, and in aortic distensibility, that is, aortic strain divided by pulse pressure; analysis of cardiac magnetic resonance imaging of 111 healthy participants has shown that nearly 80% of the total decline of aortic strain occurs before the fifth decade of age after which the decline in strain is less dramatic[6] (**Fig. 1**A); however, the small decline in aortic strain beyond 50 years of age was associated with an exponential increase in pulse wave velocity (PWV) with aging (see **Fig. 1**B).

During the same stages of life, as central arterial strain is becoming reduced, there is an *increase* in diastolic blood pressure,[7,8] which could be associated with progression of increased endothelial dysfunction with aging, leading to increased peripheral vascular resistance. Although such changes are not very well studied in normal human subjects, those with essential hypertension demonstrate eutrophic, inward remodeling of small arteries.[9,10] It is not clear whether the increase in diastolic blood pressure alters the optimal conformation of the arterial wall, making it prone to an increase in hemodynamic stress and to additional mechanical alterations beyond those resulting from simply stretching elastin fibers at higher pressures and shifting the load to the stiffer collagen fibers.

Beyond the Sixth Decade of Age: Central Arterial Mechanics and the Pulsatile Hemodynamic

Dramatic hemodynamic alterations ensue beyond the sixth decade of life, as increases in systolic blood pressure (SBP) and pulse pressure (PP) become the hallmarks of arterial aging.[8] PWV and blood pressure parameters have been shown to be strongly associated in cross-sectional and prospective studies.[11,12] The Framingham Heart Study, using data from cycle 7 to predict SBP and PWV in cycle 8, has shown that higher PWV in cycle 7 is associated with higher SBP in cycle 8[13]; however,

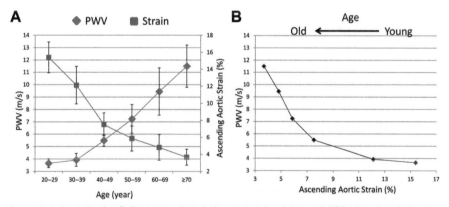

Fig. 1. Aortic strain (*red*) decreases sharply between the third and fifth decade of life after which there is a sharp increase in aortic pulse wave velocity (PWV) (*blue*) (A). Aortic strain and PWV plotted against each other showing an exponential increase in PWV with declining aortic strain with aging (B). (*Adapted from* Redheuil A, Yu WC, Wu CO, et al. Reduced ascending aortic strain and distensibility: earliest manifestations of vascular aging in humans. Hypertension 2010;55(2):323.)

the opposite was not true: SBP at cycle 7 was not associated with higher PWV in cycle 8. It is noteworthy, however, that one of the shortcomings of the Framingham Study design with a relatively short follow-up time of 7 years is that it does not address that the magnitude and the direction of the association between SBP and PWV are not addressed and could change with aging and differ by sex; merely adjusting for these variables does not inform whether these associations differed between the different categories of these variables. Hence, the findings reflect that the average associations over the age spectrum studied for both sexes.

Longitudinal Perspective on the Conundrum of Arterial Wall Stiffness, Blood Pressure, and Aging: A Vicious Cycle Between Teammates That Eventually Diverge

Indications of a vicious cycle between arterial stiffness and systolic blood pressure

The Baltimore Longitudinal Study of Aging (BLSA) is a cohort study of community-dwelling populations with extended follow-up time and multiple repeated measures of PWV and blood pressure (1988–2013). Earlier analyses from the BLSA have shown that greater PWV was associated with a larger increase in SBP with aging and predicted the incidence of hypertension.[14] Recent analysis from the BLSA, however, using linear mixed-effects models, shed light on the vicious cycle, showing that higher SBP, in a dose-dependent fashion, is also associated with a greater rate of increase in PWV; this association was more pronounced in men with accelerating rates of increase in PWV at higher SBP with advancing age.[15]

Dissociation between pulse wave velocity and systolic blood pressure trajectories

More recent insights on the longitudinal changes in PWV and SBP parameters came from the SardiNIA Study of concurrent trajectories of repeated measures of PWV and SBP; using linear mixed-effects models allows the examination of whether the longitudinal changes of these parameters over time vary by starting age.[7] This analysis demonstrated a striking dissociation in the trajectories of these parameters with advancing age, which is a dissociation more pronounced in men than women.[7] **Fig. 2** illustrate the cross-sectional differences, beginning of the splines, and the longitudinal changes (slopes of the splines) with aging (rates of changes are illustrated in the lower panels) of PWV and SBP in both men and women. In men (see **Fig. 2**) PWV increased with age at rates that increase linearly with advancing age; however, although cross-sectional SBP continues to increase, the longitudinal rates of change, although initially increasing, begin to decline with time; thus, the rates of change in SBP diverge from those of PWV by the fifth decade. A similar, but a less dramatic, divergence is observed in women (see **Fig. 2**); although PWV showed the same pattern of longitudinal changes in men with linearly increasing rates of change with advancing age, SBP increased longitudinally at a steady, rather than increasing, rate throughout the age range studied. Preliminary analyses from the BLSA using the same approach of examining the concurrent trajectories showed a similar pattern of dissociations between PWV trajectories and those of SBP and PP, which were more pronounced in men than women.[16]

Physiologic explanations for the dissociation between pulse wave velocity and the decline in systolic blood pressure with aging in men

Dissociations between the rates at which PWV and SBP change over time bring our attention again to terminology; arterial stiffness usually implies an increase in arterial opposition to flow, that is, characteristic impedance (Z_c). However, Z_c is a function of both PWV and aortic diameter squared.[17] Hence, an explanation for the dissociation between SBP and PWV longitudinal trajectories in men is an increase in aortic diameter. Preliminary analysis from the BLSA shows a greater increase in aortic root

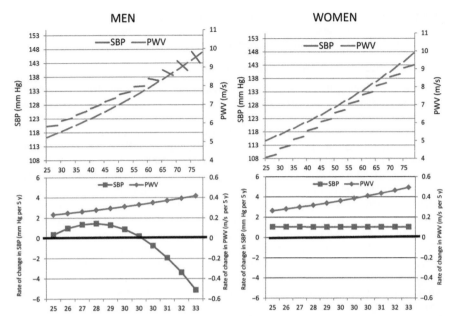

Fig. 2. Linear mixed-effects models predicted PWV and SBP values illustrating sex-specific cross-sectional differences "beginning of the splines" and the longitudinal changes (slopes of the splines) with aging (rates of changes are illustrated in the lower panels) in men and women from the SardiNIA project. (*Adapted from* Scuteri A, Morrell CH, Orru M, et al. Longitudinal perspective on the conundrum of central arterial stiffness, blood pressure, and aging. Hypertension 2014;64(6):1219–27; with permission.)

dilatation with increasing age in men than in women.[16] The net effect of increasing PWV and aortic diameter approximated by applying the water hammer equation is, in fact, a less pronounced increase in calculated Z_c in men despite their more pronounced increase in PWV, which was offset by the greater increase in diameter.[16] These results are in agreement with cross-sectional data from the Asklepios study showing that with advancing age, men have lower Z_c than women.[18] Although aortic diameter and Z_c might explain how PWV and SBP/PP trajectories would diverge, the role of wave reflection in this dissociation is not well clear and it is worth further examination.

SALT-SENSITIVE HYPERTENSION AND AGING

The incidence of hypertension and salt sensitivity increases with advancing age.[19–23] High sodium chloride (NaCl) intake in addition to its effect on blood pressure[24] increases arterial stiffness by altering vascular structure, vascular smooth muscle cell (VSMC), and endothelial cell function and producing arterial wall fibrosis.[25–27] Both clinical and experimental evidence indicate that NaCl induces hypertrophy of the arterial wall in the absence of changes in arterial pressure[26] and induces hypertrophy of cultured VSMC.[27] Excessive NaCl intake reduces the bioavailability of nitric oxide (NO) by interfering with the induction of NO synthase[28] and by elevating levels of peroxinitrite due to an increase in the reduction form of nicotinamide adenine dinucleotide phosphate (NADPH) oxidase activity, marker of oxidative stress, and production of reactive oxygen species.[29] These NaCl effects lead to hypertension by reducing arterial compliance and increasing peripheral vascular resistance (PVR)[30] and to oxidative damage to the arterial wall.[31] An age-associated decline in NO-mediated dilation becomes particularly apparent during the sixth decade, a time when PP, a barometer of large artery stiffness, begins to appreciably elevate.[32]

The Endogenous Steroids, Sodium Pump Ligands

Evidence is mounting that a NaCl-induced signaling cascade involving tissue renin angiotensin aldosterone signaling (RAAS) initiates the production of an endogenous ouabainlike substance in the brain, which then acts as a neurohormone to activate brain Angiotensin II receptor type 1 (AT1R) (**Fig. 3**).[33,34] Sympathetic signaling to the adrenal cortex leads to production of marinobufagenin (MBG), another recently discovered Na pump ligand that is an endogenous inhibitor of the alpha-1 isoform of the Na/K-ATPase (sodium-potassium adenosine triphosphatase; NKA),[35] which is the exclusive NKA isoform in renal tubules and a main isoform in VSMC (see **Fig. 3**). Inhibition of NKA in renal tubular cells leads to decreased reabsorption of Na and promotes natriuresis. However, Na-pump ligands are not only selective for renal NKA but also inhibit NKA in the vasculature, leading to arterial constriction and an increase in PVR and arterial blood pressure (see **Fig. 3**).[35–39] Interestingly, compared with normotensive control, older patients with resistant hypertension demonstrate greater blood pressure and PWV, higher plasma MBG (an NKA inhibitor), and decreased erythrocyte NKA activity.[40] In this regard, it is of note that the increase in arterial pressure induced by a chronic high NaCl intake (ie, salt-sensitive hypertension) in rodents is substantially reduced by an anti-MBG antibody.[35,41]

The age-associated increase in the secretion of Na-pump ligands, including MBG, linked to reduced renal NaCl excretion could be an explanation for the moderate

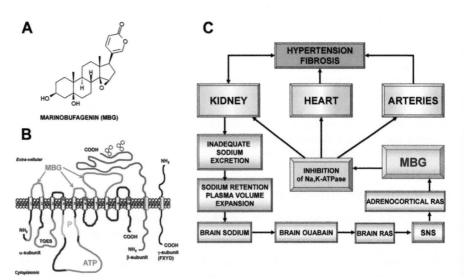

Fig. 3. Structures of marinobufagenin (MBG) (*A*) and sodium-potassium adenosine triphosphate with binding sites for MBG (*B*). Interaction between RAAS and MBG in the pathogenesis of salt-sensitive hypertension (*C*). FXYD, motif identical for all proteins in γ-subunit family; P, phosphorus ion; RAS, renin-angiotensin system; SNS, sympathetic nervous system; TGES, motif, located at the actuator domain of NKA molecule, is responsible for dephosphorylation step. (*Adapted from* Bagrov AY, Shapiro JI, Fedorova OV. Endogenous cardiotonic steroids: physiology, pharmacology, and novel therapeutic targets. Pharmacol Rev 2009;61(1): 9–38; with permission.)

increases in PVR in older persons with predominantly systolic hypertension. The effects of MBG to increase PVR in salt-sensitive hypertension may be substantially enhanced via their interaction with other vasoactive substances that are implicated in the pathogenesis of NaCl-dependent effects to increase arterial pressure. A NaCl-induced upregulation of the tissue activity of RAAS, via protein kinase C (PKC)-dependent phosphorylation of the Na/K pump, may sensitize this pump to both vasoconstrictive and NaCl-dependent growth promoting MBG effects.[42] Additionally, NaCl-dependent angiotensin II (Ang II) signaling induced a deficit in the bioavailability of endothelium-derived vasorelaxants, for example, NO and C-type natriuretic peptide, which oppose the vasopressor action of MBG but enhance its adaptive natriuretic action and may further reinforce the deleterious effects of the Na-pump ligand.

Thus, Na-pump ligands, including MBG, link high dietary salt intake to the increase in arterial stiffness and hypertension.[20,21,34,36,43] High salt intake is associated with an increase in MBG and is accompanied by marked salt sensitivity of blood pressure.[44,45] Dietary sodium restriction is an effective lifestyle approach for reducing both blood pressure and arterial stiffness in middle-aged and older individuals.[46,47] In older humans after 5 weeks of a low-salt diet versus 5 weeks of a normal salt diet a reduction in urinary MBG excretion was positively related to reductions in urinary Na excretion and arterial stiffness (**Fig. 4**).[48] Furthermore, the expression of NADPH oxidase was correlated with MBG levels, indicating that low-salt-dependent reduction in MBG may contribute to the reductions in large elastic artery stiffness and SBP through decreased oxidative stress.[48] Thus, MBG is a molecular link of increased salt sensitivity and arterial stiffness in aging.

Interaction of Marinobufagenin and Atrial Natriuretic Peptide in Age-Dependent Salt Sensitivity

In addition to MBG, high salt intake stimulates atrial natriuretic peptide (ANP) (**Fig. 5**).[49] Inhibition of renal NKA by MBG is enhanced via ANP-dependent phosphorylation of NKA, whereas, in the aorta, ANP exerts the opposite effect.[50] Vasorelaxant ANP and vasoconstrictor MBG potentiate each other's natriuretic effects, but ANP may offset the deleterious vasoconstrictor effect of MBG.[50] An imbalance of ANP-MBG signaling increases with advancing age and is a factor that underlies the phenomenon of salt sensitivity of blood pressure with aging.[50]

ANP sensitizes renal NKA to MBG inhibitory activity and reduces MBG-induced inhibition of vascular NKA via cyclic guanosine monophosphate/protein kinase

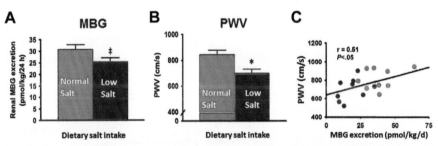

Fig. 4. Effect of low and normal dietary salt intake on urinary MBG excretion (A), aortic PWV (B), and correlation between urinary MBG and PWV (C) in older patients. Values are mean ± SE. ‡P<0.05; *P<0.01 (low salt vs. normal salt). (*Adapted from* Jablonski KL, Fedorova OV, Racine ML, et al. Dietary sodium restriction and association with urinary marinobufagenin, blood pressure, and aortic stiffness. Clin J Am Soc Nephrol 2013;8(11):1952–9; with permission.)

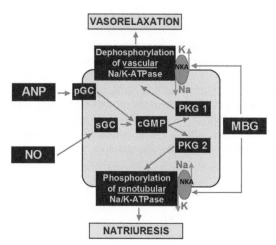

Fig. 5. Factors implicated in the modulation of cGMP-dependent phosphorylation/dephosphorylation of renal and vascular NKA. pGC, particulate guanylate cyclase; PKG, protein kinase G; sGC, soluble guanylate cyclase.

G-dependent mechanism (cGMP/PKG). Because downregulation of cGMP/PKG signaling is associated with aging, ANP does not potentiate renal effects of MBG and does not oppose vasoconstrictive effects of MBG in older rats (**Fig. 6**).[49,50]

The NaCl dependence of blood pressure in older persons with predominantly systolic hypertension can be attributed to multiple mechanisms that underlie arterial compliance and vascular resistance. Excessive dietary NaCl may also alter vascular structure and function via Ang II or Na-pump ligands–driven mechanisms (**Fig. 7**) in the setting of age-associated reductions in renal blood flow and in the ability to excrete Na. NaCl activates tissue Ang II and MBG, affects endothelial and vascular cell functions, and affects arterial structural remodeling, which results in arterial stiffening (see **Fig. 7**). NaCl also activates ANP, via a cGMP/PKG-dependent mechanism that attenuates the profibrotic effect of MBG on vascular NKA (see later discussion).[50] Remarkably, both phenomena, MBG-dependent activation of profibrotic signaling and downregulation of cGMP/PKG-dependent signaling, which accelerates the profibrotic and prohypertensive MBG effects, are the hallmarks of arterial aging (see **Fig. 6**).[50]

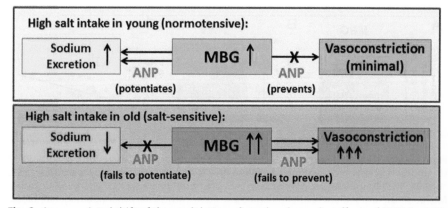

Fig. 6. Age-associated shift of the modulation of renal and vascular effects of MBG by ANP.

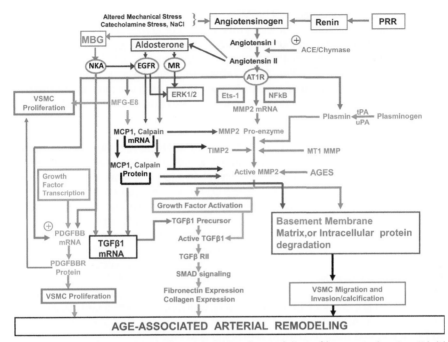

Altered Mechanical Stress
Catecholamine Stress, NaCl } → Angiotensinogen ← Renin ← PRR

Fig. 7. Pathways that participate in age-associated remodeling of large arteries. Ang II initiates both inflammatory and repair processes. ACE, angiotensin-converting enzyme; EGFR, epidermal growth factor receptor; MCP, monocyte chemoattractant protein-1; MFG-E8, milk fat globule epidermal growth factor 8; MMP, matrix metalloprotease; MT1, metallothionein 1; PDGFBB, platelet-derived growth factor-BB; TGFβ1, transforming growth factor β1; TIMP2, tissue inhibitor of metalloprotease 2; tPA, tissue plasminogen activator. (*From* Lakatta EG. The reality of aging viewed from the arterial wall. Artery Res 2013;7(2):76; with permission.)

Profibrotic MBG activity, involving MBG/NKA association, is considered to be an important therapeutic target for immunoneutralization and modulation of MBG/NKA interactions in salt sensitivity and in aging.

Excessive dietary NaCl, in fact, may be an etiologic factor in the increased central arterial stiffening that accompanies advancing age and the attendant age-associated increase in PP, as this does not occur in populations that do not consume excess NaCl.[24] The combined effects of NaCl to increase arterial stiffness and resistance progresses to the point of raising systolic pressure, in nearly half of the individuals in our society, to the current epidemiologically defined hypertensive threshold (140 mm Hg). It is imperative, therefore, that we not lose sight of the reality that the NaCl baseline diet consumed in the US population at large is 60% higher than the Dietary Approaches to Stop Hypertension recommendations[47,51] and seems to accelerate aging and to increase the likelihood of salt-sensitive hypertension.

AN AGE-ASSOCIATED INCREASE IN RENIN ANGIOTENSIN ALDOSTERONE SIGNALING IN VASCULAR SMOOTH MUSCLE CELL PROMOTES CENTRAL ARTERIAL WALL REMODELING

Age-associated changes in vascular structure/function, per se, set the stage for the pathogenesis of vascular diseases such as hypertension in older persons.[52–54] The fact that the age-associated changes in arterial wall remodeling, including proinflammation, proliferation, migration/invasion of VSMCs, elastin fragmentation, and calcification of Ang II signaling, that are observed in rats also occur across a wide range of other species, such as rabbits, nonhuman primates, and humans (see **Fig. 7**; **Table 1**), provides insights into the pathogenesis of hypertension with aging and age-associated hypertension.[52–54] **Fig. 7** and **Table 1** illustrate the proinflammatory profile of arterial wall remodeling. Components of the Ang II signaling cascade are master perpetrators of age-associated stress signaling that is linked to arterial wall remodeling.[52–54]

Proinflammation

In a hybrid Fisher 344 crossbred Brown Norway (FXBN) old rats (30 months), aortae exhibit a dramatic increase in intimal-medial thickness compared with young adults (8 months) because of increased VSMCs infiltration into the intimae, collagen deposition, calcification, and elastin fracture, which is known as arterial wall remodeling.[55–57] Arterial Ang II signaling components (see **Fig. 7**) are increased in age-associated aortic remodeling in FXBN rats, including an increased abundance of Ang II, the AT1 receptor, angiotensin-converting enzyme (ACE), and their downstream molecules aldosterone, endothelin-1, matrix metalloproteinase type II (MMP-2), calpain-1, transformation growth factor β1 (TGFβ1), monocyte chemoattractant protein-1 (MCP-1), milk fat globule epidermal growth factor (EGF)-8 (MFG-E8) in FXBN rat with aging (see **Fig. 7**).[52,55–64] In addition, aldosterone mineralocorticoid receptor (MR) activation is increased, promoting arterial wall remodeling.[65] Interestingly, aortic prorenin receptor ACE, Ang II, and AT1 receptor proteins are also upregulated in C57 and Black 6 inbred mice (C57/BL6) with aging (see **Fig. 7**).[66]

Chronic (30 days) Ang II infusion into young FXBN rats increases the intimal-medial thickness, enhances calpain-1, MMP-2, MCP-1, TGFβ1, and MFG-E8 expression or activities, collagen deposition, and elastin network breakdown in the arterial wall, mimicking arterial wall remodeling that accompanies an advancing age.[58,62,67] In other terms, in response to chronic administration of Ang II to young rats, the arterial VSMC and matrix take on the appearance of their counterparts in old rats.

Chronic ACE inhibition or AT1 receptor blockade, beginning at an early age, markedly inhibits the expression of proinflammatory molecules and delays the progression of age-associated aortic remodeling and senescence.[68,69] Interestingly, long-term AT1 receptor blockade improves endothelial function and decreases blood pressure, doubles the life span of hypertensive rats, rendering it similar to normotensives.[70] Disruption of the AT1 receptor retards arterial inflammation, promotes longevity, and improves survival after myocardial infarction in mice.[71] These findings provide strong support to the hypothesis that increased Ang II proinflammatory signaling is involved in arterial wall remodeling (see **Fig. 7**).

Proliferation

VSMCs within the aged aortic wall have an enhanced proliferation capacity compared with young cells linked to proinflammation.[60] The proliferation rate in cultured VSMCs is increased in old versus young adult rats.[59] An increase in CDK4 and PCNA, an increase in the acceleration of cell cycle S and G2 phases, a decrease in the G1/G0 phase, and an increase in platelet-derived growth factor and its receptors drive the elevated proliferative capacity in early passage of old VSMC versus young VSMC.[60]

Ang II signaling increases MFG-E8 expression in both arterial walls and VSMCs (see **Fig. 7**).[67,72] An increase in MFG-E8, a cell adhesion protein, is a signature of aging arterial walls.[60,72–74] Aortic MFG-E8 mRNA and protein levels and its integrin receptor, $a_{v}\beta_{3/5}$ (integrin alpha V beta 3/5 receptor), increase with aging.[60,72] MFG-E8 signaling via integrins activates proliferation of VSMC, proliferating cellular nuclear antigen

Table 1

Age-associated proinflammatory arterial remodeling

		Aging				Hypertension	Ang II Signaling
		Humans >56 vs <20 y	Monkeys 15–20 vs <10 y	Rats 24–30 vs 3–8 mo	Rabbits 2–6 y vs <10 mo		
Inflammation-association molecules	Local Ang II/AT1	↑	↑	↑	?	↑	↑
	ET-1	↑	?	↑	↑	↑	↑
	MMPs	↑	↑	↑	?	↑	↑
	Calpain-1	↑	↑	↑	?	↑	↑
	MCP-1/CCR2	↑	↑	↑	↑	↑	↑
	TGFβ1/TβIIR	↑	↑	↑	↑	↑	↑
	NADPH oxidase	↑	↑	↑	↑	↑	↑
	NO bioavailability	↓	↓	↓	↓	↓	↓
	TNF-α1	↑	↑	↑	↑	↑	↑
	ICAM-1	↑	↑	↑	↑	?	↑
	MFG-E8	↑	?	↑	?	↑	↑
	PDGF/PDGF-R	?	?	↑	?	↑	↑
	tPA/uPA	↑	?	↑	?	↑	↑
	AGEs/RAGE	↑	?	↑	↑	↑	↑
	IL-1/-6/-8	?	?	↑	?	?	↑
	MR	↑	↑	↑	?	↑	↑
	NF-κB	↑	?	↑	?	↑	↑
	Ets-1	?	?	↑	?	↑	↑
	SirT1	↓	?	↓	?	↓	↓
Cellular-matrix structure and function	EC dysfunction	↑	↑	↑	↑	↑	↑
	Diffuse IMT	↑	↑	↑	↑	↑	↑
	Stiffness	↑	↑	↑	↑	↑	↑
	Matrix	↑	↑	↑	↑	↑	↑
	Calcification	↑	↑	↑	?	↑	↑
	FN/collagen	↑	↑	↑	↑	↑	↑
	VSMC migration	↑	↑	↑	↑	↑	↑
	VSMC proliferation	↑	↑	↑	↑	↑	↑

Abbreviations: AGEs, advanced glycation end products; EC, endothelial cell; ET-1, endothelin-1; Ets-1, ETS Proto-Oncogene 1, Transcription Factor; FN, fibronectin; ICAM-1, intercellular adhesion molecule 1; IL, interleukin; IMT, intimal medial thickening; MCP-1, monocyte chemoattractant protein-1; MMPs, matrix metalloproteinases; MR, mineralocorticoid receptor; NF-κB, nuclear kappa B; PDGF, platelet-derived growth factor; PDGFR, platelet-derived growth factor receptor; RAGE, the receptor for advanced glycation endproducts; SIRT1, silent mating type information regulation 2 homolog; TGFβ1, transformation growth factor β1; TNF-α1, tumor necrosis factor α1; tPA, tissue plasminogen activator; uPA, urinary-type plasminogen activator.

Adapted from Wang M, Jiang L, Monticone RE, et al. Proinflammation: the key to arterial aging. Trends Endocrinol Metab 2014;25(2):74; with permission.

(PCNA), and Ki67, which are markers of cell cycle activation.[60] In young VSMC in vitro, MFG-E8 treatment triggers phosphorylated extracellular signal-regulated kinase 1/2 (p-ERK-1/2), augments levels of PCNA and CDK4, increases 5-bromodeoxyuridine incorporation, and promotes proliferation via $\alpha v \beta 5$ integrins.[60] MFG-E8 silencing, or its receptor inhibition, or the blockade of p-ERK1/2 in these cells reduces PCNA and CDK4 levels, and decelerates the cell cycle S phase, conferring a reduction in proliferative capacity.[60] Collectively, MFG-E8 coordinates the expression of cell cycle molecules and facilitates VSMC proliferation via integrin/ERK1/2 signaling (see **Fig. 7**).

Migration/Invasion

The migration/invasion of VSMCs, which is a key cellular event in age-associated diffuse intimal thickening, is driven by proinflammatory molecular signaling.[52] VSMCs from old versus young adult rats also have a 50% increase in migration potential.[59] Ang II triggers the activation of MMP-2, calpain 1, MCP-1, and MFG-E8, which play a causal role in the migration/invasion of VSMC because of its cleavage of the basement membrane and cytoskeletal remodeling (see **Fig. 7**).[58,61,62,72] In cultured young VSMCs, Ang II exposure increases VSMC migration to the level of isolated old cells.[58,62] The Ang II–mediated, age-associated increases in VSMC migration capacity is blocked by inhibition of MMP-2.[58] Calpain-1 is an intracellular Ca^{2+}-activated cysteine protease and downstream molecule of Ang II signaling cascade. Its transcription, translation, and activation are significantly upregulated in rat aortae and VSMCs in culture with aging.[55,58] Calpain-1 and MMP-2 are colocalized within old VSMC.[55] Overexpression of calpain-1 in young VSMC results in cleavage of intact vimentin (as an index of calpain-1 activity) and an increased migratory capacity, mimicking old VSMC. These actions are blocked by the MMP inhibitor, GM6001, and its inhibitor calpastatin.[58] Thus, calpain-1 and MMP-2 activation are pivotal molecular events in the age-associated arterial Ang II signaling/migration cascade of VSMC migration.

In addition, MFG-E8 plays an important role as a relay element within the Ang II/MCP-1 signaling cascade that modulates VSMC invasion with aging.[72] MCP-1 and its receptor, CCR2 (see **Fig. 7**), are upregulated in age-associated aortic remodeling.[59,61] Exposure of young VSMCs to Ang II markedly increases MFG-E8 and enhances their invasive capacity to old cell levels.[72] Treatment of VSMCs with MFG-E8 increases MCP-1 expression and VSMC invasion, and both are inhibited by the MCP-1 receptor blocker vCCI.[72] Exposure of young VSMC to MCP-1 also increases their migration, up to levels of old cells.[59] Silencing MFG-E8 substantially reduces MFG-E8 expression and VSMC invasion capacity.[72] Thus, MFG-E8, a protein secreted by VSMC, significantly increases with aging and is a pivotal relay element within the Ang II/MCP-1/VSMC invasion signaling cascade (see **Fig. 7**).

Elastin Fragmentation

Rat aortic wall elastin fraction is significantly decreased (by 60%) with advancing age, and the network of elastin is diminished.[56] The age-dependent Ang II–mediated increase in arterial MMP-2 activity is involved in the cleavage of the elastin fibrillin-1 leading to the degradation of the elastin arterial network (**Fig. 8**).[55–57,62] These age-associated changes within elastin lamina are associated with an imbalance of synthesis and degradation of tropoelastin. The level of tropoelastin production by old aortic VSMCs in vitro is markedly reduced, and tropoelastin is also degraded more rapidly in tertiary culture with increased passage number than in primary culture.[75,76] Importantly, elastin fibers are cleaved by age-associated activation of the gelatinases MMP-2/9 and elastase.[76,77] Chronic administration of a broad-spectrum MMP inhibitor, PD166793, via a daily gavage, to 16-month-old rats for 8 months markedly

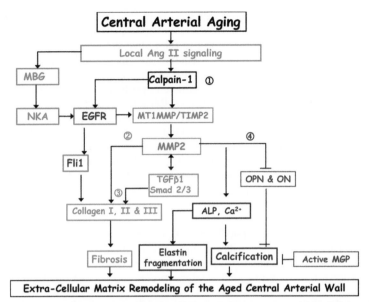

Fig. 8. Age-associated matrix remodeling of central arteries. Numerous other molecules, not shown on that diagram, have an important role in fibrosis, calcification, and elastin fragmentation. ALP, alkaline phosphatase; EGFR, EGF receptor; MGP, matrix Gla protein; MMP, matrix metalloprotease; MT1, metallothionein 1; ON, osteonectin; OPN, osteopontin; TGFβ1, transforming growth factor β1; TIMP2, tissue inhibitor of metalloprotease 2.

blunted the expected age-associated increases in aortic MMP activity and a release of fibrillin-1 and preserved the elastic fiber network integrity.[63] Importantly, degraded fibrillin-1 initiates fibrosis; ends of fractured fiber become an impetus to calcification (see **Fig. 8**).[78]

Arterial Calcification

Arterial calcification is also the calcium buildup consequence of a reparative or reactive process to chronic proinflammation. Arterial calcification, the deposition of calcium phosphate mineral, most often hydroxyapatite within or outside of arterial cells, is a salient feature of age-associated arterial remodeling (see **Fig. 8**). Old cultured VSMCs, like osteoblasts, are able to produce large amounts of bonelike substrates, including collagen II, which become bio-mineralized and calcified.[63] Overexpression of calpain-1 reduces the calcification inhibitors, osteonectin and osteopontin (OPN), and induces alkaline phosphatase activity in young VSMCs, mimicking that of old cells.[63] In addition, the activity of tissue transglutaminase (TG2), a protein crosslinking enzyme, increases in the old arterial wall and is closely associated with the reduction of NO bioavailability.[79–82] Activated TG2 upregulates calcification promoter genes, that is, *Runx2*, and downregulates the expression of calcification inhibitor genes, that is, OPN, within VSMCs and increases arterial stiffness (see **Fig. 8**).[80–82]

Arterial Fibrosis

Arterial wall fibrosis is a hallmark of aging and vascular diseases.[83,84] Arterial fibrosis is the formation of excessive extracellular fibrous tissue in a reparative or reactive process in response to chronic proinflammation (see **Figs. 7** and **8**). VSMCs are stretched via longitudinal or circumferential strain causing an age-associated increase in Ang II and TGFβ1 signaling in the arterial wall over time.[85,86] Inflammation induces tissue repair,[87] which is important in the scenario of tissue damage or blood pressure increase; TGFβ is an important player in this reparative process.[87,88] Increased aortic calpain-1–associated MMP-2 activity mediates age-associated arterial Ang II profibrotic signaling effect (see **Figs. 7** and **8**).[58] Overexpression of calpain-1 induces MMP-2 transcription, following by an increase in protein levels and activity, in part, by increasing the ratio of metallothionein 1–MMPs to tissue inhibitor of metalloprotease 2.[55] The increased MMP-2 activity of the old rat aorta colocalizes with TGFβ1.[57] The latent TGFβ1 precursor linked to fibrillin-1 and its intermediate degradation form, latent-associated protein, as well as active TGFβ1 within VSMC increase with aging via a stepwise of cleavage by MMP-2.[57] The expression of TGFβ1 receptor TGFβ receptor type II also increases with aging. Downstream receptor signaling molecules (see **Fig. 7**) of p-SMAD2, 3 and 4 increases while the medial expression of the suppressor SMAD7 is decreased with aging.[57] The effect of calpain-1–induced MMP-2 activation (see **Fig. 8**) results in increased collagen I, II, and III production in VSMCs.[55] Chronic inhibition of MMP markedly reduces arterial interstitial collagenase activity, TGFβ1 activation, the profibrogenic signaling molecule SMAD-2/3 phosphorylation, and collagen deposition.[63] Collectively, in vitro and in vivo results indicate that MMP inhibition retards age-associated arterial profibrotic signaling (see **Figs. 7** and **8**).

The Role of the Endogenous Sodium-Potassium Adenosine Triphosphate Ligand, Marinobufagenin, in Profibrotic Signaling

It is known that aging is a predominant factor for most diseases.[89] Chronic diseases even in younger ages also resemble aging by alteration of expression of genes in proinflammatory and profibrotic pathways, creating an aging profile at the genetic, molecular, cellular, and physiologic levels, especially in the cardiovascular system.[83,90–92] Fibrosis of arterial wall accompanies aging and vascular diseases.[83,90–92] Levels of the profibrotic factor, MBG, are implicated in the development of vascular fibrosis in preeclampsia, chronic renal failure, and salt-sensitive hypertension at any age.[39,93–99] Production of this steroid, MBG, is regulated by Ang II (see **Fig. 7**).[34] MBG links salt-sensitive arterial stiffness and hypertension. MBG initiates TGFβ- and Fli1 (friend leukemia integration 1 transcription factor)–dependent profibrotic signaling via binding to NKA (see **Fig. 8**).[100,101] Activation of TGFβ profibrotic signaling by MBG was demonstrated in the Dahl-S model of salt-sensitive hypertension and aging. In vivo, immunoneutralization of high MBG levels in old Dahl-S rats by an anti-MBG monoclonal antibody reverses arterial fibrosis and downregulates genes implicated in TGFβ signaling.

Fli1-dependent signaling, another profibrotic pathway, is also activated by MBG. The MBG-NKA-Src complex activates of EGF receptor (EGFR) signaling resulting in a degradation of Fli1 (a negative nuclear regulator of the procollagen-1 gene) and induction of collagen-1 synthesis (see **Fig. 8**).[101] This mechanism could be relevant to the pathogenesis of several conditions, including preeclampsia, in which elevated plasma MBG levels are associated with development of fibrosis in umbilical arteries accompanied by the reduction of Fli1.[102] Cardiovascular fibrosis activated by high endogenous MBG levels in a rat model of chronic renal disease (CRD) was reversed by immunization of these rats with monoclonal anti-MBG antibody.[103] Of note, the profibrotic effect of MBG and antifibrotic effect of anti-MBG antibody are pressure independent.[104] High NaCl intake in normotensive rats increases MBG levels and induces aortic fibrosis in the absence of a hypertensive response.[104] In this study, immunoneutralization of MBG reduces aortic fibrosis and restores the aortic relaxation.[104]

Antifibrotic effects of the MR antagonists, spironolactone, and its common metabolite, canrenone,[105] are also associated with Na-pump ligands.[106,107] The MR antagonist, canrenone, blocks the profibrotic activity of an endogenous MBG in animal models of CRD and also suppresses cardiac fibrosis in rats chronically treated by MBG in the absence of changes in aldosterone levels.[108] In addition, canrenone significantly attenuates pressure-independent profibrotic activity of MBG in cultures aortic VSMCs in vitro. Incubation of rat aortic rings with MBG reduces aortic Fli1, increases collagen-1, and attenuates relaxation of aorta. Canrenone restores aortic relaxation, restores Fli1 levels, and reduces collagen abundance in aortic wall.[40]

Older patients with resistant hypertension exhibit an increase in PWV, higher plasma MBG, and inhibited erythrocyte NKA versus normotensive age-matched control.[40] Administration of spironolactone to these patients with resistant hypertension for 6 months in addition to the conventional triple antihypertensive therapy restored NKA activity, decreased SBP and DBP, and significantly reduced PWV. These data further demonstrate the intimate relationship of MBG and arterial stiffness. Ang II–driven MBG is a novel target for MR antagonists in MBG-induced arterial remodeling and arterial stiffness. In addition, the immunoneutralization of profibrotic steroid MBG and also blocking its inhibiting effect on NKA by MR antagonists are additional approaches in treatment of salt-sensitive hypertension and conditions when heightened MBG level cause a devastating profibrotic and prohypertensive effect, which is accelerated by aging.

SUMMARY

The aforementioned evidence indicates that accelerated arterial wall remodeling via Ang II signaling within the arteries, per se, ought to be considered a type of hypertensive effect because the molecular disorder and the inflammatory milieu it creates within the arteries with advancing age are the roots of the pathophysiology of hypertension (see **Table 1**). Thus, therapies to prevent or reduce signaling that drive arterial wall remodeling may ultimately reduce the epidemic of hypertension in the older population by reducing the undisputed major risk factor for hypertension, that is, arterial aging, per se. Targeting the master perpetuators of arterial aging, that is, therapies to prevent or delay Ang II signaling–related vascular changes that accompany aging, seems to be the most promising strategy to reduce the health burden of hypertension and ultimately reduce the *prevalence* of hypertension and arterial fibrosis.

REFERENCES

1. AlGhatrif M, Lakatta EG. The conundrum of arterial stiffness, elevated blood pressure, and aging. Curr Hypertens Rep 2015;17(2):12.
2. High blood pressure fact sheet data & statistics |DHDSP|CDC. 2016. Available at: http://www.cdc.gov/dhdsp/data_statistics/fact_sheets/fs_bloodpressure.htm; http://www.ncbi.nlm.nih.gov/pubmed/16193230. Accessed May 11, 2016.
3. Colby SL, Ortman JM. Projections of the Size and Composition of the U.S. Population: 2014 to 2060, Current Population Reports, P25-1143, Washington, DC: U.S. Census Bureau; 2014.
4. Franklin SS, Jacobs MJ, Wong ND, et al. Predominance of isolated systolic hypertension among middle-aged and elderly US hypertensives: analysis based on National Health and Nutrition Examination Survey (NHANES) III. Hypertension 2001;37(3):869–74.
5. Heidenreich PA, Trogdon JG, Khavjou OA, et al. Forecasting the future of cardiovascular disease in the United States: a policy statement from the American Heart Association. Circulation 2011;123(8):933–44.

6. Redheuil A, Yu WC, Wu CO, et al. Reduced ascending aortic strain and distensibility: earliest manifestations of vascular aging in humans. Hypertension 2010; 55(2):319–26.
7. Scuteri A, Morrell CH, Orru M, et al. Longitudinal perspective on the conundrum of central arterial stiffness, blood pressure, and aging. Hypertension Dec 2014; 64(6):1219–27.
8. Franklin SS, Wt Gustin, Wong ND, et al. Hemodynamic patterns of age-related changes in blood pressure. The Framingham Heart Study. Circulation 1997; 96(1):308–15.
9. Rizzoni D, Muiesan ML, Porteri E, et al. Interrelationships between macro and microvascular structure and function. Artery Res 2010;4(4):114–7.
10. Mulvany MJ. Small artery remodelling in hypertension. Basic Clin Pharmacol Toxicol 2012;110(1):49–55.
11. Cecelja M, Chowienczyk P. Dissociation of aortic pulse wave velocity with risk factors for cardiovascular disease other than hypertension: a systematic review. Hypertension Dec 2009;54(6):1328–36.
12. Mitchell GF. Arterial stiffness and hypertension: chicken or egg? Hypertension 2014;64(2):210–4.
13. Kaess BM, Rong J, Larson MG, et al. Aortic stiffness, blood pressure progression, and incident hypertension. JAMA 2012;308(9):875–81.
14. Najjar SS, Scuteri A, Shetty V, et al. Pulse wave velocity is an independent predictor of the longitudinal increase in systolic blood pressure and of incident hypertension in the Baltimore Longitudinal Study of Aging. J Am Coll Cardiol 2008; 51(14):1377–83.
15. AlGhatrif M, Strait JB, Morrell CH, et al. Longitudinal trajectories of arterial stiffness and the role of blood pressure: the Baltimore Longitudinal Study of Aging. Hypertension 2013;62(5):934–41.
16. AlGhatrif M, Strait JB, Morrell C, et al. Attenuated aortic dilatation, not increased wall stiffness best explains the rise in pulse pressure in women with aging: results from the Baltimore Longitudinal Study of Aging. Circulation 2013;128(22):A18061.
17. Mitchell GF, Gudnason V, Launer LJ, et al. Hemodynamics of increased pulse pressure in older women in the community-based Age, Gene/Environment Susceptibility-Reykjavik Study. Hypertension 2008;51(4):1123–8.
18. Segers P, Rietzschel ER, De Buyzere ML, et al. Noninvasive (input) impedance, pulse wave velocity, and wave reflection in healthy middle-aged men and women. Hypertension 2007;49(6):1248–55.
19. Folkow B. Physiological aspects of primary hypertension. Physiol Rev 1982; 62(2):347–504.
20. Wasserstrom JA, Aistrup GL. Digitalis: new actions for an old drug. Am J Physiol Heart Circ Physiol 2005;289(5):H1781–93.
21. de Wardener HE, Clarkson EM. Concept of natriuretic hormone. Physiol Rev 1985;65(3):658–759.
22. Blanco G, Mercer RW. Isozymes of the Na-K-ATPase: heterogeneity in structure, diversity in function. Am J Physiol 1998;275(5 Pt 2):F633–50.
23. Weinberger MH, Miller JZ, Luft FC, et al. Definitions and characteristics of sodium sensitivity and blood pressure resistance. Hypertension 1986;8(6 Pt 2): II127–34.
24. De Wardener HE, MacGregor GA. Sodium and blood pressure. Curr Opin Cardiol 2002;17(4):360–7.
25. de Wardener HE, MacGregor GA. Harmful effects of dietary salt in addition to hypertension. J Hum Hypertens 2002;16(4):213–23.

26. Tobian L, Hanlon S. High sodium chloride diets injure arteries and raise mortality without changing blood pressure. Hypertension 1990;15(6 Pt 2):900–3.

27. Gu JW, Anand V, Shek EW, et al. Sodium induces hypertrophy of cultured myocardial myoblasts and vascular smooth muscle cells. Hypertension 1998; 31(5):1083–7.

28. Scuteri A, Stuehlinger MC, Cooke JP, et al. Nitric oxide inhibition as a mechanism for blood pressure increase during salt loading in normotensive postmenopausal women. J Hypertens 2003;21(7):1339–46.

29. Manning RD Jr, Hu L, Tan DY, et al. Role of abnormal nitric oxide systems in salt-sensitive hypertension. Am J Hypertens 2001;14(6 Pt 2):68S–73S.

30. Kinlay S, Creager MA, Fukumoto M, et al. Endothelium-derived nitric oxide regulates arterial elasticity in human arteries in vivo. Hypertension 2001;38(5): 1049–53.

31. Aviv A. Salt consumption, reactive oxygen species and cardiovascular ageing: a hypothetical link. J Hypertens 2002;20(4):555–9.

32. Celermajer DS, Sorensen KE, Spiegelhalter DJ, et al. Aging is associated with endothelial dysfunction in healthy men years before the age-related decline in women. J Am Coll Cardiol 1994;24(2):471–6.

33. Leenen FH, Ruzicka M, Huang BS. The brain and salt-sensitive hypertension. Curr Hypertens Rep 2002;4(2):129–35.

34. Fedorova OV, Agalakova NI, Talan MI, et al. Brain ouabain stimulates peripheral marinobufagenin via angiotensin II signalling in NaCl-loaded Dahl-S rats. J Hypertens 2005;23(8):1515–23.

35. Fedorova OV, Talan MI, Agalakova NI, et al. Endogenous ligand of alpha(1) sodium pump, marinobufagenin, is a novel mediator of sodium chloride–dependent hypertension. Circulation 2002;105(9):1122–7.

36. Hamlyn JM, Hamilton BP, Manunta P. Endogenous ouabain, sodium balance and blood pressure: a review and a hypothesis. J Hypertens 1996;14(2):151–67.

37. Fedorova OV, Shapiro JI, Bagrov AY. Endogenous cardiotonic steroids and salt-sensitive hypertension. Biochim Biophys Acta 2010;1802(12):1230–6.

38. Blaustein MP. Sodium ions, calcium ions, blood pressure regulation, and hypertension: a reassessment and a hypothesis. Am J Physiol 1977;232(5):C165–73.

39. Periyasamy SM, Liu J, Tanta F, et al. Salt loading induces redistribution of the plasmalemmal Na/K-ATPase in proximal tubule cells. Kidney Int 2005;67(5): 1868–77.

40. Fedorova OV, Emelianov IV, Bagrov KA, et al. Marinobufagenin-induced vascular fibrosis is a likely target for mineralocorticoid antagonists. J Hypertens 2015;33(8):1602–10.

41. Fedorova OV, Kolodkin NI, Agalakova NI, et al. Antibody to marinobufagenin lowers blood pressure in pregnant rats on a high NaCl intake. J Hypertens 2005;23(4):835–42.

42. Fedorova OV, Dorofeeva NA, Lopatin DA, et al. Phorbol diacetate potentiates na(+)-k(+) ATPase inhibition by a putative endogenous ligand, marinobufagenin. Hypertension 2002;39(2):298–302.

43. Bagrov AY, Shapiro JI, Fedorova OV. Endogenous cardiotonic steroids: physiology, pharmacology, and novel therapeutic targets. Pharmacol Rev 2009; 61(1):9–38.

44. Anderson DE, Fedorova OV, Morrell CH, et al. Endogenous sodium pump inhibitors and age-associated increases in salt sensitivity of blood pressure in normotensives. Am J Physiol Regul Integr Comp Physiol 2008;294(4):R1248–54.

45. Fedorova OV, Lakatta EG, Bagrov AY, et al. Plasma level of the endogenous sodium pump ligand marinobufagenin is related to the salt-sensitivity in men. J Hypertens 2015;33(3):534–41 [discussion: 541].
46. Cappuccio FP, Markandu ND, Carney C, et al. Double-blind randomised trial of modest salt restriction in older people. Lancet 1997;350(9081):850–4.
47. Gates PE, Tanaka H, Hiatt WR, et al. Dietary sodium restriction rapidly improves large elastic artery compliance in older adults with systolic hypertension. Hypertension 2004;44(1):35–41.
48. Jablonski KL, Fedorova OV, Racine ML, et al. Dietary sodium restriction and association with urinary marinobufagenin, blood pressure, and aortic stiffness. Clin J Am Soc Nephrol 2013;8(11):1952–9.
49. Fedorova OV, Kashkin VA, Zakharova IO, et al. Age-associated increase in salt sensitivity is accompanied by a shift in the atrial natriuretic peptide modulation of the effect of marinobufagenin on renal and vascular sodium pump. J Hypertens 2012;30(9):1817–26.
50. Fedorova OV, Agalakova NI, Morrell CH, et al. ANP differentially modulates marinobufagenin-induced sodium pump inhibition in kidney and aorta. Hypertension 2006;48(6):1160–8.
51. Sacks FM, Svetkey LP, Vollmer WM, et al. Effects on blood pressure of reduced dietary sodium and the Dietary Approaches to Stop Hypertension (DASH) diet. DASH-Sodium Collaborative Research Group. N Engl J Med 2001;344(1):3–10.
52. Wang M, Jiang L, Monticone RE, et al. Proinflammation: the key to arterial aging. Trends Endocrinol Metab 2014;25(2):72–9.
53. Wang M, Kim SH, Monticone RE, et al. Matrix metalloproteinases promote arterial remodeling in aging, hypertension, and atherosclerosis. Hypertension 2015; 65(4):698–703.
54. Wang M, Shah AM. Age-associated pro-inflammatory remodeling and functional phenotype in the heart and large arteries. J Mol Cell Cardiol 2015;83:101–11.
55. Jiang L, Zhang J, Monticone RE, et al. Calpain-1 regulation of matrix metalloproteinase 2 activity in vascular smooth muscle cells facilitates age-associated aortic wall calcification and fibrosis. Hypertension 2012;60(5):1192–9.
56. Wang M, Lakatta EG. Altered regulation of matrix metalloproteinase-2 in aortic remodeling during aging. Hypertension 2002;39(4):865–73.
57. Wang M, Zhao D, Spinetti G, et al. Matrix metalloproteinase 2 activation of transforming growth factor-beta1 (TGF-beta1) and TGF-beta1-type II receptor signaling within the aged arterial wall. Arterioscler Thromb Vasc Biol 2006; 26(7):1503–9.
58. Jiang L, Wang M, Zhang J, et al. Increased aortic calpain-1 activity mediates age-associated angiotensin II signaling of vascular smooth muscle cells. PLoS One 2008;3(5):e2231.
59. Spinetti G, Wang M, Monticone R, et al. Rat aortic MCP-1 and its receptor CCR2 increase with age and alter vascular smooth muscle cell function. Arterioscler Thromb Vasc Biol 2004;24(8):1397–402.
60. Wang M, Fu Z, Wu J, et al. MFG-E8 activates proliferation of vascular smooth muscle cells via integrin signaling. Aging cell 2012;11(3):500–8.
61. Wang M, Spinetti G, Monticone RE, et al. A local proinflammatory signalling loop facilitates adverse age-associated arterial remodeling. PLoS One 2011;6(2): e16653.
62. Wang M, Zhang J, Spinetti G, et al. Angiotensin II activates matrix metalloproteinase type II and mimics age-associated carotid arterial remodeling in young rats. Am J Pathol 2005;167(5):1429–42.

63. Wang M, Zhang J, Telljohann R, et al. Chronic matrix metalloproteinase inhibition retards age-associated arterial proinflammation and increase in blood pressure. Hypertension 2012;60(2):459–66.
64. Wang M, Zhang J, Walker SJ, et al. Involvement of NADPH oxidase in age-associated cardiac remodeling. J Mol Cell Cardiol 2010;48(4):765–72.
65. Krug AW, Allenhofer L, Monticone R, et al. Elevated mineralocorticoid receptor activity in aged rat vascular smooth muscle cells promotes a proinflammatory phenotype via extracellular signal-regulated kinase 1/2 mitogen-activated protein kinase and epidermal growth factor receptor-dependent pathways. Hypertension 2010;55(6):1476–83.
66. Yoon HE, Kim EN, Kim MY, et al. Age-associated changes in the vascular renin-angiotensin system in mice. Oxid Med Cell Longev 2016;2016:6731093.
67. Wang M, Fu Z, Lakatta EG, et al. Method for the diagnosis of age-associated vascular disorders. Google Patents; 2012.
68. Basso N, Cini R, Pietrelli A, et al. Protective effect of long-term angiotensin II inhibition. Am J Physiol Heart Circ Physiol 2007;293(3):H1351–8.
69. Michel JB, Heudes D, Michel O, et al. Effect of chronic ANG I-converting enzyme inhibition on aging processes. II. Large arteries. Am J Physiol 1994;267(1 Pt 2):R124–35.
70. Linz W, Heitsch H, Scholkens BA, et al. Long-term angiotensin II type 1 receptor blockade with fonsartan doubles lifespan of hypertensive rats. Hypertension 2000;35(4):908–13.
71. Benigni A, Corna D, Zoja C, et al. Disruption of the Ang II type 1 receptor promotes longevity in mice. J Clin Invest 2009;119(3):524–30.
72. Fu Z, Wang M, Gucek M, et al. Milk fat globule protein epidermal growth factor-8: a pivotal relay element within the angiotensin II and monocyte chemoattractant protein-1 signaling cascade mediating vascular smooth muscle cells invasion. Circ Res 2009;104(12):1337–46.
73. Fu Z, Wang M, Everett A, et al. Can proteomics yield insight into aging aorta? Proteomics Clin Appl 2013;7(7–8):477–89.
74. Wang M, Wang HH, Lakatta EG. Milk fat globule epidermal growth factor VIII signaling in arterial wall remodeling. Curr Vasc Pharmacol 2013;11(5):768–76.
75. Ruckman JL, Luvalle PA, Hill KE, et al. Phenotypic stability and variation in cells of the porcine aorta: collagen and elastin production. Matrix Biol 1994;14(2):135–45.
76. Antonicelli F, Bellon G, Debelle L, et al. Elastin-elastases and inflamm-aging. Curr Top Dev Biol 2007;79:99–155.
77. Cauchard JH, Berton A, Godeau G, et al. Activation of latent transforming growth factor beta 1 and inhibition of matrix metalloprotease activity by a thrombospondin-like tripeptide linked to elaidic acid. Biochem Pharmacol 2004;67(11):2013–22.
78. Kumata C, Mizobuchi M, Ogata H, et al. Involvement of matrix metalloproteinase-2 in the development of medial layer vascular calcification in uremic rats. Ther Apher Dial 2011;15(Suppl 1):18–22.
79. Chabot N, Moreau S, Mulani A, et al. Fluorescent probes of tissue transglutaminase reveal its association with arterial stiffening. Chem Biol 2010;17(10):1143–50.
80. Johnson KA, Polewski M, Terkeltaub RA. Transglutaminase 2 is central to induction of the arterial calcification program by smooth muscle cells. Circ Res 2008;102(5):529–37.
81. Santhanam L, Tuday EC, Webb AK, et al. Decreased S-nitrosylation of tissue transglutaminase contributes to age-related increases in vascular stiffness. Circ Res 2010;107(1):117–25.

82. Steppan J, Sikka G, Jandu S, et al. Exercise, vascular stiffness, and tissue trans-glutaminase. J Am Heart Assoc 2014;3(2):e000599.

83. Lakatta EG. So! What's aging? Is cardiovascular aging a disease? J Mol Cell Cardiol 2015;83:1–13.

84. Lakatta EG, Levy D. Arterial and cardiac aging: major shareholders in cardio-vascular disease enterprises: part I: aging arteries: a "set up" for vascular dis-ease. Circulation 2003;107(1):139–46.

85. Shyu KG, Chao YM, Wang BW, et al. Regulation of discoidin domain receptor 2 by cyclic mechanical stretch in cultured rat vascular smooth muscle cells. Hy-pertension 2005;46(3):614–21.

86. Li Q, Muragaki Y, Hatamura I, et al. Stretch-induced collagen synthesis in cultured smooth muscle cells from rabbit aortic media and a possible involve-ment of angiotensin II and transforming growth factor-beta. J Vasc Res 1998; 35(2):93–103.

87. Hold GL, Untiveros P, Saunders KA, et al. Role of host genetics in fibrosis. Fibro-genesis Tissue Repair 2009;2(1):6.

88. Leask A. Potential therapeutic targets for cardiac fibrosis TGF beta, angiotensin, endothelin, CCN2, and PDGF, partners in fibroblast activation. Circ Res 2010; 106(11):1675–80.

89. Kennedy BK, Berger SL, Brunet A, et al. Geroscience: linking aging to chronic disease. Cell 2014;159(4):709–13.

90. Kovacic JC, Moreno P, Hachinski V, et al. Cellular senescence, vascular dis-ease, and aging part 1 of a 2-part review. Circulation 2011;123(15):1650–60.

91. Kovacic JC, Moreno P, Nabel EG, et al. Cellular senescence, vascular disease, and aging: part 2 of a 2-part review: clinical vascular disease in the elderly. Cir-culation 2011;123(17):1900–10.

92. Harvey A, Montezano AC, Lopes RA, et al. Vascular fibrosis in aging and hyper-tension: molecular mechanisms and clinical implications. Can J Cardiol 2016; 32(5):659–68.

93. Fedorova OV, Doris PA, Bagrov AY. Endogenous marinobufagenin-like factor in acute plasma volume expansion. Clin Exp Hypertens 1998;20(5–6):581–91.

94. Fedorova OV, Anderson DE, Lakatta EG, et al. Interaction of NaCl and behav-ioral stress on endogenous sodium pump ligands in rats. Am J Physiol Regul Integr Comp Physiol 2001;281(1):R352–8.

95. Kennedy DJ, Vetteth S, Periyasamy SM, et al. Central role for the cardiotonic ste-roid marinobufagenin in the pathogenesis of experimental uremic cardiomyop-athy. Hypertension 2006;47(3):488–95.

96. Tian J, Haller S, Periyasamy S, et al. Renal ischemia regulates marinobufagenin release in humans. Hypertension 2010;56(5):914–9.

97. Kolmakova EV, Haller ST, Kennedy DJ, et al. Endogenous cardiotonic steroids in chronic renal failure. Nephrol Dial Transplant 2011;26(9):2912–9.

98. Lopatin DA, Ailamazian EK, Dmitrieva RI, et al. Circulating bufodienolide and cardenolide sodium pump inhibitors in preeclampsia. J Hypertens 1999;17(8): 1179–87.

99. Gonick HC, Ding Y, Vaziri ND, et al. Simultaneous measurement of marinobufa-genin, ouabain, and hypertension-associated protein in various disease states. Clin Exp Hypertens 1998;20(5–6):617–27.

100. Xie Z, Askari A. Na(+)/K(+)-ATPase as a signal transducer. Eur J Biochem 2002;269(10):2434–9.

101. Elkareh J, Periyasamy SM, Shidyak A, et al. Marinobufagenin induces increases in procollagen expression in a process involving protein kinase C and

Fli-1: implications for uremic cardiomyopathy. Am J Physiol Renal Physiol 2009; 296(5):F1219–26.

102. Nikitina ER, Mikhailov AV, Nikandrova ES, et al. In preeclampsia endogenous cardiotonic steroids induce vascular fibrosis and impair relaxation of umbilical arteries. J Hypertens 2011;29(4):769–76.

103. Haller ST, Kennedy DJ, Shidyak A, et al. Monoclonal antibody against marinobu-fagenin reverses cardiac fibrosis in rats with chronic renal failure. Am J Hypertens Jun 2012;25(6):690–6.

104. Grigorova YN, Juhasz O, Zernetkina V, et al. Aortic fibrosis, induced by high salt intake in the absence of hypertensive response, is reduced by a monoclonal antibody to marinobufagenin. Am J Hypertens 2016;29(5):641–6.

105. de Mendonca M, Grichois ML, Pernollet MG, et al. Antihypertensive effect of canrenone in a model where endogenous ouabain-like factors are present. J Cardiovasc Pharmacol 1988;11(1):75–83.

106. Safar ME, Blacher J, Jankowski P. Arterial stiffness, pulse pressure, and cardio-vascular disease-is it possible to break the vicious circle? Atherosclerosis 2011; 218(2):263–71.

107. Semplicini A, Serena L, Valle R, et al. Ouabain-inhibiting activity of aldosterone antagonists. Steroids 1995;60(1):110–3.

108. Tian J, Shidyak A, Periyasamy SM, et al. Spironolactone attenuates experi-mental uremic cardiomyopathy by antagonizing marinobufagenin. Hypertension 2009;54(6):1313–20.

A Reassessment of the Pathophysiology of Progressive Cardiorenal Disorders

CrossMark

Richard N. Re, MD

KEYWORDS

- Renal disease • Heart failure • Intracrine • Mineralocorticoid receptor

KEY POINTS

- Intracrines are extracellular signaling proteins that also act in the intracellular space.
- Various peptide moieties other than hormones and cytokines can display intracrine activity.
- Many intracrines exist in cardiac and renal tissues and participate in pathogenesis.
- Mineralocorticoid receptors (MRs) in heart and kidney can be activated by mineralocorticoids or by atypical mechanisms.
- Mineralocorticoid activation can amplify angiotensin II–mediated effects.

INTRODUCTION

Chronic renal disease (CRD) secondary to hypertension, diabetes, or other causes is characterized by progressive worsening of disease. A similar pattern is seen in systolic heart failure (SHF). These disorders can be the sequelae of hypertension and/or worsened by hypertension. Even if treated, these conditions worsen over time, although the reasons for this are not well understood.[1,2] It is generally assumed that an insult to the renal cortex or to the left ventricular myocardium sets in motion a chain of adaptive physiologic processes, which unfortunately also results in disease worsening. For example, loss of glomeruli is assumed to be associated with compensatory hyperfiltration in the remaining glomeruli, leading to intraglomerular hypertension and progressive glomerular dropout. Cardiac myocyte dropout after myocardial infarction is thought to lead to pressure alterations in the ventricle that result in myocyte hypertrophy, tissue remodeling, and myocyte death. Considerable data support these models as does the response to therapy. Interruption or blockade of the renin-angiotensin system (RAS) lowers intraglomerular pressure and slows the progression of diabetic

Funding: Ochsner Clinic Foundation.
The author has no conflicts of interest.
Ochsner Clinic Foundation, Division of Research, 1514 Jefferson Highway, New Orleans, LA 70121, USA
E-mail address: rre@ochsner.org

nephropathy. Cardiac resynchronization therapy improves ventricular mechanics and benefits properly selected patients with congestive heart failure.[3,4] Available therapies in general, however, do not eliminate disease progression, although they slow it. For example, attempts to stop the progression of diabetic renal disease by maximally suppressing the RAS through the combined use of angiotensin-converting enzyme (ACE) inhibitors and angiotensin type 1 (AT1) receptor blockers (ARBs) were not successful. This raises the possibility that the current view of these diseases is incomplete. The possibility that disease progression in CRD and SHF is in part cell-autonomous could provide insight into this issue. That is, local cellular responses may be contributing to disease progression over and above any actions of classic physiologic compensatory mechanisms. Surprisingly, this view is supported by the available data and, if correct, would lead to novel therapeutic options.[4,5]

In considering cell-autonomous disease progression, it is instructive to consider common chronic neurodegenerative diseases, such as Alzheimer disease, Parkinson disease, and amyotrophic lateral sclerosis.[6–8] These disorders, like CRD and SHF, are characterized by progressive cell (neuron) death and a downhill course. Although compensatory neural activity could be playing a role in the disease progression, it is becoming clear that several neuronal proteins are disordered in these disease and spread from cell to cell, thereby spreading the disorders. These proteins produce the equivalent of a locally infectious process. Because this mechanism mirrors the infectious prion spread seen in the spongiform encephalopathies, such as kuru, Creutzfeldt-Jakob disease, bovine spongiform encephalopathy (mad cow disease), and scrapie, these more common neurodegenerative disorders are arguably prionlike in their pathogenesis. Presumably, the sporadic forms of these prionlike disorders arise when a disease-specific neuron protein becomes misfolded, leading to its induction of misfolding in its normal homologues. Eventually the quantity of inclusion protein increases to the point that cell loss occurs. Spread of misfolded protein to neighboring cells, before or after cell death, leads to disease spread in the brain and progressive clinical worsening. Thus, evidence indicates that these diseases are not primarily the result of physiologic maladaptation but rather are the result of cell-autonomous processes.[6–8] These disorders, therefore, could serve as a model for disease progression in CRD and SHF.

SIGNALING PROTEIN BIOLOGY

In an effort to explore a possible cell-autonomous mode of pathogenesis for cardiorenal disease, it is instructive to review the biology of signaling proteins. The major mode of action of these factors is to bind to a cell membrane receptor with the generation of second messengers. Protein signaling action can be endocrine, paracrine, or autocrine. The author's group has also developed evidence that many signaling proteins can also act in what is termed an *intracrine mode*, meaning they can act in their cell of synthesis and/or in the interiors of target cells.[4,9–19] Moreover, they can function in a canonical mode, meaning they bind at their cognate receptors in the intracellular space, or a noncanonical mode, meaning they act without binding to their cognate receptor, for example, by binding to an alternative intracellular protein.[14–16] Angiotensin II, like other RAS components, is an intracrine. It binds to cell surface receptors, but it also binds to angiotensin II AT1 receptors on nuclear membranes and to ATI-like receptors associated with transcriptionally active euchromatin. It has also been reported to bind to angiotensin type 1 (AT1) and angiotensin type 2 (AT2) receptors on mitochondria. These actions are canonical (albeit atypical in the case of chromatin binding). There are data, however, to indicate angiotensin II also directly binds to mitochondrial electron chain proteins and causes oxidative stress. This action is noncanonical. An intracrine's action at the cell membrane may be the same as at an intracellular site, or different. For example, parathyroid hormone–related protein (PTHrP) is mitogenic for vascular smooth muscle cells when it binds to its nuclear receptor, but it inhibits cell proliferation after binding to its cell surface receptor. Intracrine peptides are varied in their chemical structure. Growth factors, hormones, enzymes, and DNA binding, protein among other moieties, have been shown to exhibit intracrine function as manifested by both extracellular and intracellular signaling/trafficking (**Table 1**).[9–18] For example, renin, angiotensinogen, and ACE exhibit intracrine action.[4,17] Moreover, the author has proposed principles of intracrine action. In particular, many intracrines have been shown to up-regulate their own synthesis or that of their signaling pathways. This, coupled with their capacity to traffic between cell interiors (either after secretion and internalization by target cells or by trafficking in exosomes), provides them the opportunity to affect the biology of a tissue, arguably placing all the cells affected in an altered state of hormonal responsiveness or differentiation, a state dependent on continued intracellular synthesis and action of an intracrine.[9–18] For example, the intracrine homeoproteins PDX-1 and Pax6 can work in this way.[19,20] The nature of intracrines and of intracrine biology in health and disease, and their possible therapeutic application, is explored elsewhere.[9–18] This biology also suggests a link between intracrine action and a possible cell-autonomous pathophysiology of progressive cardiorenal disorders.

PROGRESSIVE CARDIORENAL DISEASE

In considering the pathogenesis of progressive cardiorenal disease it is instructive to consider 1 renal disorder, diabetic nephrosclerosis (DN), in some detail and then determine to what extent observations about its pathogenesis can be applied to other disorders, such as congestive heart failure.[4,18] Diabetic nephropathy is well studied and for this reason provides adequate data for evaluation. The pathology of DN is characterized by basement membrane thickening, mesangial matrix expansion, podocyte drop out, arterial hyalinization, and glomerular sclerosis. Podocytes and mesangial cells seem to play important roles in the development of this pathologic picture.[1,4,18] Along with hyperfiltration and proteinuria, a variety of protein factors have been reported to be up-regulated in various cells during disease development. It is instructive to note that many of the peptides associated with the pathogenesis of CRD and systolic congestive heart failure are in fact intracrines. Included in this number are angiotensin II, transforming growth factor β1 (TGF-β1), PTHrP, vascular endothelial growth factor (VEGF), midkine, and renin. These factors, as well as possibly endothelin, angiotensinogen, and others, participate in disease pathogenesis and may do so through intracrine action.[1,4,18] Each of these factors is a possible candidate for therapeutic intervention. Given the known beneficial effects of RAS interruption/inhibition in CRD and congestive heart failure, the RAS, in particular angiotensin II, is a candidate for playing a major role in the pathogenesis of DN.

In exploring a possible role for intracrine physiology, several observations are instructive. First, RAS up-regulation occurs in many models of cardiorenal disorders. Exposure to elevated glucose causes up-regulate of angiotensinogen and, secondarily, of angiotensin II synthesis in cultured renal podocytes and cardiac myocytes. Elevated angiotensinogen and AT1 receptor expression occurs in some podocytes and mesangial cells in the glomeruli of streptozotocin-treated diabetic rats. Angiotensin II is up-regulated in cardiac myocytes and renal podocytes by stretch, as is angiotensin II–mediated apoptosis. Podocyte loss is seen in diabetic nephropathy and other renal disorders associated with proteinuria. Diabetic mesangial expansion

Table 1
Representative intracrines

Hormones, Cytokines	Growth Factors	DNA Binding Proteins	Enzymes	Other
Insulin	FGF (1,2,3,10)	Homeoproteins	Phosphoglucose isomerase/neuroleukin	Lactoferrin
GLP-1 (28–30)	Midkine	Amphoterin (HMGB1)	Renin/Prorenin (aspartyl-protease)	Endogenous Opioidids (Dynorphin)
Angiotensin II	VEGF	IL-33	PD-ECGF/thymidine phosphorylase	Galectins
Prolactin	NGF		Granzyme A, B	Tat
INF beta, gamma	PDGF		PLA2-I	Defensins
Interleukins	Pleiotrophin		Urokinase	SHBG
PTHrP	Proenkephalin		Lysyl-tRNA synthetase	Riboso mal Protein S 19
Oxytocin	IGF-1		Thioredoxin	Pituitary Adenylate Cyclase Activating Polypeptide
Leptin	Pigmented Epithelium- derived Factor (a serpin)		Tyrosyl-tRNA synthetase	Endostatin
Growth Hormone	Maspin (a serpin)		Pancreatic Bile Salt- Dependent Lipase	Periostin
Somatostatin	Schwannoma-derived growth factor		Trp-tRNA synthetase	Heat Shock Proteins
TRH	Leukemia Inhibiting Factor		ACE	PAI-2 (a serpin)
LHRH	Macrophage Colony- Stimulating Factor (CSF-1)		AChE-R	Reelin
VIP	Hepatopoietin		Angiogenin	PDCD5
ANP	TGF-alpha		Angiotensin-Converting Enzyme	Thrombospondin-1
Gonadotropin	Hepatopoietin		Chymase	C- Peptide
Chorionic Gonadotropin	Heregulin			STC
Angiotensin (1–7)	TGF-beta			IGF BP-3,5,6,7
Endothelin	BMP2			TCTP
Neuropeptide Y	BMP4			Wnt 13
Erythropoietin	Activin A			Oncoprotein DEK
	HB-EGF			S100B
	CTGF			

Abbreviations: AChE-R, acetylcholinesterase read-through isoform; BMP, bone morphogenetic protein; CTGF, connective tissue growth factor; FGF, fibroblast growth factor; GLP1 (28-36), glucagon-like peptide 1 fragment 28-36; HB-EGF, heparin binding epidermal growth factor-like growth factor; HMGB1, high-mobility group protein B1; IGF, insulin-like growth factor; IGF-BP, insulin-like growth factor binding protein; IL-33, interleukin-33; INF, interferon; LHRH, luteinizing hormone-releasing hormone; NGF, nerve growth factor; PAI-2, plasminogen activator inhibitor-2; PD-ECGF, platelet-derived endothelial cell growth factor; PDCD5, programmed cell death 5; PDGF, platelet derived growth factor; PLA2-I, phospholipase A2-I; PTHrP, parathyroid hormone-related protein; SHBG, sex hormone-binding globulin; STC, stanniocalcin; TCTP, translationally controlled tumor protein; TGF, transforming growth factor; TRH, thyrotropin-releasing hormone; VEGF, vascular endothelial growth factor; VIP, vasoactive intestinal polypeptide.

Data from refs.[64–72]

is characterized by the deposition of extracellular matrix and mesangial cell hyperplasia/hypertrophy. Elevated glucose up-regulates angiotensin II synthesis by mesangial cells.[4,5,18] Angiotensin II induces mesangial cell production of extracellular matrix by stimulating TGF-β1 and stimulates cell proliferation. Moreover, in some renal cells, angiotensin II can act directly at the nucleus to up-regulate TGF-β1.[4,18,21,22] In renal tubule cells, TGF-β1 up-regulates angiotensinogen. Other intracrines, such as PTHrP, VEGF, and midkine, have been shown to play important roles in progressive renal disease and, along with angiotensin, TGF-β1, angiotensinogen, renin, and endothelin, they could act in an intracrine fashion to produce disease. For example, PTHrP, an intracrine expressed in kidney and myocardium, in some systems is up-regulated by angiotensin II and by TGF-β1 and can, in turn, up-regulate TGF-β1 in renal podocytes.[4,5,18,21,22] Thus, a series of interacting, self-supporting loops could develop in progressive cardiorenal disorders; these interrelations are discussed in more detail elsewhere.[18]

Second, in multiple systems, angiotensin II up-regulates the synthesis of angiotensinogen and, therefore, can in principle establish a positive feedback loop. More specifically, angiotensin II applied to isolated hepatic cell nuclei up-regulates transcription of renin and angiotensinogen; angiotensin II has been shown to up-regulate angiotensinogen synthesis in cultured adult and neonatal cardiomyocytes. Angiotensin II up-regulates whole-kidney and renal tubular angiotensinogen. Moreover, in an in vivo study, intracellular angiotensin II has been shown to up-regulate angiotensinogen synthesis in renal proximal tubular cells and to secondarily cause hypertension. Thus, positive feedback loops in heart and kidney could well occur.[4,9,10,23–29]

Third, cardiorenal disease along with tissue up-regulation of tissue RASs can be initiated by pathologic stimuli, such as high glucose, but disease progresses even after the noxious stimulus is normalized or ameliorated. Improving glucose control only partially reduces the progression of diabetic renal disease, for example.[4,24–28]

Fourth, although interruption/blockade of the RAS is therapeutically beneficial, indicating a role for the RAS in disease pathogenesis, the benefit of RAS interruption/blockade is only partial. A variety of mechanisms have been proposed to explain the less than complete benefit provided by RAS interruption/blockade. Blockade/interruption could be incomplete, but efforts to improve therapeutic efficacy by enhancing RAS interruption/blockade by combining agents has been unsuccessful. Another possibility is that direct prorenin action at the (pro)renin receptor, independent of angiotensin II, is partially responsible for disease progression in the face of ARB or ACE inhibitor therapy.[4] This notion cannot be adequately vetted until an effective blocker of direct renin action is developed and can be tested. Evidence does suggest a direct role for prorenin in the generation of renal fibrosis.[4] The participation of direct prorenin action in these diseases, however, does not exclude intracrine action because prorenin itself is an intracrine and because prorenin's enzymatic ability to generate angiotensin II is activated by binding to its receptor. Recall that angiotensin II can up-regulate renin itself, as well as angiotensinogen, in isolated nuclei.[4] Thus, renin or prorenin could establish a renin/angiotensinogen/angiotensin II/renin loop in the intracellular space. Another possibility is that angiotensin (1-12) could serve as a generator of angiotensin II independent of renin.[4,30] These scenarios actually represent variants of the straightforward angiotensin II feedback loop, described previously: however, angiotensin II is produced, it could up-regulate angiotensinogen and lead to the creation of a positive feedback loop. Finally, other intracrines, such as TGF-β1, VEGF, PTHrP, endothelin, and midkine, are up-regulated in cardiorenal disease, and these could also form positive feedback loops, including loops that interact with one another to produce disease progression.[18,22,31–33]

The 4 observations discussed previously are consistent with an intracrine explanation of disease progression. For example, a straightforward model would involve glucose up-regulating angiotensinogen and angiotensin II production in podocytes and other cells. Angiotensin II traffics to nearby cells either after secretion and uptake or via exosomes, an established mode of intracrine trafficking. In the target cell, angiotensin II would again up-regulate angiotensinogen synthesis and intercellular trafficking would continue. In some cells, elevated intracellular angiotensin II concentrations could produce oxidative stress as well as other adverse consequences, such as the up-regulation of the intracrine TGF-β1. Up-regulated TGF-β1 can not only produce adverse consequences, such as fibrosis, it can also potentially form positive self-reinforcing loops with angiotensinogen/angiotensin II by up-regulating angiotensinogen.[4,18,32] In cardiac myocytes, up-regulation of angiotensin II up-regulates the activity of the pleiotropic protein p53, which in turn has the potential to up-regulate angiotensinogen and likely, therefore, angiotensin II synthesis; this could close a positive feedback loop and also induce apoptosis. Even if glucose stress is removed, elevated intracellular angiotensin II, and possibly TGF-β1, concentrations, once established, would persist, producing pathology over time as these intracrines traffic in glomerulus or myocardium.[4,18,24–28,32] Moreover, TGF-β1, angiotensinogen, and even renin could similarly traffic in an intracrine mode either after secretion, or more likely, in exosomes. To the extent that exosome trafficking occurs or the fluid phase trafficking of nonangiotensin II RAS intracrines occurs, angiotensin receptor blockers would be ineffective unless they acted inside cells. To the extent that noncanonical angiotensin II action is involved, for example, direct effects on mitochondrial electron chain proteins, angiotensin receptor blockers would similarly be ineffective even if they acted in the intracellular space.[14,15] Similarly, loops established by the trafficking of the angiotensin II precursor angiotensin (1-12) would be unaffected by either ARBs acting at the cell membrane or renin inhibitors acting in the cell interiors because angiotensin (1-12) can be cleaved to form angiotensin II by renin-independent mechanisms; this possibility is supported by the presence of significant amounts of angiotensin (1-12) in both heart and kidney.[28–30] Intercellular trafficking of angiotensin (1-12) could, after conversion to angiotensin II, up-regulate angiotensinogen in target cells triggering the production of a renin dependent positive loop. Alternatively, if target cells produce not only angiotensinogen but also angiotensin (1-12) a renin-independent positive loop could form. In this regard, it also is unclear how effective direct renin inhibitors, such as aliskiren, are in blocking intracellular renin activity in cell culture or in intact animals.[4,30] This schema illustrates the basic concept of intracrine disease progression. These processes could occur in myocardium after exposure to high-glucose or stretch-induced angiotensin II up-regulation and could occur in kidney in the face of high glucose or other insult.[4,5,18] Similar scenarios can be developed for the other intracrines involved in cardiorenal disorders as well as for participation of these intracrines in other disorders, such as heart failure with preserved ejection fraction (diastolic heart failure).[18]

MINERALOCORTICOID RECEPTOR

This laboratory introduced the term, intracrine, in 1984 and applied it to peptide hormones, given that steroid hormones were already known to act in cell interiors through binding to nuclear receptors.[9–17,34] Over time it became clear that some steroid hormones can act at external cell membrane receptors in a so-called nongenomic mode.[35] This means that steroid hormones, like peptide hormones, act both in cell interiors and at external cell membranes and, therefore, steroid hormones could be deemed intracrine. The authors' group has continued to apply the term exclusively to peptide hormones because it has not been demonstrated that steroid hormones operate in the feedforward loops characteristic of many peptide intracrines or that they share the other aspects of the intracrine biology described. This issue will only be determined by future research. It remains possible, however, that, just as peptide intracrine loops interact in processes, such as angiogenesis, intracellular steroid hormones could interact with peptide intracrine function.[10,16,35] This has relevance for the observation that in CRD and systolic congestive heart failure, MR antagonism has been shown to slow disease progression in a fashion that is additive (or possibly synergistic in some cases) with RAS interruption/blockade.[4,36] If the pathogenesis of these disorders is intracrine mediated, it would be expected that, given the therapeutic benefit of MR antagonists, the biology of mineralocorticoids interacts with the intracrine mechanisms driving disease progression.

It has been shown that aldosterone can be synthesized in kidney cortex and its synthesis is stimulated by angiotensin II and low salt as well as by high glucose. Angiotensin receptor blockade reduces this aldosterone up-regulation, indicating that it is angiotensin-driven. Glucose normalization in diabetic animals for 1 week causes the increase in renal aldosterone to decline to a level approximately half as great as it was in the presence of high glucose.[37,38] This is consistent with the formation of a persistent angiotensin II feedforward loop supporting aldosterone synthesis. Given the proinflammatory actions of aldosterone in the kidney, this could explain why interrupting mineralocorticoid signaling with an MR antagonist has beneficial effects. Moreover, aldosterone up-regulates angiotensin converting-enzyme in cardiac myocytes and endothelial cells.[39,40] Aldosterone synthesis has been reported in the cardiac left ventricle and this synthesis is up-regulated in heart failure, possibly as the result of increased ACE synthesis in cardiac myocytes. The investigators who made this observation suggested that it could represent a positive feedback loop in the ventricle in congestive heart failure patients.[39] Aldosterone up-regulates renin gene expression in juxtaglomerular cells and has been shown to up-regulate ACE in cardiac myocytes and endothelial cells.[41] Also, administration of the mineralocorticoid deoxycorticosterone acetate and salt produces an angiotensin-dependent hypertension with suppression of the circulating RAS but up-regulation of the brain RAS.[34,42–44] In a model of heart failure, brain aldosterone, derived from plasma, correlated with brain RAS activity as determined from ACE and angiotensin II AT1 receptor levels as well as with sympathetic activity.[45] In rats, aldosterone infusion up-regulated aortic ACE (mRNA, protein, and enzymatic activity) and up-regulated tissue angiotensin II.[46] Taken together, these data suggest that mineralocorticoids up-regulate the RAS in several tissues, such as brain, kidney, and heart. When this occurs in cells in which disease-associated up-regulation of the RAS and aldosterone is seen, such as podocytes, mesangial cells, or cardiac myocytes, a system involving the up-regulation of angiotensin II and aldosterone could develop with angiotensin II and aldosterone helping to up-regulate each other.[34,47] If angiotensin II and aldosterone up-regulation have pathologic consequences, these self-sustaining loops would produce disease. Intercellular trafficking of angiotensin II, other intracrines, or aldosterone (via extracellular vesicles or in the fluid phase) then could cause the gradual progression of disease throughout the glomerulus or myocardium even after removal of the initiating stimulus.[4,34] Moreover, aldosterone, likely acting through the MR, can up-regulate TGF-β1, thereby supporting the angiotensin II and TGF-β1 loops, discussed previously; also, high salt up-regulates TGF-β1 in the kidney and this could similarly support intracrines angiotensin II/TGF-β1 loops.[18] Because aldosterone freely enters cells, yet primary hyperaldosteronism, if treated early, is not associated with progressive renal or cardiac disease, it is not likely that the cell-to-cell trafficking of aldosterone alone can establish a pathology-producing intracrine feedforward system. Rather, aldosterone would be expected to amplify the up-regulation of an angiotensin II-driven loop, amplify the pathologic effects of angiotensin II, and produce its own pathologic effects, such as the induction of inflammation and oxidative stress.

ATYPICAL MINERALOCORTICOID RECEPTOR ACTIVATION

In animal studies cortisol, paradoxically, seems to bind to and inactivate cardiac MR. This results in protection of the myocardium from aldosterone. Oxidative stress or myocardial infarction results in cortisol becoming agonistic at ventricular MR and in that case it could produce pathology responsive to MR antagonism. Thus it has been argued that cortisol, or possibly other moieties, is responsible for activation of the MR in congestive heart failure and for the benefit derived from MR antagonism.[47-49] If that occurs, MR activation would nonetheless help up-regulate an intracrine RAS and thereby contribute to disease progression. In that case, MR action would serve as an amplifying factor of the intracrine RAS. Also, MR levels are increased in cardiac myocytes in congestive heart failure.[50] Aldosterone can up-regulate MR and this is inhibited by the MR antagonist eplerenone, indicating that this up-regulation is MR-mediated action. The AT1 receptor blocker losartan can also inhibit aldosterone-induced MR up-regulation. This implies cross-talk between the AT1 receptor and the MR.[51-53] This view is supported by the observation that angiotensin II can directly activate genomic MR activity in vascular smooth muscle cells, an effect that can be blocked by both MR antagonists and AT1 receptor blockers. This again implies cooperation between the 2 receptor types. Thus, intracrine RAS up-regulation could up-regulate MR, which, in the presence of any activating moiety and/or of activation by angiotensin II itself, would feedforward to up-regulate intracrine RAS function by up-regulating ACE and AT1 receptors. Even if cortisol is not acting as an MR agonist, angiotensin II genomic action at the MR could up-regulate ACE and AT1 receptors.[52] These mechanisms would have the same effect as angiotensin II stimulating aldosterone synthesis. Also, angiotensin II can induce oxidative stress. In cardiac myocytes, and probably in other cells as well, oxidative stress could cause cortisol to become an MR agonist, resulting in the closure of an alternative angiotensin II/MR feedforward loop.[4,51-54] Moreover, the possible participation of locally synthesized aldosterone must remains a consideration. In sum, there are multiple ways in which angiotensin II could produce a feedforward loop sensitive to MR antagonism to complement an angiotensin II/angiotensinogen feedforward loop. Thus, a feedforward MR/intracrine RAS interaction is plausible irrespective of whether aldosterone or another moiety activates the MR in disease. Finally, Rac1, a Rho family small GTPase, modulates MR activity and promotes MR nuclear translocation and the up-regulation of MR-sensitive genes. Rac1 is up-regulated by salt and is also elevated in cardiac injury induced by pressure overload and in salt-sensitive hypertension. Rac1 represents yet an additional mechanism for MR activation and its participation in renal disease and heart failure.[55]

SUMMARY

The data presented suggest that persistent intracrine positive feedback loops can develop in cardiorenal disorders, leading to intracrine trafficking, the spread of disease, and progressive loss of renal or cardiac function, even after disease initiating factors are controlled. A variety of intracrines potentially could be involved in these processes, including, among others, angiotensin II, angiotensinogen, (pro)renin, TGF-β1, VEGF, PTHrP, endothelin, and midkine.[4,5,9,10,18,21,56-59] The available data indicate that these factors have the potential to participate in positive feedback loops in certain circumstances. Although there are insufficient data to indicate in which cases those loops are driven by intracellular intracrine action, it seems that in some cases, such as angiotensin, intracellular action is important. To the extent that intracellular action of intracrines and/or their trafficking in exosomes occurs, external membrane blockers will only be partially effective. The focus in this article is the RAS because of the extensive data available linking it to the pathogenesis of these disorders, but it is likely that other intracrines, TGF-β1, VEGF, and PTHrP, in particular, participate as well.[18] Lastly, the proposed schema provides a basis for the facilitating role of the MR in augmenting disease progression.

There are several implications to this view point. First, optimal suppression of disease activity will require blockade/interruption of intracellular as well as extra-cellular intracrine signaling. The importance of intracellular intracrine action is supported by multiple studies showing that it occurs and by the inability of ACE inhibitors and ARBs to suppress disease in kidney or heart once an initiating factor like hyperglycemia is removed.[4,5,9–12,14–21,23,29,60] Second, because the RAS and other intracrine systems can up-regulate additional self-sustaining intracrine loops, optimal suppression of disease will require blockade/interruption of several intracellular intracrine actions, although given the homeostatic importance of these factors, partial blockade likely is preferable to total blockade.[18] For example, RAS activation can up-regulate TGF-β1 loops, so interruption of TGF-β1 action, at least extracellularly and probably intracellularly, will likely be required along with blockade/interruption of RAS loops. The importance of intracellular blockade is exemplified by the finding that an intracellular inhibitor of TGF-β1, unlike extracellular receptor blocking antibodies, inhibits platelet-derived growth factor-induced collagen synthesis and proliferation in pulmonary artery smooth muscle cells.[60] Third, other systems, such as mineralocorticoids and the MR, can modulate intracrine action and so provide additional therapeutic targets.[4,5,18,21]

At the same time, the proposed intracrines loops need not be exhaustive. For example, the possibility that loops involving angiotensin II up-regulation of p53 and TGF-β1 can result in cardiac myocyte drop out and cardiac fibrosis has been discussed.[4,18,24–27] But it has recently been shown that angiotensin II up-regulation of p53 phosphorylation and nuclear trafficking in cardiac microvascular endothelial cells can result in the production of a positive intracellular loop between p53 and the notch ligand Jagged1. This, in turn, has the somewhat paradoxic effect of down-regulating VEGF and contributing to inadequate angiogenesis during some forms of cardiac hypertrophy—which arguably hastens myocardial contractile dysfunction.[57,61] The point is that the intracrines involved in these various disorders may establish disease-causing networks that are as-yet unappreciated. The author coined the term, intracrine, based on angiotensin II biology and then developed principles of intracrine physiology. Now the complex ways intracrines can participate in disease are coming into focus. Moreover, given the wide tissue distribution of the intracrine factors discussed, the analysis presented, if correct, could point to similar pathobiological etiologies for diverse diseases, such as chronic progressive renal diseases, SHF, diastolic heart failure, primary pulmonary hypertension, and age-related macular degeneration.[4–16,18,21,28,29,34,60–72]

REFERENCES

1. Levey AS, Coresh J. Chronic kidney disease. Lancet 2012;379(9811):165–80.
2. Chatterjee K, Massie B. Systolic and diastolic heart failure: differences and similarities. J Card Fail 2007;13:569–76.

3. Daimee UA, Moss AJ, Biton Y, et al. Long-term outcomes with cardiac resynchronization therapy in patients with mild heart failure with moderate renal dysfunction. Circ Heart Fail 2015;8:725–32.

4. Re RN. A possible mechanism for the progression of chronic renal disease and congestive heart failure. J Am Soc Hypertens 2015;9:54–63.

5. Re RN. A mechanism for mineralocortcoid participation in renal disease and heart failure. J Am Soc Hypertens 2015;9:586–91.

6. Re RN. Could intracrine biology play a role in the pathogenesis of transmissable spongiform encephalopathies, Alzheimer's disease and other neurodegenerative diseases? Am J Med Sci 2014;347:312–20.

7. Re RN. Does intracrine amplification provide a unifying principle for the progression of common neurodegenerative disorders? Hypothesis 2015;13(1):e2.

8. Re RN. A possible mechanism for the propagation of pathological proteins in Parkinson's disease. J Parkinsons Dis Alzheimers Dis 2015;2:1–8.

9. Re RN. The intracrine hypothesis and intracellular peptide hormone action. Bioessays 2003;25:401–9.

10. Re RN, Cook JL. The intracrine hypothesis: an update. Regul Pept 2006;133:1–9.

11. Re RN, Cook JL. Senescence, apoptosis, and stem cell biology: the rationale for an expanded view of intracrine action. Am J Physiol Heart Circ Physiol 2009;297: H893–901.

12. Re RN, Cook JL. The physiological basis of intracrine stem cell regulation. Am J Physiol Heart Circ Physiol 2008;295:H447–53.

13. Re RN. Implications of intracrine hormone action for physiology and medicine. Am J Physiol Heart Circ Physiol 2003;284:H751–7.

14. Re RN, Cook JL. The mitochondrial component of intracrine action. Am J Physiol Heart Circ Physiol 2010;299:H577–83.

15. Re RN, Cook JL. Noncanonical intracrine action. J Am Soc Hypertens 2011;5: 435–48.

16. Re RN. Thirty years of intracrinology. Ochsner J 2014;14:673–80.

17. Re RN. Intrancellular renin and the nature of intracrine enzymes. Hypertension 2003;42:117–22.

18. Re RN. An expanded view of progressive cardiorenal disorders. Am J Med Sci 2016;351(6):626–33.

19. Noguchi H, Kaneto H, Weir GC, et al. PDX-1 protein containing its own antennapedia-like protein transduction domain can transduce pancreatic duct and islet cells. Diabetes 2003;52:1732–7.

20. Lesaffre B, Joliot A, Prochiantz A, et al. Direct non-cell autonomous Pax6 activity regulates eye development in the zebrafish. Neural Dev 2007;17(2):2.

21. Li XC, Zhuo JL. Intracellular ANG II directly induces in vitro transcription of TGF-beta1, MCP-1, and NHE-3 mRNAs in isolated rat renal cortical nuclei via activation of nuclear AT1a receptors. Am J Physiol Cell Physiol 2008;294:C1034–45.

22. Ortega A, Ramila D, Izquierdo A, et al. Role of the renin-angiotensin system on the parathyroid hormone-related protein overexpression induced by nephrotoxic acute renal failure in the rat. J Am Soc Nephrol 2005;16:939–49.

23. Eggena P, Zhu JH, Sereevinyayut S, et al. Hepatic angiotensin II nuclear receptors and transcription of growth-related factors. J Hypertens 1996;14:961–8.

24. Leri A, Claudio PP, Li Q, et al. Stretch-mediated release of angiotensin II induces myocyte apoptosis by activating p53 that enhances the local renin-angiotensin system and decreases the Bcl-2-to-Bax protein ratio in the cell. J Clin Invest 1998;101:1326–42.

25. Pierzchalski P, Reiss K, Cheng W, et al. p53 Induces myocyte apoptosis via the activation of the renin-angiotensin system. Exp Cell Res 1997;234:57–65.

26. Barlucchi L, Leri A, Dostal DE, et al. Canine ventricular myocytes possess a renin-angiotensin system that is upregulated with heart failure. Circ Res 2001;88:298–304.

27. Fiordaliso F, Leri A, Cesselli D, et al. Hyperglycemia activates p53 and p53-regulated genes leading to myocyte cell death. Diabetes 2001;50:2363–75.

28. Kumar R, Yong QC, Thomas CM, et al. Intracardiac intracellular angiotensin system in diabetes. Am J Physiol Regul Integr Comp Physiol 2012;302:R510–7.

29. Zhuo JL, Kobori H, Li XC, et al. Augmentation of angiotensinogen expression in the proximal tubule by intracellular angiotensin II via AT1a/MAPK/NF-κB signaling pathways. Am J Physiol Renal Physiol 2016;310(10):F1103–12.

30. Ferrario CM, Ahmad S, Nagata S, et al. An evolving story of angiotensin-II-forming pathways in rodents and humans. Clin Sci (Lond) 2014;126:461–9.

31. Czopek A, Moorhouse R, Webb DJ, et al. The therapeutic potential of endothelin receptor antagonism in kidney disease. Am J Physiol Regul Integr Comp Physiol 2016;310(5):R388–97.

32. Van Obberghen-Schilling E, Roche NS, Flanders KC, et al. Transforming growth factor beta 1 positively regulates its own expression in normal and transformed cells. J Biol Chem 1988;263:7741–6.

33. Pateder DB, Ferguson CM, Ionescu AM, et al. PTHrP expression in chick sternal chondrocytes is regulated by TGF-beta through Smad-mediated signaling. J Cell Physiol 2001;188:343–51.

34. Re RN, Bryan SE. Functional intracellular renin- angiotensin systems may exist in multiple tissues. Clin Exper Hypertens A 1984;A6(10&11):1739–42.

35. Re RN, Cook JL. An intracrine view of angiogenesis. Bioessays 2006;28:943–53.

36. Epstein M. Mineralocorticoid receptor antagonists: part of an emerging treatment paradigm for chronic kidney disease. Lancet Diabetes Endocrinol 2014;2:925–7.

37. Siragy HM, Xue C. Local renal aldosterone production induces inflammation and matrix formation in kidneys of diabetic rats. Exp Physiol 2008;93:817–24.

38. Xue C, Siragy HM. Local renal aldosterone system and its regulation by salt, diabetes, and angiotensin II type 1 receptor. Hypertension 2005;46:584–90.

39. Harada E, Yoshimura M, Yasue H, et al. Aldosterone induces angiotensin-converting-enzyme gene expression in cultured neonatal rat cardiocytes. Circulation 2001;104:137–9.

40. Sugiyama T, Yoshimoto T, Tsuchiya K, et al. Aldosterone induces angiotensin converting enzyme gene expression via a JAK2-dependent pathway in rat endothelial cells. Endocrinology 2005;146:3900–6.

41. Klar J, Vitzthum H, Kurtz A. Aldosterone enhances renin gene expression in juxtaglomerular cells. Am J Physiol Renal Physiol 2004;286:F349–55.

42. Itaya Y, Suzuki H, Matsukawa S, et al. Central renin-angiotensin system and the pathogenesis of DOCA-salt hypertension in rats. Am J Physiol 1986;251(2 Pt 2):H261–8.

43. Kubo T, Yamaguchi H, Tsujimura M, et al. Blockade of angiotensin receptors in the anterior hypothalamic preoptic area lowers blood pressure in DOCA-salt hypertensive rats. Hypertens Res 2000;23:109–18.

44. Gutkind JS, Kurihara M, Saavedra JM. Increased angiotensin II receptors in brain nuclei of DOCA-salt hypertensive rats. Am J Physiol 1988;255(3 Pt 2):H646–50.

45. Yu Y, Wei SG, Zhang ZH, et al. Does aldosterone upregulate the brain renin-angiotensin system in rats with heart failure? Hypertension 2008;51:727–33.

46. Hirono Y, Yoshimoto T, Suzuki N, et al. Angiotensin II receptor type 1-mediated vascular oxidative stress and proinflammatory gene expression in

aldosterone-induced hypertension: the possible role of local renin-angiotensin system. Endocrinology 2007;148:1688–96.

47. Funder JW. Eplerenone: hypertension, heart failure and the importance of mineralocorticoid receptor blockade. Future Cardiol 2006;2:535–41.

48. Funder JW. Mineralocorticoid receptors: distribution and activation. Heart Fail Rev 2005;10:15–22.

49. Mihailidou AS, Loan Le TY, Mardini M, et al. Glucocorticoids activate cardiac mineralocorticoid receptors during experimental myocardial infarction. Hypertension 2009;54:1306–12.

50. Yoshida M, Ma J, Tomita T, et al. Mineralocorticoid receptor is overexpressed in cardiomyocytes of patients with congestive heart failure. Congest Heart Fail 2005;11:12–6.

51. Tsai CF, Yang SF, Chu HJ, et al. Cross-talk between mineralocorticoid receptor/angiotensin II type 1 receptor and mitogen-activated protein kinase pathways underlies aldosterone-induced atrial fibrotic responses in HL-1 cardiomyocytes. Int J Cardiol 2013;169:17–28.

52. Jaffe IZ, Mendelsohn ME. Angiotensin II and aldosterone regulate gene transcription via functional mineralocortoicoid receptors in human coronary artery smooth muscle cells. Circ Res 2005;96:643–50.

53. Rautureau Y, Paradis P, Schiffrin EL. Cross-talk between aldosterone and angiotensin signaling in vascular smooth muscle cells. Steroids 2011;76:834–9.

54. Schiffrin EL. New twist to the role of the renin-angiotensin system in heart failure: aldosterone upregulates renin-angiotensin system components in the brain. Hypertension 2008;51:622–3.

55. Ayuzawa N, Nagase M, Ueda K, et al. Rac1-mediated activation of mineralocorticoid receptor in pressure overload-induced cardiac injury. Hypertension 2016;67:99–106.

56. Kosugi T, Sato W. Midkine and the kidney: health and diseases. Nephrol Dial Transplant 2012;27:16–21.

57. Zhang X, Lassila M, Cooper ME, et al. Retinal expression of vascular endothelial growth factor is mediated by angiotensin type 1 and type 2 receptors. Hypertension 2004;43:276–81.

58. Rossi GP, Sacchetto A, Cesari M, et al. Interactions between endothelin-1 and the renin-angiotensin-aldosterone system. Cardiovasc Res 1999;43(2):300–7.

59. Kohan DE. Endothelin, hypertension and chronic kidney disease: new insights. Curr Opin Nephrol Hypertens 2010;19:134–9.

60. Abeyrathna P, Kovacs L, Han W, et al. Calpain-2 activates Akt via TGFβ1-mTORC2 pathway in pulmonary artery smooth muscle cells. Am J Physiol Cell Physiol 2016;311(1):C24–34.

61. Guan A, Gong H, Ye Y, et al. Regulation of p53 by jagged1 contributes to angiotensin II-induced impairment of myocardial angiogenesis. PLoS One 2013 Oct 3; 8(10):e76529.

62. White AJ, Cheruvu SC, Sarris M, et al. Expression of classical components of the renin-angiotensin system in the human eye. J Renin Angiotensin Aldosterone Syst 2015;16(1):59–66.

63. Gao G, Li Y, Zhang D, et al. Unbalanced expression of VEGF and PEDF in ischemia-induced retinal neovascularization. FEBS Lett 2001;489(2–3):270–6.

64. Iosef C, Gkourasas T, Jia CY, et al. A functional nuclear localization signal in insulin-like growth factor binding protein-6 mediates its nuclear import. Endocrinology 2008;149:1214–26.

65. Zheng J, Wei CC, Hase N, et al. Chymase mediates injury and mitochondrial damage in cardiomyocytes during acute ischemia/reperfusion in the dog. PLoS One 2014;9(4):e94732.
66. Planque N. Nuclear trafficking of secreted factors and cell-surface receptors: new pathways to regulate cell proliferation and differentiation, and involvement in cancers. Cell Commun Signal 2006;4:7.
67. Gressner OA. Intracrine signaling mechanisms of activin A and TGF-β. Vitam Horm 2011;85:59–77.
68. Klaassen I, van Geest RJ, Kuiper EJ, et al. The role of CTGF in diabetic retinopathy. Exp Eye Res 2015;133:37–48.
69. Dai H, Zhang Y, Yuan L, et al. CTGF mediates high-glucose induced epithelial-mesenchymal transition through activation of β-catenin in podocytes. Ren Fail 2016;16:1–6.
70. Pi L, Chung PY, Sriram S, et al. Connective tissue growth factor differentially binds to members of the cystine knot superfamily and potentiates platelet-derived growth factor-B signaling in rabbit corneal fibroblast cells. World J Biol Chem 2015;6(4):379–88.
71. Duquette M, Nadler M, Okuhara D, et al. Members of the thrombospondin gene family bind stromal interaction molecule 1 and regulate calcium channel activity. Matrix Biol 2014;37:15–24.
72. Lynch JM, Maillet M, Vanhoutte D, et al. A thrombospondin-dependent pathway for a protective ER stress response. Cell 2012;149:1257–68.

Local Renin Angiotensin Aldosterone Systems and Cardiovascular Diseases

 CrossMark

Walmor C. De Mello, MD, PhD

KEYWORDS

• Local renin angiotensin • Expression • Internalization • Cardiovascular diseases

KEY POINTS

• The presence of local renin angiotensin aldosterone systems (RAAS) in the cardiovascular and renal tissues and their influence in cardiovascular and renal diseases are described.
• The fundamental role of ACE/Ang II/AT1 receptor axis activation as well the counter regulatory role of ACE2/Ang (1–7)/Mas receptor activation on cardiovascular and renal physiology and pathology are emphasized.
• Special emphasis is given to the influence of the intracrine components of the RAAS, including Ang II and renin, on the regulation of cell communication, the incidence of cardiac arrhythmias, and remodeling.
• Recent findings showing the role of intracellular Ang II on membrane potential and tone of vascular resistance vessels, in opposite to that seen with extracellular Ang II and their implications for vascular remodeling and hypertension are described.
• The presence of a local renin angiotensin system and its influence on hypertension is discussed and, finally, the hypothesis that epigenetic factors change the RAAS in utero and induce the expression of renin or Ang II inside the cells of the cardiovascular system is presented.

ON THE ROLE OF CONVENTIONAL RENIN ANGIOTENSIN ALDOSTERONE SYSTEMS

The activation of the conventional renin angiotensin aldosterone system (RAAS) plays a seminal role on the physiologic regulation of blood volume and blood pressure and it is involved on the regulation of cardiac and renal functions. Renin released from the kidney converts angiotensinogen from the liver to the decapeptide angiotensin-I, which undergoes proteolytic cleavage generating angiotensin-II (Ang II) through the activation of angiotensin-converting enzyme (ACE) (**Fig 1**). During hypertension, heart failure, and myocardial ischemia, the permanent activation of RAAS is involved in cardiac and vascular remodeling, including left ventricular hypertrophy and fibrosis.

The beneficial effects of ACE inhibitors and Ang II–type 1 receptor blockers (ARBs) in hypertensive patients and the improvement of cardiac function and remodeling in

Department of Pharmacology, School of Medicine, Medical Sciences Campus, UPR, San Juan, PR 00936, USA
E-mail address: walmor.de-mello@upr.edu

Med Clin N Am 101 (2017) 117–127
http://dx.doi.org/10.1016/j.mcna.2016.08.017
0025-7125/17/© 2016 Elsevier Inc. All rights reserved.

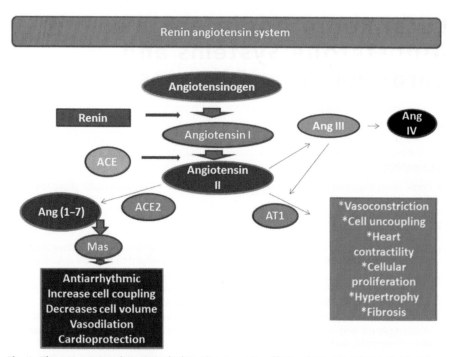

Fig. 1. The conventional RAAS including the opposite effects of Ang II and Ang (1–7) on cardiovascular pathophysiology. Furthermore, the new peptides angiotensin III (Ang III) and angiotensin IV (Ang IV) with its respective receptor (AT4) were represented.

patients with heart failure, is an indisputable evidence of the harmful effect of Ang II.[1–5] Large clinical trials like the Survival and Ventricular Enlargement (SAVE) Trial and the Veterans Administration Cooperative Study Treatment Group revealed the beneficial role of ACE inhibitors in patients with myocardial infarction as well as during hypertension.[1–8] Ang II type 1 receptor blockers also reduce the incidence of interstitial fibrosis by decreasing collagen I gene expression, which is an important factor in the etiology of left ventricular hypertrophy and diastolic dysfunction.[9]

Recent developments indicate that the classic ACE/Ang II/AT1 receptor axis is not the only signal pathway involved in the activation of RAAS, but other pathways like the ACE2/Ang (1–7)/Mas receptor axis play a fundamental role counteracting many effects of Ang II in the cardiovascular and renal systems. ACE2, an enzyme having a high homology to ACE, is able to hydrolyze Ang II to the peptide angiotensin (1–7) (Ang [1–7]),[10,11] which counteracts many effects of Ang II, including its pressor effect as well as to the proliferative and profibrotic effects of peptide.[12–17] Ang (1–7) also reduces the incidence of heart failure after myocardial infarct in rats, and in humans it increases the coronary perfusion and aortic endothelial function[18] with beneficial effect for patients with coronary insufficiency and hypertension. The electrical remodeling is also reduced by Ang (1–7) with consequent increase of the conduction velocity in the failing heart, thereby reducing the incidence of cardiac arrhythmias.[15,16]

More recently, it was found that the activation of the ACE2-Ang (1–7)-Mas receptor axis is involved in the regulation of heart cell volume.[19] The heptapeptide, for instance, decreases the cell volume and the swelling-activated chloride current (ICl$_{swell}$), an effect inhibited by ouabain what supports the view that Ang (1–7) activates the sodium pump. The reduction of cell volume induced by Ang (1–7), might be of benefit for patients with myocardial ischemia by reducing the cell swelling and decreasing the activation of ionic channels, like the potassium channel, which are responsible for alteration of cardiac excitability.[19] Although compelling evidence has been presented that ACE2 activation counteracts the effects of Ang II in cardiac and vascular muscle in animal models, its role in humans is still unclear. The overexpression of ACE2 in the failing heart, for instance, does not prevent the progress of the disease and in some animal transgenic models, overexpression of ACE2 did not influence hypertension. Studies of Rentzsch and colleagues,[20] however, using transgenic rats expressing the human ACE2 in vascular smooth muscle cells, indicated that elevated circulating levels of Ang (1–7) was associated with a 15 mm Hg decrease in mean arterial blood pressure and reduced response to Ang II.[20] These data suggest that vascular ACE2 overexpression or Ang (1–7) administration may represent novel therapeutic strategies in the treatment of hypertension and other cardiovascular diseases.

LOCAL RENIN ANGIOTENSIN ALDOSTERONE SYSTEMS AND THE INTRACRINE COMPONENT

Experimental evidence supporting the notion that local RAAS are present in different organs including the heart and kidney,[21] opened a new window in our understanding of how the RAAS contributes to local regulation of tissue and organ function. Indeed, the synthesis of several components of the RAAS in the heart[22] or their uptake from plasma,[23] makes possible the synthesis of Ang II locally. In the normal heart of pigs, as much as 75% of cardiac Ang II is synthesized locally,[24] whereas in humans the gradients of Ang II across the heart were increased in patients with congestive heart failure.[25] Not only local synthesis but rapid internalization of the Ang II-AT1 receptor complex, contributes significantly to the intracellular levels of the peptide in heart and other tissues.

To define the role of local renin angiotensin system (RAS) in cardiovascular function, transgenic animal models were generated. In some of these studies mainly related to the influence of the local system on cardiac remodeling, contradictory results were found. Because no ventricular hypertrophy or fibrosis[26] were seen, the conclusion was that cardiac remodeling is much more dependent on hemodynamic changes than on local Ang II levels. In hypertensive transgenic mice lacking the synthesis of angiotensinogen, for instance, the presence of local components of the RAS were not essential for the development of cardiac remodeling. However, in transgenic mouse lines overexpressing angiotensinogen in the heart, Ang II was increased in the cardiac muscle but not in plasma, ventricular hypertrophy was found and no change in blood pressure was seen.[27] Furthermore, the hypertrophy generated in this model, was abolished by ACE inhibitors or AT1 blockers[27] supporting the notion that a local cardiac RAs was activated. Experimental studies using low doses of aliskiren in hypertensive TGR(mRen2)27 rats, revealed a decrease in structural and electrical cardiac remodeling that was independent of blood pressure,[28] supporting the view that the renin inhibitor has a direct effect on the heart. Part of the discrepant results found in these studies is probably related to the different species used, different experimental conditions, or to the complexity of the genome.

Concerning the origin of cardiac renin in the normal heart, there is evidence that its uptake from plasma[23,24] is a major source of the enzyme, but renin expression, which was enhanced after myocardial infarction,[29,30] also has been described. A renin transcript that does not encode a secretory signal and remains inside the cell, is overexpressed during myocardial infarction,[29,30] indicating that intracellular renin has functional properties. Studies of Peters and colleagues[29,30] showed that the cytosolic renin protein exerts functions different and opposite to those of secretory renin, which increases necrotic death rates of cardiac cells while the cytosolic renin isoform protects cells from necrotic death. Evidence has been presented that the different components of the RAAS, including the peptides and receptors, are present in mitochondria or the nucleus. In the mitochondria, Ang II binds to mtAT2Rs and stimulates NO formation through mitochondrial nitric oxide synthase, suppressing mitochondrial oxygen consumption. On the other hand, nuclear Ang II can stimulate NO formation (via AT2Rs) or Ca2+ and phosphoinositol 3 kinase (PI3K) (via AT1Rs).[31]

The conceptualization of a local RAAS with its intracrine component requires the demonstration that the components of RAAS have functional properties. The functionality of intracellular renin was indeed demonstrated when renin was dialyzed into cardiac myocytes from the failing heart. In these studies, a decrease of cell communication and an increase of the inward calcium current[32,33] were found after the intracellular administration of renin or Ang II. The decrease of gap junction conductance leads to a decrease of electrical coupling and mechanical desynchronization, as well as the generation of slow conduction and cardiac arrhythmias.[34,35] More recent studies performed on the intact ventricle of normal rats, revealed that intracellular renin causes a depolarization of ventricular fibers and a decrease of the cardiac refractoriness with consequent generation of triggered activity.[32] The intimate mechanism by which intracellular renin alters cardiac excitability is related to the change of potassium current but the involvement of the intracellular renin receptor,[32,36] which when activated by renin and promotes the translocation of a transcription factor (PLZF) to the nucleus with consequent expression of several genes, cannot be discarded.[37] The intracellular localization of this receptor[37] was confirmed using different constructs and studies of mutagenesis and colocalization and experiments performed on PLZF knockout mice.[36]

Recent observations revealed that intracellular renin disrupts the exchange of chemical signals between heart cells, including the cell-to-cell diffusion of glucose.[38] Aldosterone also disrupts the process of chemical coupling between cardiac myocytes and contributes to inhibition of metabolic cooperation and heart disease.[39] The inhibition of cell-to-cell diffusion of glucose[39] elicited by aldosterone might contribute to the impairment of heart function in diabetic patients.

Previous observations revealed that the mineralocorticoid receptor (MR) activation induced by aldosterone influences the intracellular and extracellular effects of Ang II on cell volume regulation in the heart and that the cell swelling elicited by extracellular Ang II was enhanced by aldosterone, an effect inhibited by spironolactone.[40] The significant decrease in cell swelling caused by Ang II in the presence of spironolactone might indicate that the activation of stretch ionic receptors including the K(v)4.2/4.3 channels and the ICl_{swell} results in a decline in the incidence of cardiac arrhythmias (**Fig. 2**).

LOCAL RENIN ANGIOTENSIN ALDOSTERONE SYSTEMS AND THE VASCULAR SMOOTH MUSCLE PATHOPHYSIOLOGY

Some evidence is available that angiotensinogen, ACE, Ang I, and Ang II are synthesized within the vascular muscle cells and previous observations revealed the presence of renin in cultured vascular muscle,[41,42] indicating that the enzyme is expressed in these cells. The origin of vascular renin, in vivo, might be related to local production or be related to its uptake from the circulation, possibly by the (pro)renin receptor ([P]RR), which is known to play an important role in the etiology of vascular

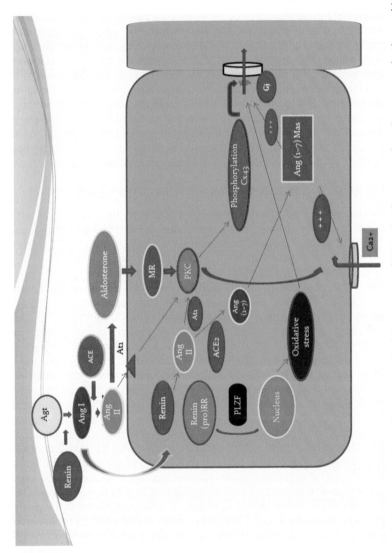

Fig. 2. Diagram shows the intracrine actions of renin, Ang II, aldosterone, and MR activation on gap junction communication and inward calcium current in cardiac muscle.

complications during hypertension and diabetes.[43,44] Although the ablation of the (P) RR in murine smooth muscle cells resulted in sclerosis in the abdominal aorta and impaired the cell recycling system, and leads to autophagic cell death,[44] the possible role of (pro)renin in cardiovascular diseases has not being supported by several experimental studies in animals.[43]

Recent findings showed that the intracellular administration of Ang II to arterial myocytes isolated from mesenteric arteries of Sprague Dawley rats increased the total potassium current and the resting potential, whereas extracellular administration of Ang II reduced the total potassium current and depolarized the smooth muscle cells.[45] These effects of intracellular Ang II were inhibited by dialyzing a protein kinase inhibitor inhibitor inside the cell together with Ang II.[45,46] Because the membrane potential of arterial myocytes is a determinant factor in the regulation of vascular tone,[47,48] the implication of these results for the regulation of vessel diameter and peripheral resistance is obvious and leads to the conclusion that endogenous or internalized Ang II in vascular resistance vessels counteracts the effect of extracellular Ang II and plays an important role on the regulation of vascular tone and peripheral resistance.[45] These findings have important implications to vascular pathology, particularly during hypertension and other vascular diseases associated with vascular remodeling.

LOCAL RENIN ANGIOTENSIN ALDOSTERONE SYSTEMS IN THE KIDNEY

All major components of the RAS are expressed or present in the kidney, and evidence is available that the levels of Ang II in the renal tissue are much higher than those in plasma.[49,51] The question, however, persists whether AGT, ACE, and AT1 receptors in the kidney contribute to blood pressure regulation and the development of hypertension.[52,53] Classically, the circulating RAS rather than the intrarenal RAS plays an essential role in the regulation of arterial blood pressure as well as during hypertension. Some studies, however, raised the possibility that tissue-bound ACE, rather than circulating ACE, is important for the regulation of blood pressure.[52] Evidence has been presented that there is an intrarenal RAS and that in renal tubuli Ang II stimulates the AT1 receptor increasing the activity of transport mechanisms involved in the reabsorption of sodium.[49–53] Ang (1–7), on the other hand, evokes natriuretic and diuretic effects and causes NO release.[54] Other studies showed that incubation of proximal tubular fluid with excess renin elicited the formation of Ang I, supporting the view that angiotensinogen was available as s substrate[55] and that when proximal tubular fluid was incubated with excess renin, the resultant formation of Ang I indicated the availability of angiotensinogen in this segment. Furthermore, tubular fluid collected from downstream segments of perfused tubules also had Ang II concentrations similar to those in nonperfused tubules, thus supporting a local origin.

Changes in levels of angiotensinogen in renal tissues may promote the activation of local RAS through mechanisms that are independent of angiotensinogen levels in the circulation. For example, in the kidney, synthesis of angiotensinogen in the proximal tubule may be augmented by Ang II[55] as part of a local, intrarenal RAS that is regulated independently of the systemic RAS. These findings, along with the demonstration that proximal tubule cells express angiotensinogen mRNA and protein in proximal tubular cells, indicate the presence of a local renal RAS.[50]

EPIGENETIC CHANGES OF THE RENIN ANGIOTENSIN ALDOSTERONE SYSTEMS AND CARDIOVASCULAR DISEASES

Epigenetic mechanisms including DNA methylation, histone modification, and microRNA alterations are involved in the cell response to environmental changes. It is

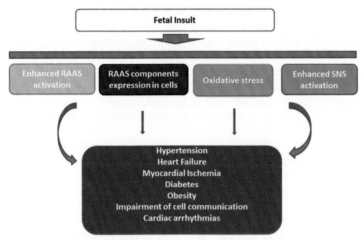

Fig. 3. The possible influence of epigenetic factors on fetal development abnormalities and the consequent generation of cardiovascular diseases later on in life. SNS, sympathetic nervous system. (*Adapted from* Alexander BT, Dasinger JH, Intapad S. Fetal programming and cardiovascular pathology. Compr Physiol 2015;5(2):997–1025.)

known, for instance, that stress during pregnancy is a cause of cardiovascular diseases, including hypertension in the newborn.[56] It is also evident that noncoding RNAs, as well chromatin-remodeling enzymes, play an important role in cardiac development and function.[57,58] According to some of these studies, the fetus would adapt for survival during gestation and a redistribution of blood flow occurs resulting in a preservation of brain circulation at the expense of other organs. In this process of fetal adaptation, changes in structure and physiology provide the explanation for higher risk for hypertension and heart diseases, including heart failure,[57] later on in life. According to Barker and Osmond,[58] cardiovascular disease has its origin in fetal life, and infant mortality during a certain period of time resembles that of death from ischemic heart disease approximately 60 years later. Other studies correlating the influence of birth weight on antihypertensive treatment showed that birth weight was associated with greater use of calcium channel blockers in black women or ACE inhibitors in men.[59–62]

Recently, we presented the hypothesis that the expression of RAAS components in the heart and vascular smooth muscle might be induced by epigenetic factors activated during pregnancy.[46] According to this hypothesis, epigenetic factors, as well as hyperglycemia, aldosterone, heart failure, or ischemia, lead to the expression of renin and Ang II inside the cardiac and vascular smooth muscle cells with consequent decrease of cell communication, impairment of metabolic cooperation, and changes in vascular smooth muscle contractility and dysfunction (**Fig 3**).

ACKNOWLEDGMENTS

This article is dedicated to Edward Frohlich for his outstanding contribution to hypertension research.

REFERENCES

1. Pfeffer MA, Pfeffer JM, Frohlich ED. Pumping ability of the hypertrophying left ventricle of the spontaneously hypertensive rat. Circ Res 1976;38:423–9.

2. Pfeffer MA, Pfeffer JM, Braunwald E. Influence of chronic captopril therapy on the infracted left ventricle of the rat. Circ Res 1985;57:84–95.

3. Pfeffer JM, Pfeffer MA, Mirsky I, et al. Regression of left ventricular hypertrophy and prevention of left ventricular dysfunction by captopril in the spontaneously hypertensive rat. Proc Natl Acad Sci U S A 1982;79:3310–4.

4. Pfeffer MA, Braunwald E, Moye LA, et al. Effect of captopril on mortality and morbidity in patients with left ventricular dysfunction after myocardial infarction. Results of the Survival and Ventricular Enlargement Trial. N Engl J Med 1992; 327:669–77.

5. Pfeffer MA, Frohlich ED. Improvements in clinical outcomes with the use of angiotensin converting enzyme inhibitors. Cross-fertilization between clinical investigations. Am J Physiol Heart Circ Physiol 2006;291:H2021–5.

6. Veterans Administration Cooperative Study Group on Antihypertensive Agents. Effects of treatment on morbidity in hypertension. Results in patients with diastolic blood pressure averaging 115 through 129 mm Hg. JAMA 1967;202:1028–34.

7. Veterans Administration Cooperative Study Group on Antihypertensive Agents. Effects of treatment on morbidity in hypertension. II. Results in patients with diastolic blood pressure averaging 90 through 114 mm Hg. JAMA 1970;213: 1143–52.

8. Frohlich ED. Risk mechanisms in hypertensive heart disease. Hypertension 1999; 34:782–9.

9. Jin Y, Han HC, Lindsey ML. ACE inhibitors to block MMP-9 activity: new functions for old inhibitors. J Mol Cell Cardiol 2007;43(6):664–6.

10. Donoghue M, Hsieh F, Baronas E, et al. Novel angiotensin converting enzyme related carboxypeptidase (ACE2) converts angiotensin I to angiotensin (1-9). Circ Res 2000;87:E1–9.

11. Tipnis SR, Hooper NM, Hyde R, et al. A human homolog of angiotensin converting enzyme. Cloning and functional expression as a captopril insensitive carboxypeptidase. J Biol Chem 2000;275:33238–43.

12. Ferrario CM, Chappell MC, Tallant EA, et al. Counterregulatory actions of angiotensin (1-7). Hypertension 1997;30:535–41.

13. Crackower MA, Sarao R, Oudit GY, et al. Angiotensin-converting enzyme 2 is an essential regulator of heart function. Nature 2002;417(6891):822–8.

14. Ferrario CM, Trask AJ, Jessup JA. Advances in biochemical and functional roles of angiotensin-converting enzyme 2 and angiotensin-(1-7) in regulation of cardiovascular function. Am J Physiol Heart Circ Physiol 2005;289:H2281–90.

15. De Mello WC, Ferrario CM, Jessup JA. Beneficial versus harmful effects of Angiotensin (1-7) on impulse propagation and cardiac arrhythmias in the failing heart. J Renin Angiotensin Aldosterone Syst 2007;8:74–80.

16. De Mello WC. Angiotensin (1–7) re-establishes impulse conduction in cardiac muscle during ischaemia-reperfusion. The role of the sodium pump. J Renin Angiotensin Aldosterone Syst 2004;5(4):203–8.

17. Zisman LS, Keller RS, Weaver B, et al. Increased angiotensin (1-7) forming activity in failing human heart ventricles: evidence for upregulation of the angiotensin converting enzyme homolog, ACE2. Circulation 2003;108:1707–12.

18. Santos RA, Ferreira AJ, Simões E. Recent advances in the angiotensin-converting enzyme 2-angiotensin (1-7)-Mas axis. Exp Physiol 2008;93(5):519–27.

19. De Mello WC. Cell swelling, impulse conduction, and cardiac arrhythmias in the failing heart. Opposite effects of angiotensin II and angiotensin (1-7) on cell volume regulation. Mol Cell Biochem 2009;330(1–2):211–7.

20. Rentzsch B, Todiras M, Iliescu R, et al. Transgenic angiotensin-converting enzyme 2 overexpression in vessels of SHRSP rats reduces blood pressure and improves endothelial function. Hypertension 2008;52(5):967–73.
21. De Mello WC, Frohlich ED. On the local cardiac renin angiotensin system. Basic and clinical implications. Peptides 2011;32:1774–9.
22. Kurdi M, De Mello WC, Booz GW. Working outside the system: an update on the unconventional behavior of the renin-angiotensin system components. Int J Biochem Cell Biol 2005;37:1357–67.
23. Danser AH, van Kats JP, Admiraal PJ, et al. Cardiac renin and angiotensins; uptake from plasma versus in situ synthesis. Hypertension 1994;24:37–48.
24. de Lannoy LM, Danser AH, Bouhuizen AM, et al. Localization and production of angiotensin II in the isolated perfused rat heart. Hypertension 1998;31:1111–7.
25. Serneri GG, Boddi M, Cecione I, et al. Cardiac angiotensin II formation in the clinical course of heart failure and its relationship with left ventricular function. Circ Res 2001;88:961–8.
26. Reudelhuber TL, Bernstein KE, Delafontaine P. Is angiotensin II a direct mediator of left ventricular hypertrophy? Hypertension 2007;49:1196–201.
27. Mazzolai L, Nussberger J, Aubert JF, et al. Blood pressure-independent cardiac hypertrophy induced by locally activated renin angiotensin system. Hypertension 1998;31:1324–30.
28. De Mello W, Rivera M, Rabell A, et al. Aliskiren, at low doses, reduces the electrical remodeling in the heart of the TGR (mRen2)27 rat independently of blood pressure. J Renin Angiotensin Aldosterone Syst 2013;14(1):23–33.
29. Clausmeyer S, Reinecke A, Farrenkopf R, et al. Tissue-specific expression of a rat renin transcript lacking the coding sequence for the prefragment and its stimulation by myocardial infarction. Endocrinology 2000;141(8):2963–70.
30. Peters J. Cytosolic (pro) renin and the matter of intracellular renin actions. Front Biosci (Schol Ed) 2013;5:198–205.
31. Abadir PM, Walston JD, Carey RM. Subcellular characteristics of functional intracellular renin-angiotensin systems. Peptides 2012;38(2):437–45.
32. De Mello WC. Intracellular renin alters the electrical properties of the intact heart ventricle of adult Sprague Dawley rats. Regul Pept 2013;181:45–9.
33. De Mello WC, Danser AHJ. Angiotensin II and the heart: on the intracrine renin-angiotensin system. Hypertension 2000;35(6):1183–8.
34. De Mello WC. Cardiac arrhythmias: the possible role of the renin-angiotensin system. J Mol Med (Berl) 2001;79(2–3):103–8.
35. De Mello WC. Is an intracellular renin-angiotensin system involved in control of cell communication in heart? J Cardiovasc Pharmacol 1994;23(4):640–6.
36. Shefe JH, Menk M, Reinemund J, et al. A novel signal transduction cascade involving direct physical interaction of the renin/prorenin receptor with the transcription factor promyelocytic zinc finger protein. Circ Res 2006;99:1355–66.
37. De Mello WC. On the pathophysiological implications of an intracellular renin receptor. Circ Res 2006;99:1285–6.
38. De Mello WC. Chemical communication between heart cells is disrupted by intracellular renin and angiotensin II: implications for heart development and disease. Front Endocrinol (Lausanne) 2015;6:72.
39. De Mello WC. Aldosterone disrupts the intercellular flow of glucose in cardiac muscle. Front Endocrinol (Lausanne) 2015;6:185.
40. De Mello WC, Gerena Y. Further studies on the effects of intracrine and extracellular angiotensin II on the regulation of heart cell volume. On the influence of aldosterone and spironolactone. Regul Pept 2010;165:200–5.

41. Dzau VJ. Vascular renin-angiotensin: a possible autocrine or paracrine system in control of vascular function. J Cardiovasc Pharmacol 1984;6(Suppl 2): S377–82.
42. Inagami T, Mizuno K, Nakamuro M, et al. The renin angiotensin system: an overview of its intracellular action. Cardiovasc Drugs Ther 1988;2:453–6.
43. Nguyen G, Muller DN. The biology of the (pro)renin receptor. J Am Soc Nephrol 2010;21(1):18–23.
44. Kurauchi-Mito A, Ichihara A, Bokuda K, et al. Significant roles of the (pro)renin receptor in integrity of vascular smooth muscle cells. Hypertens Res 2014;37(9): 830–5.
45. De Mello WC. Intracellular angiotensin II increases the total potassium current and the resting potential of arterial myocytes from vascular resistance vessels of the rat. Physiological and pathological implications. J Am Soc Hypertens 2013;7(3):192–7.
46. De Mello WC. Intracellular angiotensin II as a regulator of muscle tone in vascular resistance vessels. Pathophysiological implications. Peptides 2016;78:87–90.
47. Nelson MT, Quayle JM. Physiological roles and properties of potassium channels in arterial smooth muscle. Am J Physiol 1995;268:C799–822.
48. Gelband CH, Hume JR. [CaP]1 inhibition of K+ channels in canine renal artery. Novel mechanism for agonist induced membrane depolarization. Circ Res 1995;77:121–30.
49. Navar LG, Kobori H, Prieto MC, et al. Intrarenal renin-angiotensin system in hypertension. Hypertension 2011;57:355–62.
50. Kobori H, Nangaku M, Navar LG, et al. The intrarenal renin-angiotensin system: from physiology to the pathobiology of hypertension and kidney disease. Pharmacol Rev 2007;59(3):251–87.
51. Lu X, Roksnoer LC, Danser AH. The intrarenal renin-angiotensin system: does it exist? Implications from a recent study in renal angiotensin-converting enzyme knockout mice. Nephrol Dial Transplant 2013;28(12):2977–82.
52. Crowley SD, Gurley SB, Herrera MJ, et al. Angiotensin II causes hypertension and cardiac hypertrophy through its receptors in the kidney. Proc Natl Acad Sci U S A 2006;103(47):17985–90.
53. Gonzalez-Villalobos RA, Janjoulia T, Fletcher NK, et al. The absence of intrarenal ACE protects against hypertension. J Clin Invest 2013;123(5):2011–23.
54. Chappell MC. Non classical renin-angiotensin system and renal function. Compr Physiol 2012;2(4):2733–52.
55. Kobori H, Harrison-Bernard LM, Navar LG. Expression of angiotensinogen mRNA and protein in angiotensin II-dependent hypertension. J Am Soc Nephrol 2001; 12:431–9.
56. Bogdarina I, Welham S, King PJ, et al. Epigenetic modification of the renin angiotensin system to the fetal programming of hypertension. Circ Res 2007; 100:520.
57. Nührenberg T, Gilsbach R, Preissl S, et al. Epigenetics in cardiac development, function, and disease. Cell Tissue Res 2014;356(3):585–600.
58. Barker DJ, Osmond C. Infant mortality, childhood nutrition, and ischemic heart disease in England and Wales. Lancet 1986;1:1077–81.
59. Lackland DT, Egan BM, Syddall HE, et al. Associations between birth weight and antihypertensive medication in black and white Medicaid recipients. Hypertension 2002;39:179–83.
60. Alexander BT, Dasinger JH, Intapad S. Fetal programming and cardiovascular pathology. Compr Physiol 2015;5(2):997–1025.

61. Alexander MR, Owens GK. Owens epigenetic control of smooth muscle cell differentiation and phenotypic switching in vascular development and disease. Annu Rev Physiol 2012;74:13–40.

62. Cook JL, Re RN. Lessons from in vitro studies and a related intracellular angiotensin II transgenic mouse model. Am J Physiol Regul Integr Comp Physiol 2012;302:R482–93.

The Renin Angiotensin Aldosterone System in Obesity and Hypertension

Roles in the Cardiorenal Metabolic Syndrome

Peminda K. Cabandugama, MD[a], Michael J. Gardner, MD[a],
James R. Sowers, MD[a,b,c],*

KEYWORDS

• Obesity • Insulin resistance • Angiotensin II • Adipocyte • Hypertension

KEY POINTS

- The seminal role of hypertension in the pathogenesis of the cardiorenal metabolic syndrome (CRS) has significantly evolved over the past 5 years. The physiology of this is rooted in the concept that hypertension in the setting of obesity and CRS is partly due to the excess body mass leading to an expanded plasma volume, resulting in an increase in cardiac output.
- Impaired handling of sodium is another of the more salient features common to both hypertension and CRS. A review of the literature, which portrays that in states of insulin resistance such as with obesity, an activated systemic renin angiotensin aldosterone system (RAAS) appears to play an important role in the pathogenesis of hypertension and other components of CRS.
- Evidence shows the benefits of RAAS blockade in correcting many of the maladaptive aspects of the CRS, especially in patients with insulin resistance and obesity.
- Currently, there are inadequate guidelines for the optimal pharmacologic management of hypertension in patients with obesity and CRS and the inherent need for them be more clearly delineated.

Funding: The research of the authors is supported by funding from the National Institutes of Health (R01-HL73101 and R01-HL107910 to J.R. Sowers) and the Department of Veterans Affairs Biomedical Laboratory Research and Development Merit (0018 to J.R. Sowers).
Duality of Interest: No potential conflicts of interest relevant to this article were reported.
[a] Division of Endocrinology, Department of Medicine, Diabetes and Cardiovascular Center, University of Missouri, D109 Diabetes Center UHC, One Hospital Drive, Columbia, MO 65212, USA; [b] Department of Physiology and Pharmacology, University of Missouri, One Hospital Drive, Columbia, MO 65212, USA; [c] Harry S. Truman VA Hospital, 800 Hospital Drive, Columbia, MO 65201, USA
* Corresponding author. D109 Diabetes Center UHC, One Hospital Drive, Columbia, MO 65212.
E-mail address: sowersj@health.missouri.edu

Med Clin N Am 101 (2017) 129–137
http://dx.doi.org/10.1016/j.mcna.2016.08.009
0025-7125/17/© 2016 Elsevier Inc. All rights reserved.

medical.theclinics.com

PATHOPHYSIOLOGY

All components of the cardiorenal metabolic syndrome (CRS) are linked to metabolic abnormalities and obesity.[1–4] Hypertension, in the setting of obesity and the CRS, is partly due to an expanded plasma volume resulting in an increase in cardiac output.[5,6] A second important factor in the pathogenesis of hypertension coupled with the CRS and obesity is increased peripheral vascular resistance.[5,6] Expanded plasma volume and hyperinsulinemia lead to increased renal filtration, which affects renal sodium handling and promotes renal dysfunction characterized early by albuminuria.[5,6] The increase in vascular resistance impairs blood flow to skeletal muscle tissue, which leads to more insulin resistance and hyperinsulinemia, creating a vicious cycle that promotes more volume expansion and renal hyperfiltration.[7] In obesity-related hypertension, the expanded intravascular blood volume and increased peripheral vascular resistance, over time, lead to both concentric and eccentric left ventricular hypertrophy and impaired cardiac diastolic relaxation.[6–9]

The Contribution of Renal Sodium Handling

One of the more salient features common to both hypertension and other components of the CRS is the impaired handling of sodium. Early studies showed a direct association between increased insulin and sodium absorption through increased nephron sodium transporters. This leads to a decrease in sodium excretion and thus an increased intravascular volume.[6] There is also increasing evidence that insulin resistance in cardiovascular (CV) tissues contributes to impaired cardiac and vascular relaxation and increased CV stiffness.[5,6] More contemporary studies have delved further into this topic, elucidating the role that inflamed adipose tissue (eg, in visceral and perivascular fat) may play in hypertension associated with CRS.[10–13] This inflammation of adipose tissue likely contributes to RAAS activation related to increased pro-inflammatory adipokine secretion. The resulting systemic activation reduced activation of nitric oxide (NO) synthase and increased destruction of NO with resultant reductions in bioavailable NO in CV tissue.[10–13]

The Role of the Renin Angiotensin Aldosterone System

In states of insulin resistance such as obesity, an activated systemic RAAS is critical to the pathogenesis of hypertension and other components of the CRS.[6] Increasingly, it is apparent that expanded inflamed visceral and perivascular adipocyte tissue is key to driving RAAS activation. Adipocyte production of angiotensinogen may contribute up to 30% of circulating angiotensinogen.[12] The notion that adipocyte production of angiotensinogen contributes to an activated RAAS is strengthened by observations of angiotensinogen knockout mice being immune to developing obesity, insulin resistance, and hypertension.[14,15] In other murine studies with ablation of adipose-derived angiotensinogen, no obesity-related hypertension developed. However, some mice did go on to develop obesity.[16] This evolving research underlines the important link between adipocyte-derived angiotensinogen and HTN, particularly in the context of CRS.[17]

There is a burgeoning body of evidence indicating that adipocytes are an important source of extra-adrenal-derived aldosterone.[18] This concept is supported by the observation that obese persons, especially females, have increased circulating levels of aldosterone.[6] Recent studies have shown that aldosterone-induced mineralocorticoid receptor (MR) activation in vascular tissue can itself be an instigating factor in the promotion of vascular stiffness by promotion of oxidative stress, inflammation, maladaptive immune modulation, and fibrosis.[19,20] Therefore, this MR activation may be a therapeutic target to prevent the evolution of vascular stiffness and hypertension in diet-induced obesity.

Activation of the Sympathetic Nervous System

Multiple studies have supported the role of sympathetic nervous system (SNS) activation in obesity-related hypertension. These studies have shown that there is amplified sympathetic milieu in obese patients.[21–24] One of the mechanisms responsible for SNS-induced increases in blood pressure is via increases in the hormone leptin, which may drive SNS activation.[25] Indeed leptin deficiency, in concert with diminished SNS activation, has been associated with a propensity to postural hypotension.[26] Chronically high levels of leptin have also been shown to reduce natriuresis and lead to decreases in vascular bioavailable NO.[27–29] Thus, hyperinsulinemia, activation of the RAAS, the SNS, and hyperleptinemia may all act in a positive feedback way to promote hypertension associated with obesity, insulin resistance, and CRS.[30]

Activation of RAAS can also work in a positive feedback loop with an activated SNS as indicated (**Figs. 1** and **2**). For example, increased renal sympathetic nerve traffic promotes juxtaglomerular cell renin production, and activated RAAS promotes SNS activation. Activated RAAS effects on SNS activation include inhibition of norepinephrine reuptake in the presynaptic sympathetic nerve terminals.[31] Another contributor to increased sympathetic tone in obese patients is sleep-disordered breathing and obstructive sleep apnea (OSA), both of which are seen in many patients with CRS.[1,3] Thus, the RAAS and the SNS work in a positive feedback loop to increase hypertension in patients with obesity, insulin resistance, and the other components of CRS.[21,22,32,33]

THE ROLE OF BLOCKING RENIN ANGIOTENSIN ALDOSTERONE SYSTEM IN CARDIORENAL METABOLIC SYNDROME

Accumulating evidence has shown the benefits of RAAS blockade in correcting many of the maladaptive aspects of the CRS, especially in patients with insulin resistance

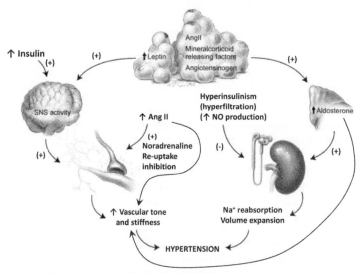

Fig. 1. Coordinated influence of obesity, insulin resistance, activation of RAAS and SNS in the pathophysiology of hypertension in CMS. (*Adapted from* Manrique C, Lastra G, Gardner M, et al. The Renin angiotensin aldosterone system in hypertension: roles of insulin resistance and oxidative stress. Med Clin North Am 2009;93(3):571; with permission.)

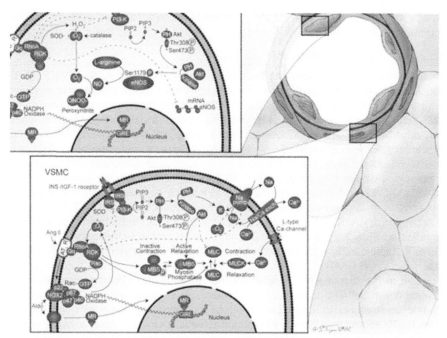

Fig. 2. (*Upper inset*) Vascular effects of insulin (INS) or insulin-like growth factor (IGF)-1 and counter-regulatory effects of AT1R and MR activation in endothelial cells. Insulin actions on the blood vessel are partially mediated by increased production of NO through phosphorylation and secondary activation of endothelial NO synthase (eNOS). AT1R activation decreases the availability of NO by way of the induction of insulin resistance, diminishing eNOS mRNA stability, and promoting NADPH oxidase-induced ROS production. Mineralocorticoids also activate NAPDH oxidase with secondary O2– production and consequent generation of peroxinitrite (ONOO–). Akt, PI3K/protein kinase B; GRE, glucocorticoid response element; Gq, G_q subunit; IRS, insulin receptor substrate; NOX2, catalytic subunit of NADPH oxidase; p22, p47, p40, and p67, subunits of NADPH oxidase; PH, pleckstrin homology domain; PIP, phosphatidylinositol phosphate; PIP2, phosphatidylinositol bisphosphate; PIP3, phosphatidylinositol (3,4,5)-trisphosphate; ROK, Rho kinase; SOD, superoxide dismutase. (*Lower inset*) Opposing effects of ANG II and aldosterone (Aldo) versus insulin/IGF-1 on VSMCs. Insulin and IGF-1 cause VSMC relaxation, whereas ANG II and mineralocorticoids cause contraction. MBS, myosin-bound serine; MLC, myosin light chain; MLCK, MLC kinase; Na/Ca exch, Na_/Ca2_ exchanger. (*From* Manrique C, Lastra G, Gardner M, et al. The Renin angiotensin aldosterone system in hypertension: roles of insulin resistance and oxidative stress. Med Clin North Am 2009;93(3):572; with permission.)

and obesity. To this point, multiple studies using angiotensin converting enzyme (ACE) inhibitors and angiotensin II-receptor blockers (ARBs) have shown their benefits in the treatment of hypertension, congestive heart failure, and coronary artery disease, as well as prevention of cardiovascular disease (CVD) and chronic kidney disease (CKD) in patients with type 2 diabetes.[34,35] The TROPHY (Trial of preventing hypertension) study, in which obese patients were randomized in a double-blinded protocol to groups receiving increasing doses of hydrochlorothiazide (12.5, 25, and 50 mg) versus lisinopril (10, 20, and 40 mg) with a diastolic goal of less than 90 mm Hg, showed some evidence of greater reduction of blood pressure with lisinopril. The statistically significant results for obese patients receiving lisinopril showed 60% had achieved the blood pressure goal compared with 43% taking hydrochlorothiazide (HCTZ).

Metabolically, it was also noted that the patients in the HCTZ arm of the study had less optimal metabolic profiles, plasma glucose levels that were significantly higher, and reduced plasma potassium when compared with the lisinopril arm.[36] Another subanalysis of patients with the metabolic syndrome in the treat to target survey compared irbesartan by itself and in combination with hydrochlorothiazide. Findings included significant reductions in blood pressure, and metabolically, irbesartan was found to alleviate the undesirable effects of HCTZ in the combination group. Moreover, there were also statistically significant improvements noted in other parameters of CRS, including waist circumference in both men and women.[37] The concept that RAAS inhibitors can improve the negative effects of CRS was shown in a trial comparing HCTZ monotherapy versus valsartan monotherapy versus a combination of the 2 in patients with the metabolic syndrome. The significant results of this study showed an increase in the A1C and triglycerides solely in the HCTZ-only arm of the study. This once again solidified the notion that the use of an RAAS antagonist was protective against the insulin resistance properties of the diuretic, when used concurrently.[38]

The Utility of Direct Renin Inhibitors and Mineralocorticoid Receptor Antagonists in Treating Hypertension in Cardiorenal Metabolic Syndrome

A caveat needs to be made when considering the role of direct renin inhibitors and MR agonists in populations with obesity and the metabolic syndrome, as these components have yet to be studied comprehensively. The ALTITUDE study (Aliskiren Trial in Type 2 Diabetes Using Cardiorenal Endpoints), which compared the addition of the renin inhibitor aliskiren versus placebo as an adjunct to an ACE inhibitor (ACE-I) or angiotensin receptor blocker (ARB), definitively showed that there was no benefit to adding aliskiren to previously established therapy. In fact, the study even had to be stopped prematurely due to greater cardiovascular events reported in the aliskiren arm of the study.[39] There are future data expected on the role of direct renin inhibitors and their role in the management of hypertension in CRS as a compendium both from the aforementioned ALTITUDE study and the ASTRONAUT study (Aliskiren Trial on Acute Heart Failure Outcomes).[40] Thus, there is no evidence currently showing the benefit of using combination RAAS blockade with ARBs plus renin or ACE inhibitors.

There is a growing body of evidence that MR agonists are efficacious in treating hypertensive populations with obesity and CRS.[3–5] This approach appears to be especially noteworthy in those patients with resistant hypertension. There are studies currently being carried out in this field. These studies are further bolstered by ongoing work that shows the direct corelation of targeting the endothelial MR to ameliorate its effect on vascular stiffness.[20]

REVIEW OF THE MOST CURRENT GUIDELINES

The most recent antihypertensive guidelines that focus specifically on the subset of patients with obesity and insulin resistance come from the 2013 European Society of Hypertension (ESH) and the European Society for Cardiology (ESC). The mainstay of initial treatment options continues to be lifestyle modification, with a greater emphasis on weight loss. The recommendation for initial pharmaceutical intervention is with either an RAAS inhibitor or a calcium channel blocker, as CRS is considered a prediabetic state, and some of the other readily available options tend to exacerbate insulin resistance in this subset of patients with hypertension.[40]

Unfortunately, the recently published eighth joint national committee (JNC 8) guidelines, also known as the 2014 Evidence-Based Guideline for the Management of High Blood Pressure in Adults, made no particular recommendations for hypertension management in patients with obesity and CRS.[41] This was in comparison to the JNC 7 guidelines, which had recommendations for patients with the CRS that focused mainly on lifestyle modification, although no mention was made about pharmaceutical interventions.[42]

A similar trend is noted with the National Institute for Health and Care Excellence (NICE) hypertension guidelines from 2011, published in collaboration with the British Hypertension Society, as well as with the Canadian Hypertension Education Program Recommendations. Both groups of guidelines tended to focus primarily on the concept of lifestyle interventions while not making any comment about pharmaceutical interventions with this subset of patients.[43,44]

SUMMARY

There are multiple factors linking hypertension and CRS. Currently, there is mounting evidence showing that RAAS and SNS activation are interactive factors that promote hypertension as well as other components of CRS. Agents that block the RAAS have been the mainstay of management with most physicians who treat this subset of patients. Even with the advent of new medications, most physicians continue to use these pharmaceutical classes because of their safety profile and long-term success.

However, the optimal pharmacologic management of hypertension in patients with obesity and CRS are yet to be definitively delineated. Most hypertension guidelines have tended to overlook the pharmacologic management of this subgroup of patients, with some focusing only on lifestyle modification interventions, while others have tended not to refer to them at all. This clearly shows a dearth in information about hypertension management in this population, and more research into the associated role of the RAAS and blockade of this system should yield more definitive material regarding optimizing hypertension treatment in this growing population.

ACKNOWLEDGMENTS

The authors would like to thank Brenda Hunter for her editorial assistance.

REFERENCES

1. Ronco C. The cardiorenal syndrome: basis and common ground for a multidisciplinary patient-oriented therapy. Cardiorenal Med 2011;1:3–4.
2. Available at: http://www.cdc.gov/nchs/data/nhis/earlyrelease/earlyrelease201602_06.pdf. Accessed June 20, 2016.
3. Hoerger TJ, Simpson SA, Yarnoff BO, et al. The future burden of CKD in the United States: a simulation model for the CDC CKD Initiative. Am J Kidney Dis 2015;65(3):403–11.
4. Landsberg L, Aronne LJ, Beilin LJ, et al. Obesity related hypertension: pathogenesis, cardiovascular risk, and treatment-a position paper of the obesity society and the American society of hypertension. Obesity (Silver Spring) 2013;21(1):8–24.
5. Aroor AR, Demarco VG, Jia G, et al. The role of tissue renin-angiotensin-aldosterone system in the development of endothelial dysfunction and arterial stiffness. Front Endocrinol (Lausanne) 2013;4:161.
6. Demarco VG, Aroor AR, Sowers JR. The pathophysiology of hypertension in patients with obesity. Nat Rev Endocrinol 2014;10:364–76.
7. Manrique C, Sowers JR. Insulin resistance and skeletal muscle vasculature: Significance, assessment and therapeutic modulators. Cardiorenal Med 2014;4:244–56.

8. Messerli FH, Christie B, DeCarvalho JG, et al. Obesity and essential hypertension. hemodynamics, intravascular volume, sodium excretion, and plasma renin activity. Arch Intern Med 1981;141(1):81–5.

9. Frohlich ED, Messerli FH, Reisin E, et al. The problem of obesity and hypertension. Hypertension 1983;5(5 Pt 2):III71–8.

10. De Faria AP, Modolo R, Fontana V, et al. Adipokines: novel players in resistant hypertension. J Clin Hypertens 2014;16(10):754–9.

11. Rahmouni K. Obesity associated hypertension: recent progress in deciphering the pathogenesis. Hypertension 2014;64:215–21.

12. Padilla J, Vierira-Potter VJ, Jia G, et al. Role of perivascular adipose tissue on vascular reactive oxygen species in type 2 diabetes: a give and take relationship. Diabetes 2015;64:1904–6.

13. Engeli S, Schling P, Gorzelniak K, et al. The adipose tissue renin-angiotensin-aldosterone system: role in the metabolic syndrome? Int J Biochem Cell Biol 2003;35:807–25.

14. Massiera F, Seydoux J, Geloen A, et al. Angiotensinogen-deficient mice exhibit impairment of diet-induced weight gain with alteration in adipose tissue development and increased locomotor activity. Endocrinology 2001;142:5220–5.

15. Yvan-Charvet L, Even P, Bloch-Faure M, et al. Deletion of the angiotensin type 2 receptor reduces adipose cell size and protects from diet-induced obesity and insulin resistance. Diabetes 2005;54:991–9.

16. Yiannikouris F, Gupte M, Putnam K, et al. Adipocyte deficiency of angiotensinogen prevents obesity-induced hypertension in male mice. Hypertension 2012; 60:1524–30.

17. Mehta PK, Griendling KK. Angiotensin II cell signaling: physiological and pathological effects in the cardiovascular system. Am J Physiol Cell Physiol 2007;292: C82–97.

18. Briones AM, Nguyen Dinh Cat A, Callera GE, et al. Adipocytes produce aldosterone through calcineurin-dependent signaling pathways: implications in diabetes mellitus-associated obesity and vascular dysfunction. Hypertension 2012;59:1069–78.

19. Bender SB, Mcgraw AP, Jaffe IZ, et al. Mineralocorticoid receptor-mediated vascular insulin resistance: an early contributor to diabetes-related vascular disease? Diabetes 2013;62(2):313–9.

20. Jia G, Habibi J, Aroor AR, et al. Endothelial mineralocorticoid receptor mediates diet-induced aortic stiffness in females. Circ Res 2016;118:935–43.

21. Troisi RJ, Weiss ST, Parker DR, et al. Relation of obesity and diet to sympathetic nervous system activity. Hypertension 1991;17:669–77.

22. Huggett RJ, Burns J, Mackintosh AF, et al. Sympathetic neural activation in nondiabetic metabolic syndrome and its further augmentation by hypertension. Hypertension 2004;44:847–52.

23. Raumouni K, Correla MI, Haynes WG, et al. Obesity associated hypertension: new insights into mechanisms. Hypertension 2005;25:9–14.

24. Haynes WG, Morgan DA, Walsh SA, et al. Receptor-mediated regional sympathetic nerve activation by leptin. J Clin Invest 1997;100:270–8.

25. Ozata M, Ozdemir IC, Licinio J. Human leptin deficiency caused by a missense mutation: multiple endocrine defects, decreased sympathetic tone, and immune system dysfunction indicate new targets for leptin action, greater central than peripheral resistance to the effects of leptin, and spontaneous correction of leptin-mediated defects. J Clin Endocrinol Metab 1999;84:3686–95.

26. Bravo PE, Morse S, Borne DM, et al. Leptin and hypertension in obesity. Vasc Health Risk Manag 2006;2(2):163–9.

27. Morgan DA, Thedens DR, Weiss R, et al. Mechanisms mediating renal sympathetic activation to leptin in obesity. Am J Physiol Regul Integr Comp Physiol 2008;295:R1730–6.
28. Cooper SA, Whaley-Connell A, Habibi J, et al. Renin-angiotensin-aldosterone system and oxidative stress in cardiovascular insulin resistance. Am J Physiol Heart Circ Physiol 2007;293:H2009–23.
29. Kazumi T, Kawaguchi A, Katoh J, et al. Fasting insulin and leptin levels are associated with systolic blood pressure independent of percentage body fat and body fat mass index. J Hypertens 1999;17:1451–5.
30. Grassi G. Renin-angiotensin-sympathetic crosstalks in hypertension: reappraising the relevance of peripheral interactions. J Hypertens 2001;19:1713–6.
31. Raasch W, Betge S, Dendorfer A, et al. Angiotensin converting enzyme inhibition improves cardiac neuronal uptake of noradrenaline in spontaneously hypertensive rats. J Hypertens 2001;19:1827–33.
32. Grassi G, Seravalle G, Cattaneo BM, et al. Sympathetic activation in obese normotensive subjects. Hypertension 1995;25:560–3.
33. Gillespie EL, White CM, Kardas M, et al. The impact of ACE inhibitors or angiotensin II type 1 receptor blockers on the development of new-onset type 2 diabetes. Diabetes Care 2005;28:2261–6.
34. Scheen AJ. Renin-angiotensin system inhibition prevents type 2 diabetes mellitus. Part 1. A meta-analysis of randomized clinical trials. Diabetes Metab 2004; 30:487–96.
35. Reisin E, Weir MR, Falkner B, et al. For the Treatment in Obese Patients with Hypertension (TROPHY) study group. Hypertension 1997;30(1):140–5.
36. Kintscher U, Bramlage P, Paar WD, et al. Irbesartan for the treatment of hypertension in patients with the metabolic syndrome: a sub analysis of the treat to target post authorization survey. Prospective, observational two armed study in 14, 200 patients. Cardiovasc Diabetol 2007;6:12.
37. Zappe DH, Sowers JR, Hsueh WA, et al. Metabolic and antihypertensive effects of combined angiotensin receptor blocker and diuretic therapy in prediabetic hypertensive patients with the cardiometabolic syndrome. J Clin Hypertens 2008; 10(12):894–903.
38. Parving HH, Brenner BM, McMurray JJ, et al. Cardiorenal end points in a trial of Aliskiren for type 2 diabetes. N Engl J Med 2012;367(23):2204–13.
39. Friedrich S, Schmieder RE. Review of direct renin inhibition by Aliskiren. J Renin Angiotensin Aldosterone Syst 2013;14(3):193–6.
40. Mancia G, Fagard R, Narkiewicz K, et al. 2013 ESH/ESC guidelines for the management of arterial hypertension: the Task Force for the management of arterial hypertension of the European Society of Hypertension (ESH) and the European Society of Cardiology (ESC). J Hypertens 2013;31:1281–357.
41. James PA, Oparil S, Carter BL, et al. 2014 Evidence based guideline for the management of high blood pressure in adults: report from the panel members appointment to the eighth Joint National Committee (JNC 8). JAMA 2014; 311(5):507–20.
42. Chobanian AV, Bakris GL, Black HR, et al. National heart, lung and blood institute joint national committee on prevention, detection, evaluation and treatment of high blood pressure; national high blood pressure education program coordinating committee. The seventh report of the joint national committee on prevention, detection, evaluation and treatment of high blood pressure: the JNC 7 report. JAMA 2003;289(19):2560–72.

43. National Clinical Guideline Centre. Hypertension: the clinical management of primary hypertension in adults: update of clinical guidelines 18 to 34. London: Royal College of Physicians; 2011.

44. Dasqupta K, Quinn RR, Zarnke KB, et al. The 2014 Canadian hypertension education program recommendations for blood pressure measurement, diagnosis, assessment of risk, prevention and treatment of hypertension. Can J Cardiol 2014;30(5):485–501.

Obesity
A Perspective from Hypertension

Dinko Susic, MD, PhD[a,†], Jasmina Varagic, MD, PhD[b,c,*]

KEYWORDS

- Obesity • Hypertension • Sodium • Sympathetic nervous system
- Renin-angiotensin-aldosterone system • Insulin resistance • Adipokines

KEY POINTS

- The prevalence of obesity-related hypertension is high worldwide and has become a major health issue.
- The mechanisms by which obesity relates to hypertensive disease are still under intense research scrutiny.
- The most recognized factors connecting obesity and hypertension are altered hemodynamics, impaired sodium homeostasis, renal dysfunction, autonomic nervous system imbalance, endocrine alterations, oxidative stress and inflammation, and vascular injury.
- Obesity-related hypertension should be recognized as a distinctive form of hypertension and specific considerations should apply in planning therapeutic approaches to treat obese individuals with high blood pressure.

INTRODUCTION

The prevalence of overweight and obesity in children and adults continues to increase worldwide and, because of their association with cardiovascular disorders, diabetes, and dyslipidemia, are becoming one of the major health issues. Obesity is often related to hypertension, either as a causative or a coexisting factor. Associations between body mass index (BMI) and arterial pressure are well established in different populations and across different age groups.[1–5] Several studies point to a direct association between overweight and obesity and hypertension in children[6,7] that increases the likelihood of hypertension burden in adult life.[8] Moreover, data from the Framingham Heart Study suggest that 78% of essential hypertension in men and 65% in

[a] Hypertension Research Laboratory, Ochsner Clinic Foundation, 1514 Jefferson Highway New Orleans, Louisiana 70121, USA; [b] Hypertension & Vascular Research, Department of Surgery, Wake Forest School of Medicine, Medical Center Boulevard, Winston-Salem, North Carolina 27157, USA; [c] Department of Physiology and Pharmacology, Wake Forest School of Medicine, Medical Center Boulevard, Winston-Salem, North Carolina 27157, USA
[†] Deceased
* Corresponding author. Hypertension & Vascular Research, Department of Surgery, Wake Forest School of Medicine, Medical Center Boulevard, Winston-Salem, NC 27157.
E-mail address: jvaragic@wakehealth.edu

Med Clin N Am 101 (2017) 139–157
http://dx.doi.org/10.1016/j.mcna.2016.08.008
0025-7125/17/© 2016 Elsevier Inc. All rights reserved.

medical.theclinics.com

women may be linked to weight gain,[2] whereas various interventions for weight loss in hypertensive obese subjects resulted in blood pressure reduction.[9–12] However, studies showing that not all obese individuals are hypertensive indicate a complex and multifactorial relationship between obesity and arterial blood pressure. Nevertheless, obesity has been identified as a strong risk factor for progression from prehypertension to more severe hypertensive disease[13–16] and maintenance of a BMI less than 25 kg/m^2 is considered crucial in primary prevention of hypertension.[9,10] Thus, this article discusses major known factors involved in the pathophysiology of obesity hypertension in an attempt to recognize a full spectrum of available treatment approaches because obesity seems to be a common underlying factor in treatment-resistant hypertension.

PATHOPHYSIOLOGY OF OBESITY-RELATED HYPERTENSION

Despite an increasing body of evidence indicating obesity as an important determinant of high blood pressure, the mechanisms by which obesity causes hypertension are still under intense research scrutiny. Among those recognized are altered hemodynamics, impaired sodium homeostasis, renal dysfunction, autonomic nervous system imbalance, endocrine alterations, oxidative stress and inflammation, and vascular injury.

Altered Hemodynamics

Obesity is a hemodynamically volume overload disease that results in increased cardiac output, which predicts development of increased arterial pressure and total peripheral resistance.[17–20] Increased cardiac output in obese people reflects the greater metabolic requirements that accompany increased adipose tissue. It is augmented by redistributing the circulating blood volume to the cardiopulmonary area, thereby resulting in an increased venous return.[17,19,21–23] In addition, increased vascular resistance caused by increased blood viscosity[24] or other changed rheological properties of red blood cells[25] could also contribute to increased blood pressure in obese hypertensive people. The left ventricle adapts to obesity-related blood volume expansion by developing eccentric hypertrophy regardless of the level of arterial pressure.[26] In the presence of hypertension, the expanded intravascular volume is superimposed on the increased peripheral resistance and resulting pressure overload.[21,22] As described by Frohlich,[22] obesity-related hypertension is a state of hyperdynamic circulation responsible for a dual overload of the left ventricle. The cardiac challenge in obesity-related hypertension is greater than the risk associated with either disease alone, carrying higher risk for cardiovascular morbidity and mortality in obese hypertensive patients. If hyperlipidemia, diabetes mellitus, or accelerated atherosclerosis are also present, as they frequently are, these individuals have an even greater risk of coronary arterial insufficiency, myocardial infarction, cardiac dysrhythmia, and sudden death.[27–29]

Impaired Sodium Homeostasis

In several epidemiologic, clinical, and experimental studies, sodium intake was positively related to blood pressure.[30,31] The association was seen in children and adolescents, and it was even stronger among those who were overweight or obese.[32] Increasing sodium intake has been identified as a potential risk factor for obesity in children and adults independent of energy intake.[33] Frohlich and colleagues[19] reported higher sodium excretion in obese patients, which could be explained by their increased food and salt intake. Increases in blood pressure caused by high salt intake have been linked to inherent inability of the kidneys to excrete their increased sodium load. However, the preponderance of clinical and experimental evidence shows that sodium has a direct effect in development of hypertension. Plasma sodium concentrations determine extracellular fluid volume, and thus affect the blood pressure. In contrast, intracellular sodium concentration may have a direct relationship with blood pressure and it was therefore suggested that the increased intracellular sodium concentrations might affect vascular smooth muscle cell (VSMC) tension, increasing blood pressure.[34,35] In *in vitro* experiments, increased sodium concentrations in the media within the physiologic range induced cellular hypertrophy in both VSMC and cardiac myocytes,[36] and decreased endothelial nitric oxide (NO) synthase (eNOS) in bovine endothelial cells.[37] In human endothelial cells, increased sodium concentrations reduced NO release and stiffened the endothelium.[38] In line with these findings, one clinical study reported that reduction of salt intake to 6 g/d improved brachial artery flow–mediated dilatation.[39] However, early reports noted that weight loss achieved by a hypocaloric diet, without reducing sodium intake, significantly decreased systolic and diastolic pressures in overweight hypertensive patients.[40] These data suggest that factors other than excessive dietary sodium intake may be involved in blood pressure increase in obese hypertensive individuals. However, in obese adolescents, a shift from a high salt intake to a low-salt diet induced greater change in blood pressure than in their lean counterparts, suggesting that hypertension in obese teenagers could also be caused by enhanced sodium sensitivity.[41]

A large body of evidence from clinical and experimental studies has indicated that obese individuals have impaired renal pressure natriuresis, such that a higher blood pressure is necessary to maintain sodium balance.[42] Several factors could be involved in blood pressure increase, including renal compression caused by visceral, retroperitoneal, and renal sinus fat,[43–46] and the effects of the activated renin-angiotensin-aldosterone system (RAAS) and sympathetic nervous system (SNS) on the kidneys. Despite sodium retention, volume expansion, and higher blood pressure, obese individuals commonly have increased plasma renin activity (PRA) and angiotensinogen levels, greater angiotensin-converting enzyme (ACE) activity, and higher concentrations of angiotensin II and aldosterone.[17,47–51] Likewise, RAAS blockade with ACE inhibitors and angiotensin type 1 (AT1) and mineralocorticoid receptor (MR) blockers decreased blood pressure in obese hypertensive patients,[47,52–55] whereas in obese experimental animals RAAS blockade attenuated sodium retention, hypertension, and glomerular filtration.[56–59] In concert, increased renal SNS activity was frequently observed in obese compared with lean persons,[60,61] which, in turn, may stimulate renin secretion and sodium reabsorption contributing to a blood pressure increase. Moreover, when compared with lean normotensive controls, obese hypertensive patients had lower concentrations of natriuretic peptides,[62,63] sometimes despite higher sodium intake.[62] These findings suggest that alterations in the natriuretic peptide system may also compromise sodium and water homeostasis in obese individuals with hypertension.

Renal Dysfunction and Structural Derangements

Along with studies addressing the effects of weight gain on cardiac structure and function, multiple studies have focused on how obesity alters the structure and function in the kidneys. Major initial renal changes associated with obesity include an increased renal blood flow and glomerular hyperfiltration,[17] probably caused by increased metabolic demands and higher tissue oxygen consumption. In addition, higher sodium reabsorption in obese individuals may exacerbate increased renal blood flow, glomerular filtration rate, and renin secretion by reducing afferent arteriolar resistance via tubuloglomerular feedback.[64] Consequently, early renal injury, manifested by glomerulomegaly, expansion of the mesangial matrix, focal segmental glomerular sclerosis, podocyte abnormalities, interstitial fibrosis, and albuminuria or proteinuria, has been reported in obese adults and obese children.[65–67] Multiple lines of evidence identified obesity as an independent risk factor in development of chronic kidney disease.[68,69] Furthermore, shifts in pressure natriuresis toward higher blood pressure, activated RAAS and SNS, and frequently comorbidities such as diabetes mellitus and dyslipidemia could amplify these early changes, eventually leading to progressive nephron loss and gradual reductions in glomerular filtration rate. This vicious circle might be accelerated further by increased salt sensitivity of blood pressure following nephron loss,[66] creating an additional challenge for optimal blood pressure control in such individuals.

Endocrine Alterations

Multiple endocrine mechanisms seem to be involved in the pathogenesis of obesity-related hypertension, among which the influence of insulin, adipokines, corticosteroids, and the RAAS have been recognized.

Insulin resistance and hyperinsulinemia, frequently associated with obesity, provide an additional functional link between obesity and hypertension. In general, insulin elicits vasodilation; however, hyperinsulinemia has been associated with an altered vascular response to insulin.[70] Thus, with insulin resistance, impaired insulin signaling in the vasculature leads to reduced NO synthase (NOS) phosphorylation and NO production, impairing vascular relaxation, whereas hyperinsulinemia increases endothelin-1 levels, favoring vasoconstriction.[71] Similarly, insulin infusion in patients with severe insulin resistance induced forearm vasoconstriction.[72] In contrast, the growth-promoting effects of insulin could contribute further to development and exacerbation of hypertension. In addition, insulin has been implicated both directly to sympathoexcitation in the central nervous system[73] and indirectly to increased muscle SNS activity through hypoglycemia and vasodilation in muscle blood vessels.[74] However, the role of insulin in sympathetic activation and development of hypertension still remains a subject of controversy. Thus, although intracerebral insulin infusion activated renal SNS in one study,[75] it did not change blood pressure in another.[76] In addition, chronic hyperinsulinemia, either caused by insulin resistance in obese rats or by exogenous insulin treatment, did not affect SNS and blood pressure in these experimental models.[77,78] Likewise, increased SNS or increased blood pressure were not necessarily observed in patients with insulinoma.[79] Nevertheless, insulin-mediated sodium retention, either by its direct effect on renal tubules[80] or by the potential activation of the renal SNS, may also contribute to the increase of blood pressure in hypertension-associated obesity.

Leptin and adiponectin belong to the family of adipokines (peptide hormones secreted from adipose tissue), which are linked to obesity-induced hypertension. While hyperleptinemia has been reported in obese individuals,[81] low levels of adiponectin were associated with adiposity.[82] Experimental studies have suggested that leptin decreased food intake and increased thermogenesis and energy expenditure through the interaction with alpha-melanocyte–stimulating hormone and its 2 receptors, MC3R and MC4R, thereby increasing sympathetic activation.[83,84] In obese individuals, leptin had no effects on food consumption or energy expenditure, but SNS effects were still present, reflecting partial leptin resistance in obese people.[81,85–88] Although mechanisms underlying leptin resistance in obesity have not been fully elucidated, reduced inhibitory effects of ghrelin on MC4R had been hypothesized in leptin-induced sympathoexcitation.[84] Low levels of ghrelin, a fasting response peptide secreted by the stomach, were identified in obese individuals,[89–91] and weight loss increased ghrelin levels.[92] Leptin-deficient mice (ob/ob), or patients with leptin gene mutations who are obese but not hypertensive, further support the possible contribution of leptin-activated SNS in the pathogenesis of obesity-induced hypertension.[93,94] In addition to SNS activation, leptin also altered NOS expression, inducing endothelial dysfunction.[95,96]

On the other hand, low levels of adiponectin in obesity were inversely related to insulin resistance,[97] and in that way adiponectin could contribute to development of hypertension in obese individuals. A role for adiponectin in reducing SNS activity has also been suggested by one study in which its infusion reduced renal SNS and blood pressure.[98] However, further studies are necessary to confirm these effects, because it is thought that adiponectin actions may involve the hypothalamus, and adiponectin concentrations in cerebrospinal fluid were much lower than in circulating plasma.[99]

Mounting evidence suggests that glucocorticoids have a role in development of hypertension-related obesity, because they increase caloric consumption; reduce energy expenditure; and promote fat accumulation, insulin resistance, and hypertension.[100,101] It was reported that the enzyme that facilitates generation of active cortisol from the inactive 11-keto form, 11β-hydroxysteroid degydrogenase-1, was increased in subcutaneous tissue of obese individuals,[102,103] suggesting that increased glucocorticoid levels in adipose tissue may be involved. Rodents overexpressing this enzyme in adipose tissue also had visceral obesity, insulin resistance, renin angiotensin system activation, and salt-sensitive hypertension that was reversed by treatment with an AT1 receptor antagonist.[104]

Angiotensin II, one of the major effector hormones of RAAS, regulates blood pressure by promoting vasoconstriction, sodium and water retention, and aldosterone production. Beside circulatory mechanism, a functional role of local RAAS has been described in many tissues and organs, including adipose tissue. Several clinical and experimental studies have characterized obesity as a state with activated circulatory RAAS reflected in increased angiotensinogen, PRA, and angiotensin II, despite significant volume expansion and sodium retention.[49–51] In turn, inappropriate angiotensin II activation may further facilitate renal sodium reabsorption, SNS activation, and insulin resistance.[105] Moreover, an activation of the RAAS in visceral adipose tissue or adipose tissue surrounding vessels may promote local functional alterations.[106,107] In agreement, several clinical trials of obese hypertensive participants reported lower blood pressure after therapy with drugs that block angiotensin II synthesis and/or action.[53–55]

Increased circulating aldosterone levels were found in obese individuals,[108] and several studies have reported that MR antagonists decreased blood pressure in obese participants with increased plasma concentrations of aldosterone.[109,110] In some studies, the blood pressure–decreasing effect of MR antagonists did not correlate with aldosterone levels, suggesting that obesity may enhance the sensitivity of MR to aldosterone. In addition, besides the well-known renal effects of aldosterone, the role of MR activation outside the kidneys in regulation of blood pressure and vascular disorders has recently been described. Aldosterone may contribute to development of endothelial dysfunction through cyclooxygenase-2 activation[111] or by activating nicotinamide adenine dinucleotide phosphate oxidase, promoting oxidative stress and reducing NO bioavailability.[112] Moreover, additional antihypertensive effects of MR antagonists in obese patients with treatment-resistant hypertension, who were already taking ACE inhibitors or AT1 receptor antagonists, suggest that MR activation has a role in blood pressure regulation independent of angiotensin II–mediated aldosterone secretion. Such a concept supports the use of MR antagonists as an adjunctive therapy to AT1 blockers or ACE or renin inhibitors to manage resistant hypertension in obese individuals.[113,114] In addition, although it was reported that plasma aldosterone levels correlated with BMI and insulin resistance in obese normotensive individuals,[109] insulin sensitivity was not improved by MR antagonism.[110] Thus, further studies are needed to fully understand the relationship between hyperaldosteronism and development of insulin resistance.

Autonomic Nervous System Dysfunction

Obesity has been associated with autonomic nervous system dysfunction reflected in decreased parasympathetic and increased sympathetic activity, both contributing to blood pressure increase. The increased heart rate and decreased heart rate variability, two important contributors to the development of hypertension,[115] reflected reduced parasympathetic tone in obese individuals.[116–118] In addition, impaired baroreflex sensitivity was reported in obese hypertensive patients,[119] favoring further sympathetic input on blood pressure regulation.

Obesity is, in general, associated with increased sympathetic activity to different tissues, including the muscle and kidney. Notably, increased SNS activity in obese individuals occurs even in those who were normotensive.[61,120,121] Increased muscle and renal SNS activity and peripheral and renal norepinephrine turnover have been observed in obese adults and obese youth.[61,122–125] In addition, free fatty acids may increase sensitivity of alpha-adrenergic receptors, contributing to arterial vasoconstriction.[126] However, although renal norepinephrine spillover was increased in obese individuals, it was not greater in those who were hypertensive compared with normotensive obese individuals, suggesting that isolated increase in renal sympathetic activity is not sufficient to initiate obesity-related hypertension.[127] In contrast, obesity is clearly associated with exaggerated sympathetic contribution to blood pressure. For example, ganglionic blockade induced greater blood pressure reduction in obese compared with lean individuals[128]; the response was doubled in obese hypertensive participants compared with obese normotensive subjects. The exaggerated sympathetic contribution to blood pressure in obese hypertensive individuals may stem from their higher muscle sympathetic activity.[124] Evidence that ganglionic blockade reduced, but did not normalize, blood pressure in obese hypertensive individuals clearly supports a role for SNS activation in the development of obesity-related hypertension but also indicates the interaction of the SNS with other pathogenic factors in creating a prohypertensive environment in obese individuals.

Vascular Injury

An increasing number of studies have shown that initiation of hypertension in obese patients depends on the development of endothelial dysfunction and vascular stiffness. Both are associated with the insulin resistance that is commonly observed in obese individuals[129,130] and precede the progression of early vascular dysfunction to hypertension.[129,131–133] In spontaneously hypertensive rats, impaired vascular reactivity to insulin was observed even before the onset of hypertension,[134] whereas obese but normotensive individuals already showed increased arterial stiffness.[129,131–133] In obesity, suppressed adiponectin production was reported,[82] which may contribute to the development of insulin resistance.[82] As mentioned earlier, impaired insulin signaling in vasculatures may alter vascular relaxation, whereas hyperinsulinemia may favor vasoconstriction.[71,135] However, lack of adiponectin may also impair vasodilation altering NOS activation, because it has been shown that adiponectin stabilized eNOS messenger RNA and promoted eNOS phosphorylation.[82] Likewise, mice lacking adiponectin showed endothelial dysfunction, vascular hypertrophy, and increased leukocyte adhesion to the endothelium; adiponectin supplementation reversed these abnormalities.[136–138] Hyperleptinemia has been reported in obese individuals,[81] and, in addition to SNS activation, leptin also altered NOS expression, inducing endothelial dysfunction.[95,96] It has also been reported that structural changes in large arteries, such as increased intima-media thickness in the carotid arteries, were associated with higher BMI in patients matched for age, sex, and blood pressure,[139] suggesting an increased risk for development of atherosclerosis, arterial stiffness, and hypertension in obese individuals. In addition, obesity-induced activation of RAAS and SNS promoting vasoconstriction and remodeling of small arteries may further amplify aortic pressures during systole, facilitating earlier return of reflected waves to the central arteries.

Oxidative Stress and Inflammation

Many studies have reported increased free oxygen radical levels and systemic inflammation as part of the pathophysiology of endothelial dysfunction, vascular hypertrophy, and consequently arterial stiffness and hypertension.[140–142] Several investigations have focused on increased levels of the markers of oxidative stress and inflammation in proportion to adiposity,[143–146] particularly to visceral adipose tissue. It has been shown that adipose tissue macrophages were principal mediators of systemic inflammation and oxidative stress.[143,147] Proinflammatory cytokines that are released from activated macrophages, such as tumor necrosis factor alpha and interleukin (IL)-6, reduced metabolic effects and promoted vascular growth effects of insulin.[148,149] In addition, activation of IL-17–secreted T-helper cells has been linked to development of hypertensive vascular injury[150] and insulin resistance.[151] In contrast, in obese rodent models, insulin resistance was associated with depletion of antiinflammatory T-regulatory cells.[152] Thus, increased levels of T-helper cells and depletion of T-regulatory cells might be linked to development of vascular dysfunction and hypertension in obese individuals. The interrelationship between oxidative stress and inflammation in obesity-induced hypertension was stressed further by the reports showing that increased levels of free radicals reduced the bioavailability of NO inducing endothelial dysfunction and augmenting inflammation as well, whereas cytokines increased the production of reactive oxygen species.[140,144]

THERAPEUTIC IMPLICATIONS

As a multifactorial disease, obesity-induced hypertension poses a significant challenge for health care providers. The major therapeutic goal, the reduction in obesity-associated cardiovascular morbidity and mortality by decreasing blood pressure, is similar to goals for other hypertensive patients. However, several specific considerations apply regarding optimal therapeutic approaches for obese individuals with high blood pressure.

Most hypertensive patients, including obese individuals, are advised to lose weight, increase physical activity, and reduce their salt intake.[153–155] Given the close link between obesity and hypertension, such changes might be even more important for obese hypertensive individuals. Moreover, obese patients who have prehypertension may benefit most if lifestyle modifications are included in the initial therapeutic approach. Weight reduction has successfully reduced blood pressure in normotensive and hypertensive obese individuals.[9–12,156,157] Likewise, dietary sodium restriction may have contributed to improved blood pressure control[158] in obese individuals. In the Treatment of Hypertension Prevention Trial, after 7 years the incidence of hypertension was significantly reduced in subjects assigned to weight loss or sodium restriction management compared with usual care.[159] The benefits of a diet rich in fresh fruits, vegetables, and low-fat dairy products (the Dietary Approach to Stop Hypertension [DASH] diet) in decreasing blood pressure were greater in obese individuals than in lean individuals consuming the same diet.[158] Furthermore, the combination of weight loss and increased physical activity may have additive effects in improved blood pressure control; aerobic exercise has reduced blood pressure in hypertensive patients,[160] even in trials in which weight loss was not significant.[161]

Despite solid evidence that lifestyle interventions are crucial in the management of obesity-induced hypertension, many patients have difficulties in maintaining healthier life and dietary habits. Thus, antiobesity medications such as a serotonin and norepinephrine reuptake inhibitor (sibutramine), an inhibitor of pancreatic lipase (orlistat), or a cannabinoid receptor-1 blocker (rimonabant) may have been useful in the management of obesity. Their effects on blood pressure ranged from a minor reduction (orlistat)[162] and no change (rimonabant)[163,164] to a blood pressure increase (sibutramine).[165] Caution was recommended when sibutramine was given to patients with uncontrolled hypertension or identified cardiovascular disease,[166] whereas rimonabant was withdrawn from the market because of reports of severe depression and suicidal thoughts.[163,164] Surgical procedures should be considered only in morbidly obese patients (BMI >40 kg/m^2) with hypertension and other comorbidities.[167] However, findings from the Swedish Obese Subjects study showed that, 10 years after bariatric surgery, weight loss, but not blood pressure reduction, was maintained,[168] raising some questions about long-term weight loss associated with blood pressure improvement.

In considering antihypertensive drugs to achieve optimal blood pressure control in obese hypertensive patients, both blood pressure–decreasing effects and the metabolic profile of agents should be taken into account. Diuretics and traditional β-blockers have not be considered as first-line therapy in obese hypertensive patients because of their side effects, including impaired glucose and lipid metabolism.[169–171] These negative effects on metabolic parameters may be less pronounced with the novel vasodilating β-blockers, carvedilol and nebivolol.[172] At present, the RAS blockers (ACE inhibitors and AT1 receptor blockers) are preferred in obese patients with hypertension, based on their cardiorenal protective effects and lower incidence of diabetes, in addition to their antihypertensive effects.[53–55,170,173,174] However, it is now generally accepted that combination therapy is usually required for targeted blood pressure accomplishment and reduction of cardiovascular risk.[175,176] Thus, calcium-channel antagonists and/or the novel vasodilating β-blockers, carvedilol and nebivolol, may be added if blood pressure is not controlled.[172,177] Because the antihypertensive effects of diuretics in obese hypertensive patients are well established[178] and their adverse metabolic effects are dose related, low doses of diuretics could be considered as additional therapy. Based on the higher aldosterone levels and PRA in obese hypertensive patients, additional approaches may involve MR antagonists and direct renin inhibitors in treatment-resistant hypertension, because they are well tolerated and effective.[47,52,109,110,179–182] In addition, studies in which increased SNS activity was targeted by sympatholytic drugs[183] or renal sympathetic denervation[184] offer a new prospect for managing resistant hypertension. However, when inhibiting SNS, a frequent potential side effect is postural hypotension and its adverse actions. In addition, commonly used drugs in hypertension treatment (eg, ACE inhibitors, AT1 receptor blockers, and statins) increase adiponectin levels. Thus, a specific therapeutic approach to increase circulating levels of adiponectin[185] may be a promising modality to achieve optimal blood pressure control in obese hypertensive patients, although further clinical studies are needed to confirm its therapeutic potential. Under all therapeutic considerations, particular attention must be directed toward potential side effects of drugs and the adverse effects of their interactions, particularly when agents of the same class are given in combination.[178,186]

SUMMARY

Obesity-related hypertension is generally considered a multifactorial disease, and most contributing factors interact with each other at multiple levels. Altered hemodynamics, renal dysfunction, and impaired sodium homeostasis seem to play significant roles in the development of hypertension in obese individuals. Autonomic nervous system imbalances and endocrine alterations also may be associated with obesity-induced hypertension, through their direct effects on vasculature or via their complex interface with other factors. In addition, oxidative stress and inflammation leading to endothelial dysfunction and vascular injury are important determinants of increased blood pressure and target organ damage in obese individuals. However, not all obese individuals are hypertensive, suggesting a complex relationship between obesity and blood pressure that is still not fully understood. Regardless, obesity-related hypertension should be recognized as a distinctive form of hypertension, and specific considerations should apply in planning therapeutic approaches to treat obese individuals with high blood pressure.

ACKNOWLEDGMENTS

The authors acknowledge the editorial assistance of Karen Klein, MA, in the Wake Forest Clinical and Translational Science Institute (UL1 TR001420; PI: McClain).

REFERENCES

1. Brown CD, Higgins M, Donato KA, et al. Body mass index and the prevalence of hypertension and dyslipidemia. Obes Res 2000;8:605–19.
2. Garrison RJ, Kannel WB, Stokes J III, et al. Incidence and precursors of hypertension in young adults: the Framingham Offspring Study. Prev Med 1987;16: 235–51.
3. Timpson NJ, Sayers A, Davey-Smith G, et al. How does body fat influence bone mass in childhood? A mendelian randomization approach. J Bone Miner Res 2009;24:522–33.
4. Weiss R, Dziura J, Burgert TS, et al. Obesity and the metabolic syndrome in children and adolescents. N Engl J Med 2004;350:2362–74.
5. Jones DW, Kim JS, Andrew ME, et al. Body mass index and blood pressure in Korean men and women: the Korean National Blood Pressure Survey. J Hypertens 1994;12:1433–7.
6. Freedman DS, Dietz WH, Srinivasan SR, et al. The relation of overweight to cardiovascular risk factors among children and adolescents: the Bogalusa Heart Study. Pediatrics 1999;103:1175–82.
7. Sorof JM, Lai D, Turner J, et al. Overweight, ethnicity, and the prevalence of hypertension in school-aged children. Pediatrics 2004;113:475–82.
8. Chen X, Wang Y. Tracking of blood pressure from childhood to adulthood: a systematic review and meta-regression analysis. Circulation 2008;117:3171–80.
9. Jones DW, Miller ME, Wofford MR, et al. The effect of weight loss intervention on antihypertensive medication requirements in the Hypertension Optimal Treatment (HOT) study. Am J Hypertens 1999;12:1175–80.
10. Stevens VJ, Obarzanek E, Cook NR, et al. Long-term weight loss and changes in blood pressure: results of the Trials of Hypertension Prevention, phase II. Ann Intern Med 2001;134:1–11.

11. Dall'Asta C, Vedani P, Manunta P, et al. Effect of weight loss through laparo-scopic gastric banding on blood pressure, plasma renin activity and aldoste-rone levels in morbid obesity. Nutr Metab Cardiovasc Dis 2009;19:110–4.

12. Neter JE, Stam BE, Kok FJ, et al. Influence of weight reduction on blood pres-sure: a meta-analysis of randomized controlled trials. Hypertension 2003;42: 878–84.

13. De MM, de SG, Roman MJ, et al. Cardiovascular and metabolic predictors of progression of prehypertension into hypertension: the Strong Heart Study. Hy-pertension 2009;54:974–80.

14. Droyvold WB, Midthjell K, Nilsen TI, et al. Change in body mass index and its impact on blood pressure: a prospective population study. Int J Obes (Lond) 2005;29:650–5.

15. Tomiyama H, Matsumoto C, Yamada J, et al. Predictors of progression from pre-hypertension to hypertension in Japanese men. Am J Hypertens 2009;22:630–6.

16. Vasan RS, Larson MG, Leip EP, et al. Assessment of frequency of progression to hypertension in non-hypertensive participants in the Framingham Heart Study: a cohort study. Lancet 2001;358:1682–6.

17. Messerli FH, Christie B, DeCarvalho JG, et al. Obesity and essential hyperten-sion. Hemodynamics, intravascular volume, sodium excretion, and plasma renin activity. Arch Intern Med 1981;141:81–5.

18. Messerli FH, Ventura HO, Reisin E, et al. Borderline hypertension and obesity: two prehypertensive states with elevated cardiac output. Circulation 1982;66: 55–60.

19. Messerli FH, Ventura HO, Reisin ED, et al. Obesity and essential hypertension. Contrib Nephrol 1982;30:116–23.

20. Messerli FH, Sundgaard-Riise K, Reisin E, et al. Disparate cardiovascular ef-fects of obesity and arterial hypertension. Am J Med 1983;74:808–12.

21. Frohlich ED, Messerli FH, Reisin E, et al. The problem of obesity and hyperten-sion. Hypertension 1983;5:III71–8.

22. Frohlich ED. Obesity and hypertension. Hemodynamic aspects. Ann Epidemiol 1991;1:287–93.

23. Reisin E, Frohlich ED, Messerli FH, et al. Cardiovascular changes after weight reduction in obesity hypertension. Ann Intern Med 1983;98:315–9.

24. Messerli FH. Cardiovascular effects of obesity and hypertension. Lancet 1982;1: 1165–8.

25. Levy Y, Elias N, Cogan U, et al. Abnormal erythrocyte rheology in patients with morbid obesity. Angiology 1993;44:713–7.

26. Messerli FH, Sundgaard-Riise K, Reisin ED, et al. Dimorphic cardiac adaptation to obesity and arterial hypertension. Ann Intern Med 1983;99:757–61.

27. Gordon T, Kannel WB. Obesity and cardiovascular diseases: the Framingham study. Clin Endocrinol Metab 1976;5:367–75.

28. Kannel WB, Brand N, Skinner JJ Jr, et al. The relation of adiposity to blood pres-sure and development of hypertension. The Framingham study. Ann Intern Med 1967;67:48–59.

29. Stamler R, Stamler J, Riedlinger WF, et al. Weight and blood pressure. Findings in hypertension screening of 1 million Americans. JAMA 1978;240:1607–10.

30. Elliott P, Stamler J, Nichols R, et al. Intersalt revisited: further analyses of 24 hour sodium excretion and blood pressure within and across populations. Intersalt Cooperative Research Group. BMJ 1996;312:1249–53.

31. Stamler J. The INTERSALT Study: background, methods, findings, and implica-tions. Am J Clin Nutr 1997;65:626S–42S.

32. Yang Q, Zhang Z, Kuklina EV, et al. Sodium intake and blood pressure among US children and adolescents. Pediatrics 2012;130:611–9.

33. Ma Y, He FJ, MacGregor GA. High salt intake: independent risk factor for obesity? Hypertension 2015;66:843–9.

34. Friedman SM. The relation of cell volume, cell sodium and the transmembrane sodium gradient to blood pressure. J Hypertens 1990;8:67–73.

35. Friedman SM, McIndoe RA, Tanaka M. The relation of blood sodium concentration to blood pressure in the rat. J Hypertens 1990;8:61–6.

36. Gu JW, Anand V, Shek EW, et al. Sodium induces hypertrophy of cultured myocardial myoblasts and vascular smooth muscle cells. Hypertension 1998; 31:1083–7.

37. Li J, White J, Guo L, et al. Salt inactivates endothelial nitric oxide synthase in endothelial cells. J Nutr 2009;139:447–51.

38. Oberleithner H, Riethmuller C, Schillers H, et al. Plasma sodium stiffens vascular endothelium and reduces nitric oxide release. Proc Natl Acad Sci U S A 2007; 104:16281–6.

39. Dickinson KM, Clifton PM, Keogh JB. A reduction of 3 g/day from a usual 9 g/day salt diet improves endothelial function and decreases endothelin-1 in a randomised cross_over study in normotensive overweight and obese subjects. Atherosclerosis 2014;233:32–8.

40. Reisin E, Frohlich ED. Effects of weight reduction on arterial pressure. J Chronic Dis 1982;35:887–91.

41. Rocchini AP, Key J, Bondie D, et al. The effect of weight loss on the sensitivity of blood pressure to sodium in obese adolescents. N Engl J Med 1989;321:580–5.

42. Hall JE. Mechanisms of abnormal renal sodium handling in obesity hypertension. Am J Hypertens 1997;10:49S–55S.

43. Chandra A, Neeland IJ, Berry JD, et al. The relationship of body mass and fat distribution with incident hypertension: observations from the Dallas Heart Study. J Am Coll Cardiol 2014;64:997–1002.

44. Chughtai HL, Morgan TM, Rocco M, et al. Renal sinus fat and poor blood pressure control in middle-aged and elderly individuals at risk for cardiovascular events. Hypertension 2010;56:901–6.

45. Foster MC, Hwang SJ, Porter SA, et al. Fatty kidney, hypertension, and chronic kidney disease: the Framingham Heart Study. Hypertension 2011;58:784–90.

46. Sugerman H, Windsor A, Bessos M, et al. Intra-abdominal pressure, sagittal abdominal diameter and obesity comorbidity. J Intern Med 1997;241:71–9.

47. Calhoun DA. Hyperaldosteronism as a common cause of resistant hypertension. Annu Rev Med 2013;64:233–47.

48. Engeli S, Sharma AM. The renin-angiotensin system and natriuretic peptides in obesity-associated hypertension. J Mol Med (Berl) 2001;79:21–9.

49. Kidambi S, Kotchen JM, Grim CE, et al. Association of adrenal steroids with hypertension and the metabolic syndrome in blacks. Hypertension 2007;49: 704–11.

50. Massiera F, Bloch-Faure M, Ceiler D, et al. Adipose angiotensinogen is involved in adipose tissue growth and blood pressure regulation. FASEB J 2001;15: 2727–9.

51. Ruano M, Silvestre V, Castro R, et al. Morbid obesity, hypertensive disease and the renin-angiotensin-aldosterone axis. Obes Surg 2005;15:670–6.

52. de SF, Muxfeldt E, Fiszman R, et al. Efficacy of spironolactone therapy in patients with true resistant hypertension. Hypertension 2010;55:147–52.

53. Dorresteijn JA, Schrover IM, Visseren FL, et al. Differential effects of renin-angiotensin-aldosterone system inhibition, sympathoinhibition and diuretic therapy on endothelial function and blood pressure in obesity-related hypertension: a double-blind, placebo-controlled cross-over trial. J Hypertens 2013;31: 393–403.
54. Grassi G, Seravalle G, Dell'Oro R, et al. Comparative effects of candesartan and hydrochlorothiazide on blood pressure, insulin sensitivity, and sympathetic drive in obese hypertensive individuals: results of the CROSS study. J Hypertens 2003;21:1761–9.
55. Reisin E, Weir MR, Falkner B, et al. Lisinopril versus hydrochlorothiazide in obese hypertensive patients: a multicenter placebo-controlled trial. Treatment in Obese Patients with Hypertension (TROPHY) study group. Hypertension 1997;30:140–5.
56. Alonso-Galicia M, Brands MW, Zappe DH, et al. Hypertension in obese Zucker rats. Role of angiotensin II and adrenergic activity. Hypertension 1996;28: 1047–54.
57. Boustany CM, Brown DR, Randall DC, et al. AT1-receptor antagonism reverses the blood pressure elevation associated with diet-induced obesity. Am J Physiol Regul Integr Comp Physiol 2005;289:R181–6.
58. de Paula RB, da Silva AA, Hall JE. Aldosterone antagonism attenuates obesity-induced hypertension and glomerular hyperfiltration. Hypertension 2004;43: 41–7.
59. Robles RG, Villa E, Santirso R, et al. Effects of captopril on sympathetic activity, lipid and carbohydrate metabolism in a model of obesity-induced hypertension in dogs. Am J Hypertens 1993;6:1009–15.
60. Carlyle M, Jones OB, Kuo JJ, et al. Chronic cardiovascular and renal actions of leptin: role of adrenergic activity. Hypertension 2002;39:496–501.
61. Vaz M, Jennings G, Turner A, et al. Regional sympathetic nervous activity and oxygen consumption in obese normotensive human subjects. Circulation 1997;96:3423–9.
62. Asferg CL, Nielsen SJ, Andersen UB, et al. Relative atrial natriuretic peptide deficiency and inadequate renin and angiotensin II suppression in obese hypertensive men. Hypertension 2013;62:147–53.
63. Wang TJ, Larson MG, Levy D, et al. Impact of obesity on plasma natriuretic peptide levels. Circulation 2004;109:594–600.
64. Hall ME, do Carmo JM, da Silva AA, et al. Obesity, hypertension, and chronic kidney disease. Int J Nephrol Renovasc Dis 2014;7:75–88.
65. Amann K, Benz K. Structural renal changes in obesity and diabetes. Semin Nephrol 2013;33:23–33.
66. Hall JE, Henegar JR, Dwyer TM, et al. Is obesity a major cause of chronic kidney disease? Adv Ren Replace Ther 2004;11:41–54.
67. Henegar JR, Bigler SA, Henegar LK, et al. Functional and structural changes in the kidney in the early stages of obesity. J Am Soc Nephrol 2001;12:1211–7.
68. Burton JO, Gray LJ, Webb DR, et al. Association of anthropometric obesity measures with chronic kidney disease risk in a non-diabetic patient population. Nephrol Dial Transplant 2012;27:1860–6.
69. Hsu CY, McCulloch CE, Iribarren C, et al. Body mass index and risk for end-stage renal disease. Ann Intern Med 2006;144:21–8.
70. Hall JE, Brands MW, Zappe DH, et al. Hemodynamic and renal responses to chronic hyperinsulinemia in obese, insulin-resistant dogs. Hypertension 1995; 25:994–1002.

71. Montagnani M, Quon MJ. Insulin action in vascular endothelium: potential mechanisms linking insulin resistance with hypertension. Diabetes Obes Metab 2000; 2:285–92.

72. Gudbjornsdottir S, Elam M, Sellgren J, et al. Insulin increases forearm vascular resistance in obese, insulin-resistant hypertensives. J Hypertens 1996;14:91–7.

73. Landsberg L. Diet, obesity and hypertension: an hypothesis involving insulin, the sympathetic nervous system, and adaptive thermogenesis. Q J Med 1986;61:1081–90.

74. Anderson EA, Balon TW, Hoffman RP, et al. Insulin increases sympathetic activity but not blood pressure in borderline hypertensive humans. Hypertension 1992;19:621–7.

75. Muntzel MS, Morgan DA, Mark AL, et al. Intracerebroventricular insulin produces nonuniform regional increases in sympathetic nerve activity. Am J Physiol 1994;267:R1350–5.

76. Liu J, da Silva AA, Tallam LS, et al. Chronic central nervous system hyperinsulinemia and regulation of arterial pressure and food intake. J Hypertens 2006;24: 1391–5.

77. Johansson ME, Andersson IJ, Alexanderson C, et al. Hyperinsulinemic rats are normotensive but sensitized to angiotensin II. Am J Physiol Regul Integr Comp Physiol 2008;294:R1240–7.

78. Verma S, Leung YM, Yao L, et al. Hyperinsulinemia superimposed on insulin resistance does not elevate blood pressure. Am J Hypertens 2001;14:429–32.

79. Scherrer U, Owlya R, Trueb L. Sympathetic-nerve activity before and after resection of an insulinoma. N Engl J Med 1996;335:1240–2.

80. Nizet A, Lefebvre P, Crabbe J. Control by insulin of sodium potassium and water excretion by the isolated dog kidney. Pflugers Arch 1971;323:11–20.

81. de Court M, Zimmet P, Hodge A, et al. Hyperleptinaemia: the missing link in the, metabolic syndrome? Diabet Med 1997;14:200–8.

82. Wang ZV, Scherer PE. Adiponectin, cardiovascular function, and hypertension. Hypertension 2008;51:8–14.

83. Hall JE, Brands MW, Hildebrandt DA, et al. Role of sympathetic nervous system and neuropeptides in obesity hypertension. Braz J Med Biol Res 2000;33: 605–18.

84. Matsumura K, Tsuchihashi T, Fujii K, et al. Neural regulation of blood pressure by leptin and the related peptides. Regul Pept 2003;114:79–86.

85. Considine RV, Sinha MK, Heiman ML, et al. Serum immunoreactive-leptin concentrations in normal-weight and obese humans. N Engl J Med 1996;334:292–5.

86. Correia ML, Haynes WG, Rahmouni K, et al. The concept of selective leptin resistance: evidence from agouti yellow obese mice. Diabetes 2002;51:439–42.

87. Rahmouni K, Morgan DA, Morgan GM, et al. Role of selective leptin resistance in diet-induced obesity hypertension. Diabetes 2005;54:2012–8.

88. Myers MG, Cowley MA, Munzberg H. Mechanisms of leptin action and leptin resistance. Annu Rev Physiol 2008;70:537–56.

89. Oner-Iyidogan Y, Kocak H, Gurdol F, et al. Circulating ghrelin levels in obese women: a possible association with hypertension. Scand J Clin Lab Invest 2007;67:568–76.

90. Zhang S, Zhang Q, Zhang L, et al. Expression of ghrelin and leptin during the development of type 2 diabetes mellitus in a rat model. Mol Med Rep 2013;7: 223–8.

91. Wang WM, Li SM, Du FM, et al. Ghrelin and obestatin levels in hypertensive obese patients. J Int Med Res 2014;42:1202–8.

92. Hansen TK, Dall R, Hosoda H, et al. Weight loss increases circulating levels of ghrelin in human obesity. Clin Endocrinol (Oxf) 2002;56:203–6.

93. Mark AL, Shaffer RA, Correia ML, et al. Contrasting blood pressure effects of obesity in leptin-deficient ob/ob mice and agouti yellow obese mice. J Hypertens 1999;17:1949–53.

94. Ozata M, Ozdemir IC, Licinio J. Human leptin deficiency caused by a missense mutation: multiple endocrine defects, decreased sympathetic tone, and immune system dysfunction indicate new targets for leptin action, greater central than peripheral resistance to the effects of leptin, and spontaneous correction of leptin-mediated defects. J Clin Endocrinol Metab 1999;84:3686–95.

95. Knudson JD, Payne GA, Borbouse L, et al. Leptin and mechanisms of endothelial dysfunction and cardiovascular disease. Curr Hypertens Rep 2008;10: 434–9.

96. Korda M, Kubant R, Patton S, et al. Leptin-induced endothelial dysfunction in obesity. Am J Physiol Heart Circ Physiol 2008;295:H1514–21.

97. Weyer C, Funahashi T, Tanaka S, et al. Hypoadiponectinemia in obesity and type 2 diabetes: close association with insulin resistance and hyperinsulinemia. J Clin Endocrinol Metab 2001;86:1930–5.

98. Tanida M, Shen J, Horii Y, et al. Effects of adiponectin on the renal sympathetic nerve activity and blood pressure in rats. Exp Biol Med (Maywood) 2007;232: 390–7.

99. Kos K, Harte AL, da Silva NF, et al. Adiponectin and resistin in human cerebrospinal fluid and expression of adiponectin receptors in the human hypothalamus. J Clin Endocrinol Metab 2007;92:1129–36.

100. Kellendonk C, Eiden S, Kretz O, et al. Inactivation of the GR in the nervous system affects energy accumulation. Endocrinology 2002;143:2333–40.

101. Whitworth JA, Schyvens CG, Zhang Y, et al. Glucocorticoid-induced hypertension: from mouse to man. Clin Exp Pharmacol Physiol 2001;28:993–6.

102. Lindsay RS, Wake DJ, Nair S, et al. Subcutaneous adipose 11 beta-hydroxysteroid dehydrogenase type 1 activity and messenger ribonucleic acid levels are associated with adiposity and insulinemia in Pima Indians and Caucasians. J Clin Endocrinol Metab 2003;88:2738–44.

103. Michailidou Z, Coll AP, Kenyon CJ, et al. Peripheral mechanisms contributing to the glucocorticoid hypersensitivity in proopiomelanocortin null mice treated with corticosterone. J Endocrinol 2007;194:161–70.

104. Masuzaki H, Yamamoto H, Kenyon CJ, et al. Transgenic amplification of glucocorticoid action in adipose tissue causes high blood pressure in mice. J Clin Invest 2003;112:83–90.

105. Kurukulasuriya LR, Stas S, Lastra G, et al. Hypertension in obesity. Med Clin North Am 2011;95:903–17.

106. Engeli S, Negrel R, Sharma AM. Physiology and pathophysiology of the adipose tissue renin-angiotensin system. Hypertension 2000;35:1270–7.

107. Szasz T, Bomfim GF, Webb RC. The influence of perivascular adipose tissue on vascular homeostasis. Vasc Health Risk Manag 2013;9:105–16.

108. Bentley-Lewis R, Adler GK, Perlstein T, et al. Body mass index predicts aldosterone production in normotensive adults on a high-salt diet. J Clin Endocrinol Metab 2007;92:4472–5.

109. Garg R, Hurwitz S, Williams GH, et al. Aldosterone production and insulin resistance in healthy adults. J Clin Endocrinol Metab 2010;95:1986–90.

110. Garg R, Kneen L, Williams GH, et al. Effect of mineralocorticoid receptor antagonist on insulin resistance and endothelial function in obese subjects. Diabetes Obes Metab 2014;16:268–72.
111. Blanco-Rivero J, Cachofeiro V, Lahera V, et al. Participation of prostacyclin in endothelial dysfunction induced by aldosterone in normotensive and hypertensive rats. Hypertension 2005;46:107–12.
112. Sanz-Rosa D, Oubina MP, Cediel E, et al. Eplerenone reduces oxidative stress and enhances eNOS in SHR: vascular functional and structural consequences. Antioxid Redox Signal 2005;7:1294–301.
113. Jordan J, Yumuk V, Schlaich M, et al. Joint statement of the European Association for the Study of Obesity and the European Society of Hypertension: obesity and difficult to treat arterial hypertension. J Hypertens 2012;30:1047–55.
114. Landsberg L, Aronne LJ, Beilin LJ, et al. Obesity-related hypertension: pathogenesis, cardiovascular risk, and treatment–a position paper of The Obesity Society and The American Society of Hypertension. Obesity (Silver Spring) 2013; 21:8–24.
115. Shaltout HA, Rose JC, Chappell MC, et al. Angiotensin-(1-7) deficiency and baroreflex impairment precede the antenatal Betamethasone exposure-induced elevation in blood pressure. Hypertension 2012;59:453–8.
116. Arone LJ, Mackintosh R, Rosenbaum M, et al. Autonomic nervous system activity in weight gain and weight loss. Am J Physiol 1995;269:R222–5.
117. Hirsch J, Leibel RL, Mackintosh R, et al. Heart rate variability as a measure of autonomic function during weight change in humans. Am J Physiol 1991;261: R1418–23.
118. Van Vliet BN, Hall JE, Mizelle HL, et al. Reduced parasympathetic control of heart rate in obese dogs. Am J Physiol 1995;269:H629–37.
119. Grassi G, Seravalle G, Dell'Oro R, et al. Adrenergic and reflex abnormalities in obesity-related hypertension. Hypertension 2000;36:538–42.
120. Grassi G, Seravalle G, Cattaneo BM, et al. Sympathetic activation in obese normotensive subjects. Hypertension 1995;25:560–3.
121. Scherrer U, Randin D, Tappy L, et al. Body fat and sympathetic nerve activity in healthy subjects. Circulation 1994;89:2634–40.
122. Davy KP, Hall JE. Obesity and hypertension: two epidemics or one? Am J Physiol Regul Integr Comp Physiol 2004;286:R803–13.
123. Rumantir MS, Vaz M, Jennings GL, et al. Neural mechanisms in human obesity-related hypertension. J Hypertens 1999;17:1125–33.
124. Lambert E, Straznicky N, Schlaich M, et al. Differing pattern of sympathoexcitation in normal-weight and obesity-related hypertension. Hypertension 2007;50: 862–8.
125. Lambert E, Sari CI, Dawood T, et al. Sympathetic nervous system activity is associated with obesity-induced subclinical organ damage in young adults. Hypertension 2010;56:351–8.
126. Stepniakowski KT, Goodfriend TL, Egan BM. Fatty acids enhance vascular alpha-adrenergic sensitivity. Hypertension 1995;25:774–8.
127. Esler M, Straznicky N, Eikelis N, et al. Mechanisms of sympathetic activation in obesity-related hypertension. Hypertension 2006;48:787–96.
128. Shibao C, Gamboa A, Diedrich A, et al. Autonomic contribution to blood pressure and metabolism in obesity. Hypertension 2007;49:27–33.
129. Aroor AR, Demarco VG, Jia G, et al. The role of tissue renin-angiotensin-aldosterone system in the development of endothelial dysfunction and arterial stiffness. Front Endocrinol (Lausanne) 2013;4:161.

130. Sandoo A, van Zanten JJ, Metsios GS, et al. The endothelium and its role in regulating vascular tone. Open Cardiovasc Med J 2010;4:302–12.

131. Cavalcante JL, Lima JA, Redheuil A, et al. Aortic stiffness: current understanding and future directions. J Am Coll Cardiol 2011;57:1511–22.

132. Femia R, Kozakova M, Nannipieri M, et al. Carotid intima-media thickness in confirmed prehypertensive subjects: predictors and progression. Arterioscler Thromb Vasc Biol 2007;27:2244–9.

133. Liao D, Arnett DK, Tyroler HA, et al. Arterial stiffness and the development of hypertension. The ARIC study. Hypertension 1999;34:201–6.

134. Li R, Zhang H, Wang W, et al. Vascular insulin resistance in prehypertensive rats: role of PI3-kinase/Akt/eNOS signaling. Eur J Pharmacol 2010;628:140–7.

135. Kim JA, Montagnani M, Koh KK, et al. Reciprocal relationships between insulin resistance and endothelial dysfunction: molecular and pathophysiological mechanisms. Circulation 2006;113:1888–904.

136. Cao Y, Tao L, Yuan Y, et al. Endothelial dysfunction in adiponectin deficiency and its mechanisms involved. J Mol Cell Cardiol 2009;46:413–9.

137. Ouedraogo R, Gong Y, Berzins B, et al. Adiponectin deficiency increases leukocyte-endothelium interactions via upregulation of endothelial cell adhesion molecules in vivo. J Clin Invest 2007;117:1718–26.

138. Matsuda M, Shimomura I, Sata M, et al. Role of adiponectin in preventing vascular stenosis. The missing link of adipo-vascular axis. J Biol Chem 2002; 277:37487–91.

139. Kotsis VT, Stabouli SV, Papamichael CM, et al. Impact of obesity in intima media thickness of carotid arteries. Obesity (Silver Spring) 2006;14:1708–15.

140. Sprague AH, Khalil RA. Inflammatory cytokines in vascular dysfunction and vascular disease. Biochem Pharmacol 2009;78:539–52.

141. Chae CU, Lee RT, Rifai N, et al. Blood pressure and inflammation in apparently healthy men. Hypertension 2001;38:399–403.

142. Schnabel R, Larson MG, Dupuis J, et al. Relations of inflammatory biomarkers and common genetic variants with arterial stiffness and wave reflection. Hypertension 2008;51:1651–7.

143. Faber DR, van der Graaf Y, Westerink J, et al. Increased visceral adipose tissue mass is associated with increased C-reactive protein in patients with manifest vascular diseases. Atherosclerosis 2010;212:274–80.

144. Furukawa S, Fujita T, Shimabukuro M, et al. Increased oxidative stress in obesity and its impact on metabolic syndrome. J Clin Invest 2004;114:1752–61.

145. Gletsu-Miller N, Hansen JM, Jones DP, et al. Loss of total and visceral adipose tissue mass predicts decreases in oxidative stress after weight-loss surgery. Obesity (Silver Spring) 2009;17:439–46.

146. Pou KM, Massaro JM, Hoffmann U, et al. Visceral and subcutaneous adipose tissue volumes are cross-sectionally related to markers of inflammation and oxidative stress: the Framingham Heart Study. Circulation 2007;116:1234–41.

147. Cancello R, Tordjman J, Poitou C, et al. Increased infiltration of macrophages in omental adipose tissue is associated with marked hepatic lesions in morbid human obesity. Diabetes 2006;55:1554–61.

148. Aroor AR, Mandavia CH, Sowers JR. Insulin resistance and heart failure: molecular mechanisms. Heart Fail Clin 2012;8:609–17.

149. Rocha VZ, Folco EJ. Inflammatory concepts of obesity. Int J Inflam 2011;2011: 529061.

150. Kalupahana NS, Moustaid-Moussa N, Claycombe KJ. Immunity as a link between obesity and insulin resistance. Mol Aspects Med 2012;33:26–34.

151. Ohshima K, Mogi M, Jing F, et al. Roles of interleukin 17 in angiotensin II type 1 receptor-mediated insulin resistance. Hypertension 2012;59:493–9.
152. Zhong J, Rao X, Braunstein Z, et al. T-cell costimulation protects obesity-induced adipose inflammation and insulin resistance. Diabetes 2014;63: 1289–302.
153. Mancia G, Fagard R, Narkiewicz K, et al. 2013 ESH/ESC guidelines for the management of arterial hypertension: the Task Force for the Management of Arterial Hypertension of the European Society of Hypertension (ESH) and of the European Society of Cardiology (ESC). Eur Heart J 2013;34:2159–219.
154. Eckel RH, Jakicic JM, Ard JD, et al. 2013 AHA/ACC guideline on lifestyle management to reduce cardiovascular risk: a report of the American College of Cardiology/American Heart Association Task Force on Practice Guidelines. J Am Coll Cardiol 2014;63:2960–84.
155. Jensen MD, Ryan DH, Apovian CM, et al. 2013 AHA/ACC/TOS guideline for the management of overweight and obesity in adults: a report of the American College of Cardiology/American Heart Association Task Force on Practice Guidelines and The Obesity Society. J Am Coll Cardiol 2014;63:2985–3023.
156. The Trials of Hypertension Prevention Collaborative Research Group. The effects of nonpharmacologic interventions on blood pressure of persons with high normal levels. Results of the Trials of Hypertension Prevention, Phase I. JAMA 1992;267:1213–20.
157. Whelton PK, Appel LJ, Espeland MA, et al. Sodium reduction and weight loss in the treatment of hypertension in older persons: a randomized controlled trial of nonpharmacologic interventions in the elderly (TONE). TONE Collaborative Research Group. JAMA 1998;279:839–46.
158. Appel LJ, Brands MW, Daniels SR, et al. Dietary approaches to prevent and treat hypertension: a scientific statement from the American Heart Association. Hypertension 2006;47:296–308.
159. He J, Whelton PK, Appel LJ, et al. Long-term effects of weight loss and dietary sodium reduction on incidence of hypertension. Hypertension 2000;35:544–9.
160. Paffenbarger RS Jr, Hyde RT, Wing AL, et al. The association of changes in physical-activity level and other lifestyle characteristics with mortality among men. N Engl J Med 1993;328:538–45.
161. Whelton SP, Chin A, Xin X, et al. Effect of aerobic exercise on blood pressure: a meta-analysis of randomized, controlled trials. Ann Intern Med 2002;136: 493–503.
162. Torgerson JS, Hauptman J, Boldrin MN, et al. XENical in the prevention of diabetes in obese subjects (XENDOS) study: a randomized study of orlistat as an adjunct to lifestyle changes for the prevention of type 2 diabetes in obese patients. Diabetes Care 2004;27:155–61.
163. Pi-Sunyer FX, Aronne LJ, Heshmati HM, et al. Effect of rimonabant, a cannabinoid-1 receptor blocker, on weight and cardiometabolic risk factors in overweight or obese patients: RIO-North America: a randomized controlled trial. JAMA 2006;295:761–75.
164. Van Gaal LF, Scheen AJ, Rissanen AM, et al. Long-term effect of CB1 blockade with rimonabant on cardiometabolic risk factors: two year results from the RIO-Europe Study. Eur Heart J 2008;29:1761–71.
165. Scholze J, Grimm E, Herrmann D, et al. Optimal treatment of obesity-related hypertension: the Hypertension-Obesity-Sibutramine (HOS) study. Circulation 2007;115:1991–8.

166. Poirier P, Giles TD, Bray GA, et al. Obesity and cardiovascular disease: pathophysiology, evaluation, and effect of weight loss: an update of the 1997 American Heart Association scientific statement on obesity and heart disease from the Obesity Committee of the Council on Nutrition, Physical Activity, and Metabolism. Circulation 2006;113:898–918.

167. Clinical guidelines on the identification, evaluation, and treatment of overweight and obesity in adults–the evidence report. National Institutes of Health. Obes Res 1998;6(Suppl 2):51S–209S.

168. Sjostrom L, Narbro K, Sjostrom CD, et al. Effects of bariatric surgery on mortality in Swedish obese subjects. N Engl J Med 2007;357:741–52.

169. Jacob S, Rett K, Henriksen EJ. Antihypertensive therapy and insulin sensitivity: do we have to redefine the role of beta-blocking agents? Am J Hypertens 1998; 11:1258–65.

170. Mancia G, Grassi G, Zanchetti A. New-onset diabetes and antihypertensive drugs. J Hypertens 2006;24:3–10.

171. Pischon T, Sharma AM. Use of beta-blockers in obesity hypertension: potential role of weight gain. Obes Rev 2001;2:275–80.

172. Kaiser T, Heise T, Nosek L, et al. Influence of nebivolol and enalapril on metabolic parameters and arterial stiffness in hypertensive type 2 diabetic patients. J Hypertens 2006;24:1397–403.

173. Dahlof B, Devereux RB, Kjeldsen SE, et al. Cardiovascular morbidity and mortality in the Losartan Intervention for Endpoint reduction in hypertension study (LIFE): a randomised trial against atenolol. Lancet 2002;359:995–1003.

174. Scheen AJ. Prevention of type 2 diabetes mellitus through inhibition of the renin-angiotensin system. Drugs 2004;64:2537–65.

175. Black HR, Elliott WJ, Neaton JD, et al. Baseline characteristics and early blood pressure control in the CONVINCE trial. Hypertension 2001;37:12–8.

176. Cushman WC, Ford CE, Cutler JA, et al. Success and predictors of blood pressure control in diverse North American settings: the Antihypertensive and Lipid-lowering Treatment to Prevent Heart Attack Trial (ALLHAT). J Clin Hypertens (Greenwich) 2002;4:393–404.

177. Pepine CJ, Handberg EM, Cooper-DeHoff RM, et al. A calcium antagonist vs a non-calcium antagonist hypertension treatment strategy for patients with coronary artery disease. The International Verapamil-Trandolapril Study (INVEST): a randomized controlled trial. JAMA 2003;290:2805–16.

178. Frohlich ED. Clinical management of the obese hypertensive patient. Cardiol Rev 2002;10:127–38.

179. Byrd JB, Brook RD. A critical review of the evidence supporting aldosterone in the etiology and its blockade in the treatment of obesity-associated hypertension. J Hum Hypertens 2014;28:3–9.

180. Jansen PM, Danser JA, Spiering W, et al. Drug mechanisms to help in managing resistant hypertension in obesity. Curr Hypertens Rep 2010;12:220–5.

181. Jordan J, Engeli S, Boye SW, et al. Direct renin inhibition with aliskiren in obese patients with arterial hypertension. Hypertension 2007;49:1047–55.

182. Schmieder RE, Philipp T, Guerediaga J, et al. Aliskiren-based therapy lowers blood pressure more effectively than hydrochlorothiazide-based therapy in obese patients with hypertension: sub-analysis of a 52-week, randomized, double-blind trial. J Hypertens 2009;27:1493–501.

183. Sanjuliani AF, de Abreu VG, Francischetti EA. Selective imidazoline agonist moxonidine in obese hypertensive patients. Int J Clin Pract 2006;60:621–9.

184. Esler MD, Krum H, Sobotka PA, et al. Renal sympathetic denervation in patients with treatment-resistant hypertension (the Symplicity HTN-2 trial): a randomised controlled trial. Lancet 2010;376:1903–9.

185. Phillips SA, Kung JT. Mechanisms of adiponectin regulation and use as a pharmacological target. Curr Opin Pharmacol 2010;10:676–83.

186. Ferrario CM. Addressing the theoretical and clinical advantages of combination therapy with inhibitors of the renin-angiotensin-aldosterone system: antihypertensive effects and benefits beyond BP control. Life Sci 2010;86:289–99.

Patient Management of Hypertensive Subjects without and with Diabetes Mellitus Type II

 CrossMark

Michel E. Safar, MD[a,*], Jacques Blacher, MD, PhD[a],
Athanase D. Protogerou, MD, PhD[b]

KEYWORDS

- Hypertension management • Blood pressure • Arterial stiffness • Wave reflection

KEY POINTS

- Antihypertensive drug treatment should include not only the reduction of steady and pulsatile pressures, but also of the increased stiffness gradient relating carotid and brachial arteries.
- Blood pressure measurements should have to include not only systolic and diastolic pressure but also evaluations of carotid-femoral aortic stiffness and carotid wave reflections.
- Antihypertensive drug treatment should be associated with the reduction of the progression of aortic stiffness with age, particularly in comorbid events associated with diabetes mellitus.

INTRODUCTION

Cardiovascular diseases are among the leading causes of death worldwide. Data from multicenter trials have established the importance of office blood pressure (BP) measurement using conventional brachial cuff BP techniques.[1] Studies focusing on brachial BP in treated hypertensive patients have shown that, although diastolic blood pressure (DBP) frequently reaches levels close to 90 mm Hg, systolic BP (SBP) has a tendency to remain higher than 140 mm Hg during treatment. Thus, more recent antihypertensive strategies should focus on SBP, which is closely correlated with cardiovascular risk and events. Arterial pulse pressure (PP), the difference between SBP and

The authors have nothing to disclose.
[a] Centre de Diagnostic et de Thérapeutique, Hôpital Hôtel Dieu, 1 place du Parvis Notre-Dame, Paris 75004, France; [b] Hypertension Center and Cardiovascular Research Laboratory, 1st Department of Propaedeutic Medicine, Laiko Hospital, Medical School, National and Kapodistrian University of Athens, Athens, Greece
* Corresponding author.
E-mail address: michel.safar@aphp.fr

Med Clin N Am 101 (2017) 159–167
http://dx.doi.org/10.1016/j.mcna.2016.08.014
0025-7125/17/© 2016 Elsevier Inc. All rights reserved.

medical.theclinics.com

DBP, also tends to increase with age and is an independent cardiovascular risk factor.[2] This report addresses the basic mechanisms underlying SBP and PP.

Treated hypertensive patients still have considerable residual cardiovascular (CV) risk.[3] Alterations in vascular mechanics within the microcirculation and macrocirculation may well contribute to explain any fluctuations in CV risk that cannot be identified solely from brachial BP measurements. In this context, several important points must be considered. First, BP waves differ markedly between central and peripheral sites of the arterial tree because brachial SBP is higher than central SBP, leading to a significant stiffness gradient, whereas the differences between DBP and mean arterial pressure (MAP) differ only slightly. Second, the reduction of SBP by antihypertensive medication is not distributed continuously along the arterial tree, due to the complex aspects of central BP, which largely depend on arterial diameter and stiffness as well as pressure wave reflections.[4] Last, data from the REASON and other studies have shown that central BP lowering is responsible for reducing cardiac hypertrophy and cardiovascular outcomes when compared with peripheral BP lowering.[4,5] Thus, current speculation, epidemiologic data, and recent advances in technology each raise the difficulty to optimize the assessement and reduction of CV risk. In this regard, risk due to elevated BP is more valid by measuring local BP at those sites where the CV organ damage or events occur, particularly within central (aorta and carotid) arteries.

Abnormal plasma lipids and glucose disorders, atherosclerosis, smoking, abdominal obesity, psychosocial factors, and dietary habits are the main cardiovascular risk factors with both sexes and at all ages, worldwide. These factors are frequently associated with hypertension[6] and require specific attention, particularly with respect to diabetes and atherosclerosis. Because these factors each play a significant role in reducing the CV risk of treated hypertensive patients, it is fitting that they should be discussed in this report.

This review therefore addresses 3 major questions: (1) What are the main pathophysiological differences between central and brachial BP and what are the most appropriate techniques for assessing them? (2) What are the main characteristics of antihypertensive agents when used alone or in combination therapies? (3) What is the role of associated factors such as diabetes mellitus and how do they affect treatment of hypertensive patients? Analysis of these observations will undoubtedly provide clearer insight into brachial and central CV risk in clinical practice.

PATIENT MANAGEMENT AND BASIC APPROACH TO THE CENTRAL AND BRACHIAL BLOOD PRESSURE

In a conventional approach of vascular mechanics,[7–9] the arterial system is seen as a steady flow system in vessels, as deduced from the steady levels of cardiac output, MAP, and total peripheral resistance. This classic interpretation is consistent with flow conditions in the microcirculation, the necessity of maintaining optimal oxygen and nutrient delivery to tissues, and the objective of minimizing BP fluctuations.[7] However, this model does not take into consideration that blood flow is pulsatile and not constant, and that arterial homeostasis is modulated by this flow condition. In recent years, epidemiologic studies have shown that increased pulsatility, as assessed by PP, is a powerful predictor of CV risk.[2] The arterial stiffness gradient, as well as the presence of branching points and potential calcification, generates a multitude of pressure wave reflections along the arterial bed. This report indicates that the final pattern of the recorded arterial pressure wave, at any distinct location along the arterial tree, results from the summation of the forward and backward propagating pressure waves. Arterial stiffness and pulse wave velocity (PWV), as well as pressure wave reflections, are therefore closely related and are among the principal factors affecting the arterial pressure waveforms.[8]

In young healthy individuals, central (aortic) SBP is lower than peripheral (brachial) SBP, whereas MAP and DBP remain almost steady throughout the length of the arterial tree. This hemodynamic pattern, known as SBP or PP amplification, is considered to be primarily a result of the arterial stiffness gradient (central stiffness is normally below brachial stiffness) and pressure wave reflections along the vascular bed. In older individuals ($\geq$60 years), PP amplification is reduced as a consequence of increased aortic stiffness and the early return of reflected waves in the central arteries. Therefore, the relative "timing" of pressure waves merging (ie, forward-traveling or backward-traveling waves) can be considered as a third main factor that defines central BP. This aspect has been elegantly described in past studies that applied to incremental pacing.[7-9] The augmentation index (AI), which is the currently used index to describe the relative increase in central BP due to pressure wave reflections, incorporates both the magnitude and the timing of reflected pressure waves and, therefore, depends on both arterial stiffness and heart rate.[8]

This description of arterial mechanics provides a model that attempts to explain how heart rate, left ventricular ejection time, stroke volume, the distance of the reflected site (ie, body height), and PWV all interplay to define the timing of the forward-traveling and backward-traveling pressure waves within the central arteries. These interactions appear to have a greater impact on the genesis of central rather than peripheral pressures, revealing the well-described effect of height and gender on central BP. The relative contribution of each of these factors is particularly difficult to delineate with currently available technology, because the parameters described are all closely interrelated and would appear to be modulated by the autonomic nervous system, neuro-hormonal factors (eg, renin-angiotensin-aldosterone system [RAAS], sex hormones), and systemic inflammation. A dissociation of PWV and AI may appear in various circumstances, such as insulin resistance, inflammation, or the aging process. Whether this dissociation has a clinical impact and whether pressure wave reflections or large artery stiffness are main determinants of central BP are yet to be determined. Two major approaches are without doubt important criteria for such studies: the estimation of central pressure waveforms by direct, noninvasive measurements in the carotid artery; and the application of generalized transfer functions for indirect estimation of aortic pressure waveforms based on pressure wave measurements in the radial artery. Although both procedures are worthy of consideration, each requires cautious interpretation, as is widely documented in the literature.[8] Finally, mechanical factors in hypertension should no longer be restricted to measurements of SBP and DBP alone and should include a number of other important variables (**Table 1**). One most important factor is the stiffness gradient, which is constantly increased stiffness in the aorta most typically observed in the elderly in contrast to the practically unchanged stiffness observed at the peripheral arterial level (eg, brachial artery).

NEW CONCEPTS OF ANTIHYPERTENSIVE DRUG STRATEGIES

Any antihypertensive agent requires the presence of absolute or relative arteriolar vasodilation to occur for BP to be reduced. However, changes in large arteries are also important to consider in the mechanism(s) of cardiovascular progression and development of complications.

Table 1	
Indexes of arterial stiffness and related parameters	
Term	**Definition (units)**
Stroke change in diameter	Change in diameter during systole = systolic diameter (Ds) − diastolic diameter (Dd) (mm)
Stroke change in lumen area	Change in lumen area during systole, $\Delta A = \pi(Ds^2 - Dd^2)/4$ (mm²) with D = internal diameter
Wall cross-sectional area (WCSA)	Surface of a cross-section of the arterial wall, $WCSA = \pi(De^2 - Di^2)/4$ (mm²) with De, external diameter and Di, internal diameter, measured in diastole
Elastic properties of the artery as a whole	
Cross-sectional distensibility coefficient (DC)	Relative change in lumen area during systole for a given pressure change, $DC = \Delta A/A\ \Delta P$ (kPa⁻¹), with ΔP = local pulse pressure
Cross-sectional compliance coefficient (CC)	Absolute change in lumen area during systole for a given pressure change, $CC = \Delta A/\Delta P$ (m²kPa⁻¹), with ΔP = local pulse pressure
Peterson elastic modulus	Inverse of distensibility coefficient: the pressure change driving an increase in relative lumen area. Peterson = $A\ \Delta P/\Delta A$ (kPa)
Elastic properties of the arterial wall material	
Young's elastic modulus or incremental elastic modulus	$E_{inc} = [3(1 + A/WCSA)]/DC$ (kPa)

From Nichols WW, O'Rourke MF. McDonald's blood flow in arteries. In: Theoretical, experimental and clinical principles. 4th edition. London: Edward Arnold; 2006. p. 175–7.

Angiotensin Blockade and Factors Reversing Arterial Stiffness in Long-Term Antihypertensive Protection

Several randomized, double-blind studies,[7–9] obtained particularly in individuals with high plasma renin levels, have shown that pharmacologic agents that modulate the RAAS produce 3 major long-term arterial changes: large artery stiffness can be reduced independently of BP changes; carotid and aortic wave reflections may be delayed and/or attenuated; and most importantly, systolic BP and PP may be reduced to a greater extent in central than in peripheral arteries. Presence of the endothelium appears to be an important prerequisite for the interpretation of resulting changes in compliance and distensibility (particularly with RAAS blockers).[10] Thus, promotion of NO-dependent pathways may be mainly obtained with preservation of bradykinin and stimulation of the B2-bradykinin receptor. In a population of hypertensive diabetic patients, the angiotensin-converting enzyme (ACE) inhibitor perindopril was shown to reverse aortic stiffness in a dose-dependent manner and independently of changes in BP.[11] In this respect, several meta-analyses have indicated that, whereas AT-1 receptor antagonism may indeed favor a rapid and potentially sudden decrease in BP, ACE inhibitors tend to lower BP more smoothly as a consequence of a progressive decrease in angiotensin II concentrations and an increase in bradykinin levels.

The REASON study[4] was the first to conduct a long-term assessment of interactions among PP, arterial stiffness, and wave reflections with RAAS blockers. In this double-blind study, the perindopril/indapamide combination was shown to reduce central and peripheral SBP and PP to a greater extent than atenolol, despite similar reductions in

DBP and MAP. In addition, with the perindopril/indapamide combination, central BP reductions were greater than those observed in peripheral BP. The CAFE study showed similar results.[5] Together, these findings underscore the view that brachial SBP and PP should not be used as a proxy for central aortic SBP and PP. In contrast, reducing central BP with ACE inhibitors is likely to be associated with better clinical outcomes. Central BP control has indeed been shown to have a significant independent impact on mortality. In addition, other trials[7–9] showed that greater control of BP variability with the perindopril/amlodipine combination compared with the atenolol/thiazide combination was also associated with improved outcomes. In hypertension, it appears that not only should BP be normalized, but also that the balance between BP reduction and the degree of BP variability must be closely monitored.

Therapeutic Combinations Involving Thiazide Diuretics and Calcium Channel Blockers

In patients with low-renin hypertension, further reduction of plasma renin concentration levels through RAAS inhibition may be not useful. Low-renin hypertension could be expected to gain considerable benefit from pharmacologic compounds such as diuretics and calcium channel blockers (CCBs) that promote natriuresis, and would be less likely to experience a reflex increase in renin levels.[12] Studies have shown that patients with low renin at baseline respond better to treatment with diuretics or CCBs than to AT1 receptor blockers.[12] Low-renin hypertension is particularly prevalent among black and elderly patients, and these populations also have been shown to respond best to diuretics and CCBs. As low-renin hypertension has been estimated to affect 30% of patients with essential hypertension, these observations are of crucial importance in clinical practice.[12]

Elderly patients tend to have less-active renin-angiotensin systems as well as stiffened arteries. The progressive remodeling and dilation of proximal large elastic arteries as well as rarefaction of the microcirculation lead to increased peripheral PP and disturbed wave reflections. These factors contribute to increased PP and SBP and these patients are more widely preexposed to rapid onset of CV disease, with a notably higher frequency of stroke in comparison with younger patients. A recent meta-analysis[13] has shown that diuretic/CCB combination therapies were significantly more effective than comparators in reducing the incidence of stroke in 4 studies including 30,791 patients demonstrating a significant 23% reduction in relative risk for stroke (hazard ratio 0.77; confidence interval 0.64–0.92), as well as a significantly reduced incidence of coronary events. This therapeutic strategy is therefore likely to prove a valuable alternative to RAAS blockers. In this context, it is important to note that amlodipine, a long-acting, L-type CCB, blocks transmembrane calcium influx into vascular smooth muscle cells, thereby promoting vasodilation of small arteries and reduced BP.[7–9] Amlodipine also causes calcium release and inhibition of vascular smooth muscle cell proliferation, a key event in the pathogenesis of atherosclerosis. Finally, amlodipine reduces progression of carotid artery intima-media thickness and angina in patients with coronary artery disease.

Indapamide, is a sustained-release, lipophilic diuretic with mild, but significant, natriuretic activity and modest hypokalemia. Indapamide also reduces total peripheral resistance. Unlike hydrochlorothiazide (HCTZ), the drug selectively reduces SBP and arterial stiffness in hypertensive individuals, thereby decreasing heart load and PP[14] associated with a significant increase in PP amplification. Indapamide has 2 important properties. First, when compared with HCTZ, the drug has superoxide radical anion scavenging properties and, second, its effect on glycosaminoglycans, in spontaneously hypertensive rats receiving a long-term high-sodium diet was associated with reduced carotid arterial hyaluronan and increased aortic wall stiffness. Both of these properties have been reduced by indapamide.[15]

Therapeutic Combinations of Diuretics and Calcium or Angiotensin Blockade

Interestingly, the CV benefits of a triple-drug antihypertensive combination were first reported in a subgroup analysis in the ADVANCE trial. Patients treated with the combination of perindopril, indapamide, and a CCB experienced a 28% reduction in all-cause mortality, as compared with the 14% reduction in the overall trial with the dual combination of perindopril/indapamide resulting in similar BP reductions versus the comparator.[16] On the basis of 26 trials involving 152,290 participants including 30,295 individuals with moderately reduced renal function, Ninomiya and colleagues[17] showed that BP-lowering regimens (compared with placebo) reduced the risk of major CV events by approximately one-sixth per 5-mm Hg reduction in SBP in patients with or without reduced renal function. Results were similar irrespective of whether BP was reduced by regimens based on ACE inhibitors, CCB, or diuretics/beta-blockers. These findings were more favorable than several other combination therapies (**Table 2**). A recent meta-analysis (including more than 20,000 individuals) demonstrated that combination therapies comprising angiotensin and calcium blockade were superior to other combinations in preventing cardiac and renal events.[18]

COMBINATION OF ANTIHYPERTENSIVE AND NONANTIHYPERTENSIVE STRATEGIES FOR HYPERTENSIVE PATIENTS WITH DIABETES MELLITUS

In a population of hypertensive patients divided into those with and without type 2 diabetes, aortic stiffness was compared between these 2 groups having the same MAP. Aortic stiffness was shown to be significantly greater in the diabetic than in the nondiabetic patients having the same MAP level.[19] In nondiabetic individuals, the factors associated with increased stiffness were age, heart rate, and MAP; whereas, in those patients with diabetes itself, pressure of diabetes and its duration were the major factors to consider.

Studies involving the duration of diabetes have shown this characteristic feature was associated with increased arterial stiffness through different possibilities. First,

Table 2
Comparison of the drug effects on pulse wave velocity (PWV) and wave reflection of various antihypertensive drug classes

	PWV	Wave Reflection
Angiotensin-converting enzyme inhibitor	Increase	Significantly decrease
Angiotensin receptor blockers	Decrease	Significantly decrease
Aldosterone antagonists	Unchanged	Decrease
Thiazides	Unchanged	Unchanged
Calcium channel blocker: dihydropyridine	Decrease	Significantly decrease
Calcium channel blocker: verapamil	Decrease	Significantly decrease
Alpha-blockers	Unchanged	Significantly decrease
Beta-blockers: nonvasodilating	Decrease	Increase
Beta-blockers: vasodilating	Decrease	Decrease
Nitrates	Unchanged	Decrease

Drugs can "increase" or "decrease" a given parameter, which, in some cases, remain "unchanged."
Data from Refs.[7–9]

in diabetic individuals, insulin therapy and/or diabetes duration were associated with increased arterial stiffness resulting from significant positive interactions between duration and age, but not MAP. Second, clinical studies, mainly involving patients with metabolic syndrome, as defined on the basis of the International Diabetes Federation criteria,[20] have shown that diabetes affected both the small and large arteries independent of MAP but affected precapillary alterations that reduce the effective length of the arterial system, thus contributing to increased PP.[20] Taken together, each of these studies suggests that the association of diabetes with hypertension per se contributes to exacerbate pulsatility as a consequence of the increased aortic stiffness observed in diabetic subjects.

Further treatment strategies are necessary to reduce PP. First, specific data concerning identified therapeutic agents that reduce arterial stiffening should be obtained that include angiotensin or calcium blockade. Second, lifestyle modifications would be necessary (particularly with respect to considering the role of nutrition and other risks of obesity).[21] Third, to achieve the goal of reducing CV risk, certain oral antidiabetic agents could be considered and potentially combined with statins.[21] Indeed, the synergy between the antihypertensive agents, perindopril and amlodipine, and atorvastatin was particularly manifest in the ASCOT trial in which a 53% reduction in cardiovascular events was observed.

SUMMARY AND PERSPECTIVES

In the past, our understanding of hypertension was influenced by 2 main contributing factors: epidemiologic results and pharmacologic research. Based on these findings, a number of therapeutic trials were conducted to improve our understanding of treatment effects and to prevent potential complications. Many antihypertensive drug therapies were believed to cover all aspects of hypertension, thus enabling them to be widely used. It was even believed that one single, lifelong therapeutic strategy could "per se" improve consistently total CV risk in most hypertensive subjects.

At the present time, this basic analysis no longer applies. First, the main difficulty of the drug treatment of hypertension is the concept of "residual risk,"[3] which, until recently, was greatly underestimated and still requires further investigation, particularly to account for the ever-increasing factor of life expectancy. Second, potential complications of drug therapy have come to light, such as those observed with combinations of various angiotensin antagonists, and also the subtle relations between hypertension and sleep apnea or even cancer. Third, investigations into the hemodynamic parameters of hypertension were previously limited to the calculation of total peripheral resistance. Progressively, BP variability and pulsatile arterial hemodynamics, such as aortic stiffness and wave reflections, have become more widely studied in human beings, which can be measured using easily applicable noninvasive vascular techniques. The aim of the present review was designed to provide the exciting potential of these procedures in the development of drug therapies for hypertension and their crucial role in CV risk reduction.

REFERENCES

1. Safar ME, Toto-Moukouo JJ, Bouthier JA, et al. Arterial dynamics, cardiac hypertrophy, and antihypertensive treatment. Circulation 1987;75(1 Pt 2):I156–61.
2. Blacher J, Staessen JA, Girerd X, et al. Pulse pressure not mean pressure determines cardiovascular risk in older hypertensive patients. Arch Intern Med 2000; 160(8):1085–9.

3. Blacher J, Evans A, Arveiler D, et al. Residual cardiovascular risk in treated hypertension and hyperlipidaemia: the PRIME Study. J Hum Hypertens 2010; 24(1):19–26.

4. London GM, Asmar RG, O'Rourke MF, et al, REASON Project Investigators. Mechanism(s) of selective systolic blood pressure reduction after a low-dose combination of perindopril/indapamide in hypertensive subjects: comparison with atenolol. J Am Coll Cardiol 2004;43:92–9.

5. Williams B, Lacy PS, Thom SM, et al, Cafe Investigators, Anglo-Scandinavian Cardiac Outcomes Trial Investigators, CAFE Steering Committee and Writing Committee. Differential impact of blood pressure-lowering drugs on central aortic pressure and clinical outcomes: principal results of the Conduit Artery Function Evaluation (CAFE) study. Circulation 2006;113(9):1213–25.

6. Franklin SS, Larson MG, Khan SA, et al. Does the relation of blood pressure to coronary heart disease risk change with aging? The Framingham Heart Study. Circulation 2001;103(9):1245–9.

7. Safar ME, Levy BI, Struijker-Boudier H. Current perspectives on arterial stiffness and pulse pressure in hypertension and cardiovascular diseases. Circulation 2003;107:2864–9.

8. Nichols WW, O'Rourke MF. McDonald's blood flow in arteries. Theoretical, experimental and clinical principles. 4th edition. London: Edward Arnold; 2006. p. 49–94, 193–233, 339–402, 435–502.

9. Protogerou AD, Papaioannou TG, Blacher J, et al. Central blood pressures: do we need them in the management of cardiovascular disease? Is it a feasible therapeutic target? J Hypertens 2007;25(2):265–72.

10. Levy BI, Benessiano J, Poitevin P, et al. Endothelium-dependent mechanical properties of the carotid artery in WKY and SHR. Role of angiotensin converting enzyme inhibition. Circ Res 1990;66(2):321–8.

11. Tropeano AI, Boutouyrie P, Pannier B, et al. Brachial pressure-independent reduction in carotid stiffness after long-term angiotensin-converting enzyme inhibition in diabetic hypertensives. Hypertension 2006;48(1):80–6.

12. Sever PS, Messerli FH. Hypertension management 2011: optimal combination therapy. Eur Heart J 2011;32(20):2499–506.

13. Rimoldi SF, Ott SR, Rexhaj E, et al. Effect of patent foramen ovale closure on obstructive sleep apnea. J Am Coll Cardiol 2015;65(20):2257–8.

14. London G, Schmieder R, Calvo C, et al. Indapamide SR versus candesartan and amlodipine in hypertension: the X-CELLENT Study. Am J Hypertens 2006;19(1): 113–21.

15. Et-Taouil K, Schiavi P, Levy BI, et al. Sodium intake, large artery stiffness, and proteoglycans in the spontaneously hypertensive rat. Hypertension 2001;38(5): 1172–6.

16. Chalmers J, Arima H, Woodward M, et al. Effects of combination of perindopril, indapamide, and calcium channel blockers in patients with type 2 diabetes mellitus: results from the action in diabetes and vascular disease: preterax and diamicron controlled evaluation (ADVANCE) trial. Hypertension 2014;63(2):259–64.

17. Blood Pressure Lowering Treatment Trialists' Collaboration, Ninomiya T, Perkovic V, Turnbull F, et al. Blood pressure lowering and major cardiovascular events in people with and without chronic kidney disease: meta-analysis of randomised controlled trials. BMJ 2013;347:f5680.

18. Rimoldi SF, Messerli FH, Chavez P, et al. Efficacy and safety of calcium channel blocker/diuretics combination therapy in hypertensive patients: a meta-analysis. J Clin Hypertens (Greenwich) 2015;17(3):193–9.

19. Safar ME, Balkau B, Lange C, et al. Hypertension and vascular dynamics in men and women with metabolic syndrome. J Am Coll Cardiol 2013;61(1):12–9.
20. Czernichow S, Greenfield JR, Galan P, et al. Macrovascular and microvascular dysfunction in the metabolic syndrome. Hypertens Res 2010;33(4):293–7.
21. Dengo AL, Dennis EA, Orr JS, et al. Arterial destiffening with weight loss in overweight and obese middle-aged and older adults. Hypertension 2010;55(4): 855–61.

Oxidative Stress and Hypertensive Diseases

Roxana Loperena, BSc[a], David G. Harrison, MD[b],*

KEYWORDS

- Superoxide • Hydrogen peroxide • NADPH oxidase • Vascular • Renal
- Sympathetic nerves • Dendritic cells

KEY POINTS

- Oxidative stress is considered a major mechanism in hypertension.
- Formation of reactive oxygen species contributes to dysfunction in the vasculature, the kidney, and the central nervous system.
- Recent evidence supports a role of reactive oxygen species in inflammation in hypertension.

INTRODUCTION

It has become clear that reactive oxygen species (ROS) contribute to the development of hypertension via myriad effects. ROS are essential for normal cell function; however, they mediate pathologic changes in the brain, the kidney, and blood vessels that contribute to the genesis of chronic hypertension. There is also emerging evidence that ROS contribute to immune activation in hypertension. In this review, we discuss these events and how they coordinate to contribute to hypertension and its consequent end-organ damage.

REACTIVE OXYGEN SPECIES

ROS are formed by oxidation-reduction reactions in which one molecule is reduced by removal of an electron, which is then transferred to a recipient molecule. ROS can be divided into 2 major groups: free radicals and nonradical derivatives. Free radicals possess an unpaired electron in their outer orbital, which makes them highly reactive. These include superoxide ($O_2^{\cdot-}$), the hydroxyl radical ($OH^{\cdot}$), lipid peroxy-radicals

[a] Department of Molecular Physiology and Biophysics, Vanderbilt University School of Medicine, 2220 Pierce Drive, Room 536 Robinson Research Building, Nashville, TN 37232, USA;
[b] Division of Clinical Pharmacology, Department of Medicine, Vanderbilt University Medical Center, Vanderbilt University, 2220 Pierce Drive, Room 536 Robinson Research Building, Nashville, TN 37232, USA
* Corresponding author.
E-mail address: david.g.harrison@vanderbilt.edu

Med Clin N Am 101 (2017) 169–193
http://dx.doi.org/10.1016/j.mcna.2016.08.004
0025-7125/17/© 2016 Elsevier Inc. All rights reserved.

(LOO·) and alkoxy-radicals (LO·). Nitric oxide (NO) is also a free radical, and often is referred to as a reactive nitrogen species. Nonradical ROS include hydrogen peroxide (H_2O_2), peroxynitrite $(ONOO^-)$, hypochlorous acid $(HOCl^-)$, and reactive carbonyls. These do not possess unpaired electrons, and are more stable with a longer half-life but have strong oxidant properties.

PHYSIOLOGIC ROLES OF REACTIVE OXYGEN SPECIES

Although originally considered toxic by-products of cellular metabolism, ROS are now recognized to have signaling roles that are critical for normal cell function, including proliferation, differentiation, aging, host defense, and repair processes. Recent studies show that ROS, including H_2O_2, may drive prosurvival signaling and protect from the aging process.[1] As a part of innate immunity, ROS not only contribute to host defense via respiratory bursts in phagocytes, but also by signaling chemotaxis of inflammatory cells to sites of infection or injury. Related to this, ROS also participate in tissue repair and remodeling by inducing expression of matrix metalloproteinases (MMPs).[2] These responses, which are vital for normal cell function, become exaggerated in disease states and promote pathologic processes.

OXIDATIVE STRESS

The term oxidative or oxidant stress traditionally refers to an imbalance between the production of ROS and antioxidant defenses. This can lead to an increase in ambient levels of ROS that can damage various cellular components, including DNA, proteins, and lipids. This traditional definition of oxidant stress has been modified, because it is now clear that such an imbalance might be localized to subcellular compartments, such the mitochondria, the nucleus, or localized at the cellular membrane. Localized alterations of ROS production in the mitochondria can affect energy homeostasis, whereas localized ROS production in the nucleus can affect transcriptional events and epigenetic control. Extracellular ROS can participate in outside in signaling and affect cellular function.

MAJOR REACTIVE OXYGEN SPECIES MOLECULES
Superoxide Radical

Superoxide, produced by 1-electron reduction of molecular oxygen, can act both as an oxidant and as a reductant in biological systems, depending on the redox potential of the molecule with which it is reacting. Superoxide is important, as it serves as the progenitor for many other biologically relevant ROS, including hydrogen peroxide (H_2O_2), the hydroxyl radical (HO·), and peroxynitrite $(OONO^-)$, which forms on reaction of $O_2{}^{·-}$ with NO.

Hydrogen Peroxide

Hydrogen peroxide is formed by dismutation of $O_2{}^{·-}$, which can occur either spontaneously or can be catalyzed by the superoxide dismutases (SODs). In contrast to $O_2{}^{·-}$, H_2O_2 is relatively stable under physiologic conditions. Because it is uncharged and lipophilic, H_2O_2 can readily diffuse across membranes and thus can react with targets in organelles and cells apart from where it is formed. In this regard, H_2O_2 has been implicated as a signaling molecule that can, among other actions, promote vasodilatation, activate gene transcription, modify phosphatase activity, and activate other sources of ROS. As part of the antioxidant defense mechanisms, catalase and glutathione peroxidase (Gpx) can further reduce H_2O_2 to H_2O. Myeloperoxidase catalyzes the reaction of H_2O_2 with the chloride ion to generate hypochlorous acid ($HOCl^-$), which is a strong oxidant with high reactivity. Other peroxidases use alternate anions to generate other oxidants. Some of these reactions are illustrated in **Fig. 1**.

Hydroxyl Radical

Hydroxyl is formed when $O_2^{\cdot-}$ reacts with H_2O_2 in the Haber-Weiss reaction in which $O_2^{\cdot-}$ donates 1 electron to H_2O_2. Hydrogen peroxide can also accept 1 electron from the Ferrous cation (Fe^{2+}) in the Fenton reaction to generate $OH\cdot$ and a Ferric cation (Fe^{3+}). The hydroxyl radical is a highly reactive oxidant that can attack a variety of bio-molecules including lipids, proteins, and DNA.

Peroxynitrite

As mentioned previously, $OONO^-$ is the product of the spontaneous reaction between $O_2^{\cdot-}$ and NO. This reaction is essentially diffusion limited, with a rate that has been estimated to be 9×10^9 mols $\times$ s^{-1}. At physiologic pH, $OONO^-$ exists in the proton-ated form, HOONO or peroxynitrous acid, which is uncharged and can diffuse across cell membranes. Moreover, HONOO undergoes homolysis to yield hydroxyl, and in fact might serve as a more important source of this radical that the Fenton reaction mentioned previously. Like hydroxyl, $OONO^-$ is a very strong oxidant and can react with lipids, DNA, and proteins. Peroxynitrite can react with and modify proteins and other cellular structures causing oxidative damage to these macromolecules. In particular, $OONO^-$ modifies protein tyrosine residues to form 3-nitrotyrosine, a biomarker for $OONO^-$ in tissues and blood.

Reactive Carbonyls

Carbonyls are highly reactive molecules that contain a carbon atom double bonded to an oxygen atom (C=O). These are formed both enzymatically and nonenzymatically from lipids, sugars, and proteins, and include reactive aldehydes and advanced glyca-tion end products. These have been extensively reviewed elsewhere,[3] but are highly reactive and can modify macromolecules, such as proteins and DNA, forming cross-links and altering both structure and function. Reactive carbonyls accumulate with aging, increased oxidative stress, and in the setting of various diseases, and likely underlie the pathogenesis of these diseases. An example is isolevuglandin-modification of lysines, which as noted later in this article, produces protein modifica-tions that lead to immune activation in hypertension.[4]

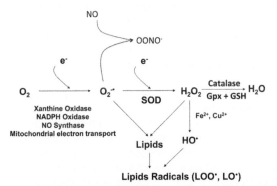

Fig. 1. Sources and formation of ROS in mammalian cells that are relevant to hypertension.

SOURCES OF REACTIVE OXYGEN SPECIES
Nicotinamide Adenine Dinucleotide Phosphate Oxidase

The nicotinamide adenine dinucleotide phosphate (NADPH) oxidases are major sources of ROS in mammalian cells. The NADPH oxidase was first identified in professional phagocytes as a multi-subunit enzyme complex responsible for the oxidative burst used to kill invading microorganisms. The catalytic subunit of the neutrophil oxidase is also referred to as gp91^{phox}, due to its apparent molecular weight and because it is extensively glycosylated. Subsequently, it was discovered that there are 6 related proteins, which have been named the Nox enzymes, termed Nox 1 to 5 and the 2 Duox enzymes. These vary in tissue distribution, function, and regulatory mechanisms. Nox1 exists in colon, muscle, prostate, uterus, and blood vessels and plays important roles in host defense and blood pressure regulation. As noted previously, Nox2 is found in phagocytes, where it is responsible for the oxidative burst. It is also present in endothelial cells, tubular cells of the kidney, and in other immune cells. Nox3 is present in fetal tissue and in the inner ear, where it is essential for vestibular function. Nox4, expressed in kidneys, vessels, and bone, is involved in vasoregulation and erythropoietin synthesis. Nox5, not present in rodents, is a Ca^{2+}-dependent homolog that is activated in response to intracellular Ca_2^+ mobilization in lymph nodes, testes, and blood vessels. Nox5 is also expressed in atherosclerotic lesions and seems to accumulate in more complex lesions.[5] Duox1/2 are distant Nox homologs involved in hormone biosynthesis in the thyroid.

Nox 1 through 4 require the small docking subunit p22^{phox} for function and stability. In addition, the various Nox enzymes are activated on translocation of cytoplasmic subunits. For Nox2, these include p47^{phox}, p67^{phox}, p40^{phox}, and the small g protein rac. For Nox1, alternate subunits, termed NoxA1 and NoxO1, can substitute for p47^{phox} and p67^{phox}. Poldip2 associates with Nox4 and positively regulates its activity and cellular functions.[6] Factors that cause assembly of these cytoplasmic units with the membrane components include inflammatory cytokines, growth factors, mechanical forces, and various G-protein–coupled receptor agonists. Of particular importance to cardiovascular disease, ang II activates the NADPH oxidases via the AT1 receptor and stimulation of a signaling pathway involving c-Src, protein kinase C (PKC), phospholipase D (PLD), and phospholipase A_2 (PLA$_2$).[7]

The NADPH oxidases use an Fe^{2+}-containing heme group in their catalytic center as a means of electron transfer. This center should be able to perform only 1-electron reductions of oxygen, and thus the major initial product of these enzymes should be $O_2^{\cdot-}$. Surprisingly, the most measurable product of Nox4 and the Duox enzymes seems to be H_2O_2. In the case of Nox4, this has been attributed to structural characteristics that retard the release of $O_2^{\cdot-}$ until it spontaneously dismutes to H_2O_2.[8] We have also found that Nox5 seems to predominately release H_2O_2.[5]

Studies of rodents lacking or overexpressing components of the NADPH oxidase have been most revealing in demonstrating a role of these enzymes in hypertension. Mice lacking p47^{phox}, a cytosolic component essential for activation of Nox2, are protected against ang II and DOCA-salt hypertension.[9,10] Overexpression p22^{phox}, the small docking subunit of the Nox enzymes in vascular smooth muscle enhanced the hypertensive response to ang II and aging. Mice overexpressing Nox1 develop augmented hypertension when given a chronic infusion of ang II, and mice lacking this enzyme are protected against ang II–induced hypertension.[11,12] Recently, Nox4 has been shown to play a role in salt-sensitive hypertension in rats.[13] The role of Nox4 of modulating renal sodium transport is discussed more completely later in this article. Overexpression of human Nox5 in the podocytes of increases albuminuria and causes a proportional increase in baseline blood pressure.[14]

NITRIC OXIDE SYNTHASE UNCOUPLING AND TETRAHYDROBIOPTERIN

The nitric oxide synthase (NOS) enzymes are the endogenous sources of NO in mammalian cells. NO has myriad effects on cardiovascular function, including modulation of vascular tone, blood pressure, sympathetic outflow, renal renin release, and renal sodium excretion. In the absence of their critical cofactor tetrahydrobiopterin (BH_4), or their substrate L-arginine, the NOS enzymes become uncoupled, such that they produce $O_2{}^{\cdot-}$ rather than NO. NOS uncoupling has been documented as a source of ROS in diseases such as hypertension, atherosclerosis, and diabetes and following ischemia and reperfusion injury. In several of these diseases, oral supplementation of BH_4 reverses NOS uncoupling, and improves endothelial function. Importantly, oral BH_4 blunts the elevation of blood pressure in angiotensin II– and salt-induced hypertension in animals and has been shown to lower blood pressure in humans with hypertension.[15–17] There seems to be interplay between overproduction of NO by inflammatory monocytes and uncoupling of the endothelial cell isoform of NOS.[18] Treatment with a tetrahydrobiopterin precursor reduces the pressor response and increase in sympathetic outflow that occurs in response to hand grip in subjects with chronic kidney disease.[19] Moreover, administration of BH_4 also prevents the development of endothelium dysfunction, vascular inflammation, and atherosclerosis induced by disturbed flow.[20,21] Acute and short-term administration of BH_4 improves endothelial function in humans with rheumatoid arthritis.[22] There is also convincing evidence that eNOS uncoupling occurs in humans with obstructive sleep apnea, leading to increased vascular superoxide production and endothelial dysfunction.[23] Thus, reversing NOS uncoupling is an attractive approach to improve endothelium function and prevent the pathogenesis of vascular diseases.

A major cause of NOS uncoupling is oxidation of tetrahydrobiopterin by oxidants, such as peroxynitrite. Interestingly, ROS produced by the NADPH oxidase play a role in this process, and mice lacking the NADPH oxidase are protected against tetrahydrobiopterin oxidation in the setting of hypertension.[10]

XANTHINE OXIDASE

Xanthine oxidoreductase (XOR) is another important source of ROS in mammalian cells. XOR exists in 2 forms, including xanthine dehydrogenase (XDH) and xanthine oxidase (XO). XDH transfers electrons from hypoxanthine and xanthine to nicotinamide adenine dinucleotide (NAD^+) yielding NADH and uric acid, whereas XO transfers electrons to oxygen from these same substrates to generate $O_2{}^{\cdot-}$ and H_2O_2. The cellular ratio of XO to XDH is therefore critical in modulating ROS production by these enzymes. XDH is converted to XO when a critical cysteine residue is oxidized by peroxynitrite.[24] This conversion is also favored in several pathophysiological settings, including inflammation,[25] hypoxia,[26] and radiation exposure,[27] and likely contributes to increased ROS production and in these situations. XO has been shown to contribute to experimental hypertension in animal models,[28–30] and there is accumulating evidence supporting a role of xanthine oxidase in human hypertension.[31–33] Although a recent study found no significant effect of the xanthine oxidase inhibitor allopurinol in blood pressure control in hypertensive humans,[34] a prior retrospective analysis of a large database showed that treatment with allopurinol was associated with a small (2.1 mm Hg) reduction of systolic blood pressure.[35] A carefully controlled randomized trial showed that 4 weeks of treatment of adolescents with allopurinol reduced systolic pressure by 6 mm Hg, whereas the placebo group had no change in pressure.[35] These effects of allopurinol could be due to lowering of uric acid, which is known to activate the inflammasome, or due to inhibition of xanthine oxidase. In one study, allopurinol markedly lowered blood pressure in obese adolescents with prehypertension, whereas the uricosuric agent probenecid had no effect.[36] These findings implicate XO, and potential ROS derived from this enzyme, as having an important role in adolescent prehypertension.

MITOCHONDRIA

The mitochondria are responsible for most ATP production in the cell. These organelles contain 5 enzyme complexes that comprise the electron transport chain. Electrons are transported sequentially from NADH through complexes I to V, the site of ATP generation. During normal mitochondrial function, this electron transfer from one complex to the next is efficient and there is minimal loss or leak from electron transport; however, in various disease states, electron leak is increased and can lead to reduction of oxygen and formation of $O_2{}^{\cdot-}$ and H_2O_2. Electron leak can occur at complexes I to IV, but occurs predominantly at complexes I and III due to defects in these complexes. These defects can include changes in their levels, posttranslational modifications like glutathionylation, or nitration. A recurring paradigm is that oxidative damage to mitochondrial DNA promotes deficiency in components of the electron transport chain, promoting electron leak. An important phenomenon is reverse electron transport, which occurs particularly in complex I in various pathophysiological states. Mitochondrial dysfunction is a major source of cellular ROS production in various pathophysiological states. Importantly, ROS from the NADPH oxidase have been shown to enter the mitochondria and promote electron leak and ROS production from the electron transport chain in hypertension.[37] Of note, antioxidants target the mitochondria and have proven effective in both preventing and reversing experimental hypertension.[38] Mitochondrial cyclophilin D (CypD) plays a critical role in opening of membrane transition pore, which depolarizes the mitochondria and enhances ROS production by this organelle. Recently it was found that pharmacologic inhibition or deletion of CypD in mice prevents ang II–induced hypertension.[39] Mitochondrial DNA fragments, indicative of mitochondrial damage, are increased in the urine of hypertensive humans and directly correlate with markers of renal injury in these individuals.[40]

ANTIOXIDANT DEFENSE MECHANISMS

Antioxidants are molecules that prevent the oxidation of other molecules often by being oxidized themselves. Due to our oxygen-rich atmosphere, all living organisms, including bacteria, plants, and animals, have adapted and developed enzymatic and nonenzymatic defenses against chronic oxidative stress. In mammalian cells, the major intracellular antioxidant enzymes include superoxide dismutase, catalase and glutathione peroxidase. As mentioned previously, SOD catalyzes the dismutation of $O_2{}^{\cdot-}$ to H_2O_2 and molecular O_2. Catalase and glutathione peroxidase further decompose H_2O_2 into H_2O and O_2. Glutathione peroxidase requires glutathione as a cosubstrate, yielding oxidized glutathione (GSSG) on reaction. In addition to H_2O_2, glutathione peroxidase also reduces lipid hydroperoxides to their respective alcohols and thus protects the cell membrane from lipid peroxidation. Glutathione peroxidase is also protective against $OONO^-$, which it efficiently reduces to nitrite.[41] Unlike $O_2{}^{\cdot-}$ or H_2O_2, the there are no enzymatic antioxidants that scavenge hydroxyl, but a variety of nonenzymatic antioxidants, including vitamin C (ascorbic acid), vitamin E (α-tocopherol), and glutathione, react with and eliminate this radical.

Mammalian cells have the capacity to modulate their antioxidant levels by transcriptional modulators such as Nrf2 and DJ-1. The former is a transcription factor that binds to the antioxidant response element of many genes, including the glutathione-S transferases, heme oxygenase 1, and glutamate-cysteine ligase, which controls glutathione synthesis.[42] Nrf2 is activated in the setting of oxidative stress, and moves to the nucleus to induce these and other important antioxidant genes. DJ-1 is a recently discovered protein that has antioxidant properties, and translocates to either the nucleus or the mitochondria on oxidative stress.[43] As discussed later in this article, DJ-1 plays a major role in the response of proximal tubular cells to dopamine, and ultimately regulates blood pressure.[44]

LIMITATIONS OF ANTIOXIDANT THERAPY

Although basic studies have strongly supported a role of ROS in cell dysfunction and animal models of disease, clinical trials with high-dose antioxidants have been disappointing. Numerous large clinical trials have failed to show beneficial effects of either vitamin C or vitamin E supplementation in cancer, cardiovascular disease, and neurodegenerative diseases.[45] A very recent meta-analysis of 50 randomized trials including almost 300,000 patients confirmed the futility of treatment with a variety of antioxidants in cardiovascular disease.[46] In hypertensive subjects, a few small trials initially showed benefit,[47,48] but, later large clinical trials, including the SU.VI.MAX study, showed no improvement in blood pressure with antioxidant therapy.[49,50] Surprisingly, large doses of beta-carotene, vitamin A, and vitamin E have paradoxically worsened cardiovascular outcomes in some studies.[51,52] The failure of antioxidants in humans might reflect the low rate constant of vitamins such as E and C with superoxide and related ROS, the inability to target subcellular sites in which ROS are formed, and that some ROS have beneficial effects. Prevention of ROS generation by inhibiting specific enzymatic sources might be more efficient than nonspecific antioxidants such as vitamins C and E. In this regard, a recent study showed that a Nox 1 inhibitor is effective in reducing atherosclerosis in mice with experimental diabetes.[53] It is also possible that these trials were negative because they did not target patients who actually have oxidative stress. As an example, the effect of vitamin E versus placebo was studied on cardiovascular outcomes in almost 1500 middle-aged diabetic patients with the haptoglobin 2/2 genotype.[54] The 2/2 genotype is associated with a reduction of the antioxidant properties of haptoglobin and therefore these patients were deemed to be at risk for oxidative stress. Vitamin E reduced all cardiovascular events, myocardial infarction, and stroke by 50% in this population. Because of this striking benefit of vitamin E, the study was stopped prematurely. It is also possible that more potent, catalytic agents, such as tempol, or targeted agents, such as mito-Tempol, which scavenges radicals specifically in the mitochondria, would have greater efficacy. This topic has been reviewed recently.[55]

Another drawback to the use of individual antioxidants is that individual agents are unlikely able to replenish deficiencies in multiple endogenous antioxidants that might be encountered in a disease like hypertension or caused by long-standing dietary indiscretion. For example, treatment with vitamin E would not be expected to restore selenium or ascorbate levels. In contrast, consumption of a diet rich in antioxidants might have a beneficial effect. As an example, the dietary approach to stop hypertension (DASH) study showed that a diet high in fruits and vegetables had a striking benefit in control of blood pressure.[56] Likewise, a recent study showed that grape seed extract, which contains numerous potential nutrients, was also effective in lowering blood pressure in subjects with prehypertension.[57]

POTENTIAL ROLES OF REACTIVE OXYGEN SPECIES IN HYPERTENSION

A large body of literature has shown that excessive production of ROS contributes to hypertension and that scavenging of ROS decreases blood pressure. Despite the evidence that oxidative stress contributes to hypertension, the mechanisms involved are not well understood. Hypertension is associated with increased ROS production by multiple organs, including the brain, the vasculature, and the kidney, all of which are likely important. A major problem is that we currently lack a complete understanding of which of these organs or cell types predominate in the genesis of hypertension or if there is important interplay between them that causes this disease. In the following section, we discuss evidence that ROS in the central nervous system (CNS), the kidney, and the vasculature contribute to hypertension, and we review recent data showing that the adaptive immunity is activated by oxidative events and can contribute to hypertension by interacting with these organs.

RENAL OXIDATIVE STRESS AND HYPERTENSION

There is ample evidence supporting that ROS generated in the kidney and its blood vessels contribute to the development and maintenance of hypertension. Virtually all cells in the kidney, including vessels, glomeruli, podocytes, interstitial fibroblasts, the medullary thick ascending limb (mTAL), the macula densa, the distal tubule, and the collecting duct express components of the NADPH oxidase, and various stimuli have been shown to activate these. Several of the effects of ROS in the kidney are summarized in **Fig. 2**. For purposes of discussion, we first focus on oxidative events in the renal cortex and then in the medulla.

Several studies have examined the effect of various hypertensive stimuli on the renal cortex and how these are modulated by ROS. The structures that are targets of oxidant stress include the afferent arteriole, the glomerulus, the proximal tubule, and the cortical collecting duct (CCD). As with other vessels, an increase in $O_2^{\cdot-}$ in

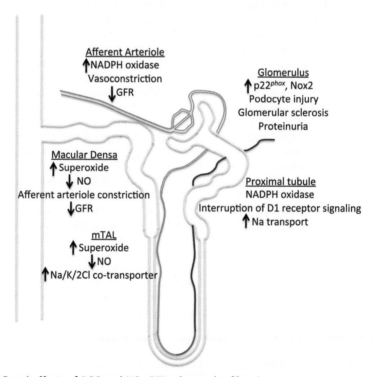

Fig. 2. Renal effects of ROS and NO. GFR, glomerular filtration rate.

the afferent arteriole can oxidatively degrade NO, which would enhance afferent arteriolar vasoconstriction and reduce glomerular filtration rate. Indeed, studies in rabbits have shown that ang II–induced hypertension increases expression of the NADPH oxidase subunit p22^{phox}, activates the NADPH oxidase and causes endothelial dysfunction in afferent arterioles.[58] Studies of isolated afferent arterioles have also shown that $O_2^{\cdot-}$ generated by the NADPH oxidase potentiates intracellular calcium.[59] ROS are also generated in the afferent arterioles of spontaneous hypertensive rats and in the kidney of animals in response to other vasoconstrictors such as endothelin-1 (ET-1) and thromboxane prostanoids.[60,61] A recent study has shown that $O_2^{\cdot-}$ enhances afferent arteriolar myogenic tone, while H_2O_2 inhibits this via actions on voltage-gated potassium channels.[62] These findings illustrate the complexity of attempting to scavenge all ROS to improve renal perfusion.

Podocyte injury causes proteinuria and is a precursor to glomerulosclerosis. Moreover, proteinuria seems to promote further podocyte injury in a feed-forward fashion. Dahl salt-sensitive rats demonstrate upregulation of glomerular p22^{phox} and Nox2 and the antioxidant tempol reduces glomerular sclerosis and proteinuria in these animals.[63,64] Recent evidence has implicated a role of plasminogen in stimulating expression of Nox2 and Nox4 in podocytes and causing podocyte injury.[65] Ang II also stimulates mitochondria ROS generation and induces podocyte autophagy.[66] Oxidative injury impairs the crosstalk between nephrin and caveolin-1 in podocytes, leading to disruption of glomerular filtration barrier.[67] ROS also mediate mesangial cell proliferation, migration, and extracellular matrix deposition, features characteristic of glomerulosclerosis induced by angiotensin II or aldosterone.[68] Mice lacking p47^{phox} are protected against the development of glomerulosclerosis and albuminuria following either Adriamycin injection or 5/6 nephrectomy, supporting a role of the NADPH oxidase in this common form of glomerular injury.[69]

Components of the NADPH oxidase exist in lipid rafts within epithelial cells of the proximal tubule, where they are maintained in an inactive state. Dopamine-1 (D1) receptor agonists inhibit, whereas disruption of lipid rafts and angiotensin II stimulate the proximal tubule NADPH oxidase function.[70,71] ROS from the NADPH oxidase modulate sodium transport via altering Na/K-ATPase and Na/H exchange-3 (NHE-3) function on the basal and apical membranes of the proximal tubular cells, respectively.[72,73] Deletion of the dopamine D2 receptor (D2R) inhibits ROS production in renal proximal tubular cells and leads to hypertension, supporting a role of ROS in the proximal tubule in blood pressure control.[44]

An important mechanism by which ROS in the cortex modulates sodium reuptake and blood pressure is via tubuloglomerular feedback. This is mediated by an interaction of the macula densa of the thick ascending limb as it makes contact with its own glomerulus in the cortex. Sodium concentration is sensed by the macula densa via its apical Na/K/2Cl cotransporter, which in turn stimulates NO produced by the neuronal NOS. This promotes dilatation of afferent arterioles and increases glomerular filtration.[74,75] Increases in $O_2^{\cdot-}$ in macula densa can inactivate NO, leading to afferent arteriolar vasoconstriction and a reduction of glomerular filtration rate.[76] An elegant study of isolated, single nephrons by Nouri and colleagues[77] showed that in vivo RNA silencing of the NADPH oxidase subunit p22^{phox} enhances single tubular glomerular filtration in angiotensin II–treated rats but not in control rats. By either including or excluding the distal tubule, these investigators showed that this effect was likely mediated by ROS produced in the macula densa.

The epithelial Na$^+$ channel (ENaC) mediates final tubular adjustment of Na$^+$ reabsorption in the CCD.[78] Angiotensin II activates the NADPH oxidase in the CCD, stimulating ENaC activity.[79] This is likely mediated by aldosterone, the principal regulator of ENaC activity. Aldosterone induces superoxide generation in A6 epithelial cells, which in turn reduces inhibition of ENaC by NO.[80] A similar pathway modulates ENaC activity in response to insulin, the insulinlike growth factor, and the epidermal growth factor.[81]

Oxidative stress also modulates sodium reabsorption and blood pressure in the renal medulla. As in the blood vessel, there is a balance between $O_2^{\cdot-}$ and NO produced by epithelial cells of the medullary thick ascending limb (mTAL) and the pericytes of the vasa recta. NO synthase activity is higher in the renal medulla than in the cortex, likely contributing to independent regulation of medullary and cortical perfusion.[82] Cowley's group has shown that NO released by cells of the mTAL promotes dilation of the adjacent vasa recta, increasing medullary flow. This augments interstitial Starling forces and promotes sodium movement to the tubule and thus natriuresis and diuresis.[83,84] Activation of the NADPH oxidase in the medulla has the opposite effect: promoting vasa recta vasoconstriction, sodium movement into the vasa recta, reducing natriuresis and increasing blood pressure. A growing body of evidence indicates that medullary $O_2^{\cdot-}$ affects sodium transport.[85,86] Superoxide enhances Na/K/2Cl cotransporter activity via a protein kinase C activation in mTAL preparations.[87] Infusion of angiotensin II in vivo mimics this effect and administration of the O_2^- scavenger tempol prevents this.[88] NO has the opposite effect on NaCl transport in the mTAL. NO generated by eNOS inhibits the Na/K/2Cl cotransporter and NHE-3 in isolated thick ascending limb.[89] This inhibitory effect on the Na/K/2Cl cotransporter is mediated by phosphodiesterase-mediated degradation of cyclic AMP while NO directly inhibits NHE-3.[90] Of interest, increased sodium delivery to cells of the mTAL stimulates H_2O_2 production by the mitochondria, and this is linked to vasodilatation of the nearby vasa recta.[91]

The role of ROS in control of renal perfusion and sodium handling likely illustrates a normal physiologic role of these molecules and shows that they are not uniformly deleterious. The kidney must retain sodium and water during times of salt deprivation, and in land-dwelling mammals, survival would be impossible without this. It is therefore likely that generation of $O_2^{\cdot-}$ and other ROS within the kidney play a crucial role in this important physiologic process.

REACTIVE OXYGEN SPECIES, THE CENTRAL NERVOUS SYSTEM, AND HYPERTENSION

It is now obvious that the CNS is essential for production and maintenance of most forms of experimental hypertension, principally by enhancing sympathetic efferent outflow. Even the hypertension caused by hormones, such as angiotensin II and aldosterone, which have myriad systemic effects, is importantly mediated by actions in the CNS.[92,93] As an illustration of this, the development of many forms of experimental hypertension is prevented by destruction of a region of the forebrain surrounding the anteroventral third cerebral ventricle (AV3V) in rodents.[94,95] This region includes the median preoptic eminence, the organum vasculosum of the lateral terminalis, and the preoptic periventricular nucleus (**Fig. 3**).[96] Following AV3V lesioning, virtually all of the central actions of angiotensin II, including drinking behavior, vasopressin secretion, and increased sympathetic outflow, are diminished or eliminated. These portions of the forebrain are connected to other regions involved in central cardiovascular regulation. Important among these are the subfornical organ (SFO) and the organum vasculosum of the lamina terminalis (OVLT), which are circumventricular organs (CVO) lacking a blood-brain barrier. Other CVOs include the median eminence and the area postrema. Hormones in the periphery can act on these regions, modulating neuronal input into cardiovascular control centers in the midbrain and hindbrain,

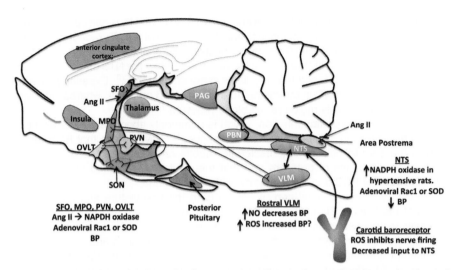

Fig. 3. Sites in the brain implicated in hypertension. Shown also are documented actions of ROS and NO to modulate central control of blood pressure (BP). PAG, periaqueductal gray; PBN, parabrachial nucleus; PVN, paraventricular nucleus; SON, supraoptic nucleus.

including the parabrachial nucleus, the nucleus tractus solitarius (NTS), and the rostral ventral lateral medulla (VLM) (see **Fig. 3**).

There is strong evidence that signaling in these brain centers and their influence on blood pressure is modulated by local production of ROS.[97] Intracerebroventricular (ICV) injection of an adenovirus encoding SOD attenuates the hypertension caused by either local injection or systemic infusion of angiotensin II.[98] Zimmerman and colleagues[99] showed that angiotensin II stimulates $O_2{}^{\cdot-}$ production in cultured neurons and that this increases intracellular calcium. Peterson and colleagues,[100] using selective small-interfering RNA–expressing adenoviruses, have shown that Nox2 and Nox4 have different roles in the SFO, such that both are linked to blood pressure regulation, but only Nox2 modulates drinking behavior. Lob and colleagues[101] used Cre-Lox technology to delete p22^{phox} in the SFO and showed that this completely abrogated the hypertensive response to long-term infusion of angiotensin II.

There is also evidence that ROS derived from the NADPH oxidase enhances nerve firing within the hypothalamus. ICV injection of angiotensin II increases NADPH oxidase–mediated $O_2{}^{\cdot-}$ production not only in the SFO but also in anterior hypothalamic nuclei such as the median preoptic eminence and in the paraventricular nucleus of the hypothalamus.[102] These effects were blocked by the NADPH oxidase inhibitor apocynin, as were the hemodynamic effects of centrally administered angiotensin II. Thus, angiotensin II and its effects on the NADPH oxidase seem to coordinate activation of several forebrain centers to promote a hypertensive response.

Signaling between the forebrain and the hindbrain pontomedullary cardiovascular control centers is also important for blood pressure control. The NTS is such a hindbrain nucleus that receives input from the CVO and relays inhibitory stimuli from baroreceptors. Angiotensin II augments ROS production by the NADPH oxidase in neurons from the NTS, and this in turn activates L-type calcium channel activity and neuronal firing.[103] NADPH oxidase is increased in the NTS of stroke-prone, spontaneously hypertensive rats.[104] H_2O_2 causes delayed hyperexcitability of NTS neurons via actions on barium sensitive potassium channels. This might be expected to enhance sympathetic outflow in vivo.[105]

As discussed previously, NO can be consumed by $O_2{}^{\cdot-}$ and thus can act as a radical scavenger. NO produced in response to ang II stimulation of the AT_2 receptor limits the effects of $O_2{}^{\cdot-}$ in the medial NTS and thus inhibits L-type channel activation.[106] NO has a similar role in the ventral lateral medulla, which lies below the NTS and receives and sends signals to the NTS and thus regulates sympathetic tone.[107] Experimental interventions that increase NO in the rostral VLM lower blood pressure, whereas increase in oxidative stress in this region raises blood pressure.[108,109]

ROS modulate baroreflex function, which is commonly abnormal in the setting of chronic hypertension. Studies by Li and colleagues[110] have shown that ROS generated in the carotid bulb of atherosclerotic rabbits reduce carotid sinus nerve responses to elevations of pressure and that this could be mimicked by exogenous administration of ROS and prevented by ROS scavenging.

Efferent sympathetic renal nerves govern both the vasculature and tubular segments of the kidney. Stimulation of the renal sympathetic nerves promotes afferent arteriolar vasoconstriction and renin release and increases Na+ reabsorption.[111] Alpha1 adrenergic receptor activation enhances ROS generation and constriction of the afferent arterioles, reducing renal blood flow in angiotensin II–infused rabbits.[112] In contrast, β1 adrenergic receptor activation inhibits ROS generation and promotes vasodilation.[113] In keeping with these important roles of renal sympathetic nerves in controlling renal ROS production, renal denervation blunts blood pressure elevation in multiple experimental hypertensive models, including angiotensin II–induced, DOCA-salt, and 2 kidney one clip hypertension, as well as spontaneous hypertensive rat (SHR) and SHR stroke-prone (SHRSP) rats.[114] The role of renal denervation to control human hypertension remains a topic of debate.

A consequence of renal denervation is ablation of the renal afferent nerves. These are mainly located in the renal pelvis and are activated by various physical and chemical stimuli.[115] During kidney injury, increased input from these afferent nerves activates central sympathetic nuclei in a ROS-dependent manner.[116] For instance, renal denervation prevents release of norepinephrine from the posterior hypothalamic nuclei and blood pressure elevation following kidney injury induced intrarenal phenol injection.[117] Intrarenal phenol injection increases NADPH oxidase expression in the central nuclei and this is prevented by ICV injection of the SOD mimetic tempol or PEG-SOD. Interestingly, a vitamin E–fortified diet blunts the increase of sympathetic nerve activity and hypertension in response to intrarenal phenol injection.[118] These data indicate that ROS modulate both efferent and afferent renal nerve activity and therefore promote development of hypertension.

VASCULAR OXIDATIVE STRESS AND HYPERTENSION

Elevated vascular ROS promote the development of hypertension in various animal models, including angiotensin II–induced and DOCA-salt hypertension,[9,119,120] Dahl salt-sensitive hypertension, and the SHR.[121–123] Humans with hypertension have alterations of vascular reactivity. The several mechanisms by which ROS modulate the vasculature are illustrated in **Fig. 4**.

The endothelium regulates vascular tone via releasing of endothelium-derived relaxing factors (EDRFs) and endothelium-derived contractile factors. Oxidative stress causes imbalanced production and bioavailability of these molecules, leading to endothelial dysfunction. NO is one of the most important mediators of endothelium-dependent relaxation in blood pressure regulation. The major mechanism for alteration of NO bioavailability when $O_2{}^{\cdot-}$ is increased is that this radical rapidly reacts with NO, as discussed previously. Uncoupling of endothelial NOS,

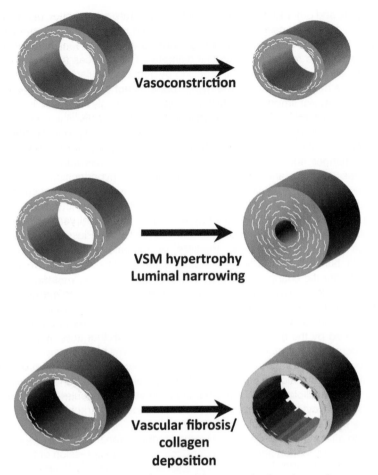

Fig. 4. Mechanisms by which ROS and NO modulate vascular function and structure in hypertension. VSM, vascular smooth muscle.

due to deprivation of its cofactor tetrahydrobiopterin, results in reduced NO release, increased $O_2{}^{\cdot-}$ production, impaired endothelium-dependent relaxation, and elevated arterial pressure. Similarly, a lack of the eNOS substrate L-arginine also reduces NO bioavailability and impairs NO-induced dilation. L-arginine is the substrate for both eNOS and arginase, and increased arginase activity reduces the local bioavailability of L-arginine.[124] Interestingly, peroxynitrite and hydrogen peroxide increase the expression and activity of arginase in endothelial cells, potentially contributing to endothelial dysfunction.[125]

Oxidation of membrane fatty acids and in particular arachidonic acid can lead to formation of F_2-isoprostanes, which are present in the blood of patients with oxidative stress (eg, those with hypercholesterolemia or diabetes, and cigarette smokers). Importantly, plasma F2-isoprostanes are increased in animals with experimental hypertension and in humans with renovascular hypertension.[126,127] These oxidatively modified fatty acids act on prostaglandin H/thromboxane receptors to enhance vasoconstriction.

Superoxide and other ROS can also affect the structure and function of the vascular media. An important consequence of ROS formation is vascular smooth muscle hypertrophy. Eutrophic vascular remodeling leads to an increase in medial thickness at the expense of a reduction in luminal diameter. This reduces the cross-sectional area of the effective vasculature, increasing systemic vascular resistance.[128] H_2O_2 seems to be a major mediator of the hypertrophic effect of angiotensin II in cultured cells,[129] and vascular smooth muscle hypertrophy is strikingly increased in mice over-expressing the NADPH oxidase in the vascular smooth muscle.[130]

Vascular ROS also stimulate the production of collagen and fibronectin both in vitro and in vivo,[131,132] and removal of vascular ROS prevents these fibrotic changes.[133,134] Structural changes such as these in resistance vessels could add to the increased systemic vascular resistance that occurs in established hypertension and, therefore, worsen the disease.[135,136] In larger central arteries, this leads to loss of the Windkessel effect, and increases pulse wave velocity. In population studies, increased pulse wave velocity precedes the development of hypertension by several years. There is substantial evidence that ROS contribute to vascular stiffening. Plasma levels of myeloperoxidase and F_2-isoprostanes, markers of oxidation, correlate with arterial stiffening in humans.[137] Studies in experimental animals have shown that ROS contribute to fibrotic changes in several tissues including blood vessels.[138,139]

Endothelium-dependent hyperpolarization represents an NO-independent mechanism of vasodilatation that is particularly important in resistance vessels.[140] The nature of the endothelium-derived hyperpolarizing factor (EDHF) remains a topic of study, but H_2O_2 produced by the mitochondria is clearly one EDHF that acts by activating the Ca++-dependent potassium (BK) channel.[141] This seems to be an important mechanism of flow-mediated vasodilatation in human coronary arterioles. The production of H_2O_2 is mediated by calcium entry into endothelial cells through the transient receptor potential (TRP) vanilloid type 4 (TRPV4) channel in several vascular beds.[142] Another EDHF is likely a cytochrome p450 epoxide metabolite of arachidonic acid, which also opens the TRPV4 channel.[143,144]

H_2O_2 also affects the NO–cyclic guanosine monophosphate pathway. H_2O_2 acutely stimulates NO production and over the long term induces expression of the endothelial NO synthase (NOS3).[119,145,146] H_2O_2 also activates protein kinase G (PKG) by inducing cross-linking 2 alpha subunits of this enzyme via disulfide bond formation, and therefore promotes vasodilation independent of NO.

REACTIVE OXYGEN SPECIES, INFLAMMATION, AND HYPERTENSION

Diverse stimuli common to the hypertensive milieu, including angiotensin II, aldosterone, catecholamines, increased vascular stretch, and endothelin promote ROS production, which then increases expression of proinflammatory molecules that cause rolling, adhesion, and transcytosis of inflammatory cells.[147,148] As a result, there is a striking accumulation of inflammatory cells in the vessel and kidney.[149–151] In keeping with this, there is an increase in plasma markers of inflammation in hypertensive humans.[152,153] Although macrophages are commonly considered important in the genesis of cardiovascular disease, increasing evidence has accumulated suggesting that the adaptive immune response and, in particular, T lymphocytes are important in hypertension. Mice and rats lacking the *Rag1* gene are partly protected against the blood pressure elevation and renal damage caused by angiotensin II or salt.[154–156] Effector T cells enter the kidney and the perivascular fat, where they release cytokines that promote salt retention and vasoconstriction, ultimately promoting hypertension. These cells mediate their effect by producing cytokines that potently affect vascular and renal function, including tumor necrosis factor–α, interferon-γ and interleukin (IL)-17A (**Fig. 5**). Mice lacking IL-17A do not sustain angiotensin II–induced hypertension, and treatment with soluble IL-17C lowers blood pressure and prevents oxidative stress in experimental preeclampsia.[157,158] IL-17A directly evokes endothelial dysfunction and ROS production in isolated vessels and causes hypertension when infused in mice.[159] Recent data indicate that IL-17A modulates expression and function of the sodium hydrogen exchanger 3 and sodium chloride cotransporter in renal tubular epithelial cells, thus promoting sodium reuptake by these cells.[160] IL-17A also promotes aortic stiffening and directly stimulates production of collagen by aortic fibroblasts.[161]

Recently, we identified a novel mechanism linking oxidative events and immune activation in hypertension. This involves formation of isolevuglandins (isoLGs), which are a form of reactive carbonyl produced on oxidation of fatty acids and phospholipids. These react rapidly with lysines on proteins and we found that hypertension increases formation of isoLG-modified proteins in monocyte-derived dendritic cells of mice and in monocytes of humans. These modified proteins seem immunogenic (**Fig. 6**).[4] We have found that isoLG-modified peptides are presented in major histocompatibility complexes and can promote T-cell activation. Chronic vascular oxidant stress also seems to enhance formation of these and their accumulation in dendritic cells.[162]

The observation that circulating cells, including T cells and monocytes, are important in the genesis of hypertension might help provide a unifying link between oxidative events in the CNS, the vasculature, and the kidney. These interactions, illustrated in **Fig. 6**, are dependent on ROS formation in all of these sites. Centrally, in the SFO, and other CVOs, NADPH oxidase activation increases neuronal firing and sympathetic nerve outflow to peripheral lymphoid tissues, leading to T-cell activation.[163] In

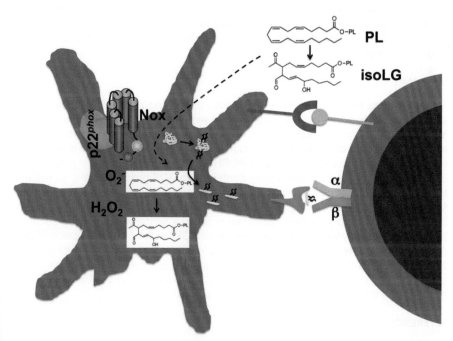

Fig. 5. Formation of isoLGs in antigen-presenting cells and modification of self-proteins leading to T-cell activation.

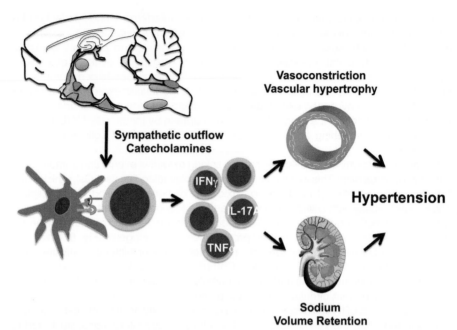

Fig. 6. Interplay between immune activation, the CNS, the vasculature, and the kidney in hypertension. IFN, interferon; TNF, tumor necrosis factor.

dendritic cells, ROS lead to isoLG formation and modification of self-proteins. ROS in the kidney and vessels initiates signal that cause T cell homing and infiltration.[149] Finally, cytokines released by T cells diffuse to renal and vascular cells, promoting further NADPH oxidase activation, sodium retention, and vasoconstriction, leading to overt hypertension.

SUMMARY

This review has summarized some of the data supporting a role of ROS and oxidant stress in hypertension. There is evidence that hypertensive stimuli, such as high salt and angiotensin II, promote production of ROS in the brain, the kidney, and the vasculature and that each of these sites contributes either to hypertension or to the untoward sequelae of this disease. Although the NADPH oxidase in these various organs is a predominant source, other enzymes likely contribute to ROS production and signaling in these tissues. A major clinical challenge is that the routinely used antioxidants are ineffective in preventing or treating cardiovascular disease and hypertension. This is likely because these drugs are either ineffective or act in a nontargeted fashion, such that they remove not only injurious but also beneficial ROS involved in normal cell signaling. An important and relatively new concept is that inflammatory cells contribute to hypertension in a ROS-dependent fashion. Future studies are needed to understand the interaction of inflammatory cells with the CNS, the kidney, and the vasculature and how this might be interrupted to provide therapeutic benefit.

REFERENCES

1. Liochev SI. Reactive oxygen species and the free radical theory of aging. Free Radic Biol Med 2013;60:1–4.

2. Shin MH, Moon YJ, Seo JE, et al. Reactive oxygen species produced by NADPH oxidase, xanthine oxidase, and mitochondrial electron transport system mediate heat shock-induced MMP-1 and MMP-9 expression. Free Radic Biol Med 2008; 44:635–45.
3. Semchyshyn HM. Reactive carbonyl species in vivo: generation and dual biological effects. ScientificWorldJournal 2014;2014:417842.
4. Kirabo A, Fontana V, de Faria AP, et al. DC isoketal-modified proteins activate T cells and promote hypertension. J Clin Invest 2014;124:4642–56.
5. Guzik TJ, Chen W, Gongora MC, et al. Calcium-dependent NOX5 nicotinamide adenine dinucleotide phosphate oxidase contributes to vascular oxidative stress in human coronary artery disease. J Am Coll Cardiol 2008;52:1803–9.
6. Lyle AN, Deshpande NN, Taniyama Y, et al. Poldip2, a novel regulator of Nox4 and cytoskeletal integrity in vascular smooth muscle cells. Circ Res 2009;105: 249–59.
7. Seshiah PN, Weber DS, Rocic P, et al. Angiotensin II stimulation of NAD(P)H oxidase activity: upstream mediators. Circ Res 2002;91:406–13.
8. Takac I, Schroder K, Zhang L, et al. The E-loop is involved in hydrogen peroxide formation by the NADPH oxidase Nox4. J Biol Chem 2011;286:13304–13.
9. Landmesser U, Cai H, Dikalov S, et al. Role of p47(phox) in vascular oxidative stress and hypertension caused by angiotensin II. Hypertension 2002;40:511–5.
10. Landmesser U, Dikalov S, Price SR, et al. Oxidation of tetrahydrobiopterin leads to uncoupling of endothelial cell nitric oxide synthase in hypertension. J Clin Invest 2003;111:1201–9.
11. Dikalova A, Clempus R, Lassegue B, et al. Nox1 overexpression potentiates angiotensin II–induced hypertension and vascular smooth muscle hypertrophy in transgenic mice. Circulation 2005;112:2668–76.
12. Gavazzi G, Banfi B, Deffert C, et al. Decreased blood pressure in NOX1-deficient mice. FEBS Lett 2006;580:497–504.
13. Cowley AW Jr, Yang C, Zheleznova NN, et al. Evidence of the importance of Nox4 in production of hypertension in Dahl salt-sensitive rats. Hypertension 2016;67:440–50.
14. Holterman CE, Thibodeau JF, Towaij C, et al. Nephropathy and elevated BP in mice with podocyte-specific NADPH oxidase 5 expression. J Am Soc Nephrol 2014;25:784–97.
15. Harrison DG, Chen W, Dikalov S, et al. Regulation of endothelial cell tetrahydrobiopterin pathophysiological and therapeutic implications. Adv Pharmacol 2010;60:107–32.
16. Chen W, Li L, Brod T, et al. Role of increased guanosine triphosphate cyclohydrolase-1 expression and tetrahydrobiopterin levels upon T cell activation. J Biol Chem 2011;286:13846–51.
17. Porkert M, Sher S, Reddy U, et al. Tetrahydrobiopterin: a novel antihypertensive therapy. J Hum Hypertens 2008;22:401–7.
18. Kossmann S, Hu H, Steven S, et al. Inflammatory monocytes determine endothelial nitric-oxide synthase uncoupling and nitro-oxidative stress induced by angiotensin II. J Biol Chem 2014;289:27540–50.
19. Lin AM, Liao P, Millson EC, et al. Tetrahydrobiopterin ameliorates the exaggerated exercise pressor response in patients with chronic kidney disease: a randomized controlled trial. Am J Physiol Renal Physiol 2016;310:F1016–25.
20. Li L, Chen W, Rezvan A, et al. Tetrahydrobiopterin deficiency and nitric oxide synthase uncoupling contribute to atherosclerosis induced by disturbed flow. Arterioscler Thromb Vasc Biol 2011;31:1547–54.

21. Hofmeister LH, Lee SH, Norlander AE, et al. Phage-display-guided nanocarrier targeting to atheroprone vasculature. ACS Nano 2015;9:4435–46.

22. Maki-Petaja KM, Day L, Cheriyan J, et al. Tetrahydrobiopterin supplementation improves endothelial function but does not alter aortic stiffness in patients with rheumatoid arthritis. J Am Heart Assoc 2016;5(2):e002762.

23. Varadharaj S, Porter K, Pleister A, et al. Endothelial nitric oxide synthase uncoupling: a novel pathway in OSA induced vascular endothelial dysfunction. Respir Physiol Neurobiol 2015;207:40–7.

24. Sakuma S, Fujimoto Y, Sakamoto Y, et al. Peroxynitrite induces the conversion of xanthine dehydrogenase to oxidase in rabbit liver. Biochem Biophys Res Commun 1997;230:476–9.

25. Friedl HP, Till GO, Ryan US, et al. Mediator-induced activation of xanthine oxidase in endothelial cells. FASEB J 1989;3:2512–8.

26. Sohn HY, Krotz F, Gloe T, et al. Differential regulation of xanthine and NAD(P)H oxidase by hypoxia in human umbilical vein endothelial cells. Role of nitric oxide and adenosine. Cardiovasc Res 2003;58:638–46.

27. Kale RK. Post-irradiation free radical generation: evidence from the conversion of xanthine dehydrogenase into xanthine oxidase. Indian J Exp Biol 2003;41: 105–11.

28. Suzuki H, DeLano FA, Parks DA, et al. Xanthine oxidase activity associated with arterial blood pressure in spontaneously hypertensive rats. Proc Natl Acad Sci U S A 1998;95:4754–9.

29. Swei A, Lacy F, Delano FA, et al. A mechanism of oxygen free radical production in the Dahl hypertensive rat. Microcirculation 1999;6:179–87.

30. Shirakura T, Nomura J, Matsui C, et al. Febuxostat, a novel xanthine oxidoreductase inhibitor, improves hypertension and endothelial dysfunction in spontaneously hypertensive rats. Naunyn Schmiedebergs Arch Pharmacol 2016; 389(8):831–8.

31. Cardillo C, Kilcoyne CM, Cannon RO 3rd, et al. Xanthine oxidase inhibition with oxypurinol improves endothelial vasodilator function in hypercholesterolemic but not in hypertensive patients. Hypertension 1997;30:57–63.

32. Butler R, Morris AD, Belch JJ, et al. Allopurinol normalizes endothelial dysfunction in type 2 diabetics with mild hypertension. Hypertension 2000;35:746–51.

33. Kohagura K, Tana T, Higa A, et al. Effects of xanthine oxidase inhibitors on renal function and blood pressure in hypertensive patients with hyperuricemia. Hypertens Res 2016;39(8):593–7.

34. Segal MS, Srinivas TR, Mohandas R, et al. The effect of the addition of allopurinol on blood pressure control in African Americans treated with a thiazide-like diuretic. J Am Soc Hypertens 2015;9:610–9.e1.

35. Feig DI, Soletsky B, Johnson RJ. Effect of allopurinol on blood pressure of adolescents with newly diagnosed essential hypertension: a randomized trial. JAMA 2008;300:924–32.

36. Soletsky B, Feig DI. Uric acid reduction rectifies prehypertension in obese adolescents. Hypertension 2012;60:1148–56.

37. Doughan AK, Harrison DG, Dikalov SI. Molecular mechanisms of angiotensin II-mediated mitochondrial dysfunction: linking mitochondrial oxidative damage and vascular endothelial dysfunction. Circ Res 2008;102:488–96.

38. Dikalova AE, Bikineyeva AT, Budzyn K, et al. Therapeutic targeting of mitochondrial superoxide in hypertension. Circ Res 2010;107:106–16.

39. Itani HA, Dikalova AE, McMaster WG, et al. Mitochondrial cyclophilin D in vascular oxidative stress and hypertension. Hypertension 2016;67:1218–27.

40. Eirin A, Saad A, Tang H, et al. Urinary mitochondrial DNA copy number identifies chronic renal injury in hypertensive patients. Hypertension 2016;68(2):401–10.
41. Arteel GE, Briviba K, Sies H. Protection against peroxynitrite. FEBS Lett 1999; 445:226–30.
42. Kansanen E, Kuosmanen SM, Leinonen H, et al. The Keap1-Nrf2 pathway: mechanisms of activation and dysregulation in cancer. Redox Biol 2013;1:45–9.
43. Duan X, Kelsen SG, Merali S. Proteomic analysis of oxidative stress-responsive proteins in human pneumocytes: insight into the regulation of DJ-1 expression. J Proteome Res 2008;7:4955–61.
44. Cuevas S, Zhang Y, Yang Y, et al. Role of renal DJ-1 in the pathogenesis of hypertension associated with increased reactive oxygen species production. Hypertension 2012;59:446–52.
45. Lonn E, Bosch J, Yusuf S, et al. Effects of long-term vitamin E supplementation on cardiovascular events and cancer: a randomized controlled trial. JAMA 2005;293:1338–47.
46. Myung SK, Ju W, Cho B, et al. Efficacy of vitamin and antioxidant supplements in prevention of cardiovascular disease: systematic review and meta-analysis of randomised controlled trials. BMJ 2013;346:f10.
47. Duffy SJ, Gokce N, Holbrook M, et al. Treatment of hypertension with ascorbic acid. Lancet 1999;354:2048–9.
48. Mullan BA, Young IS, Fee H, et al. Ascorbic acid reduces blood pressure and arterial stiffness in type 2 diabetes. Hypertension 2002;40:804–9.
49. Czernichow S, Bertrais S, Blacher J, et al. Effect of supplementation with antioxidants upon long-term risk of hypertension in the SU.VI.MAX study: association with plasma antioxidant levels. J Hypertens 2005;23:2013–8.
50. Kim MK, Sasaki S, Sasazuki S, et al. Lack of long-term effect of vitamin C supplementation on blood pressure. Hypertension 2002;40:797–803.
51. Miller ER 3rd, Pastor-Barriuso R, Dalal D, et al. Meta-analysis: high-dosage vitamin E supplementation may increase all-cause mortality. Ann Intern Med 2005;142:37–46.
52. Bjelakovic G, Nikolova D, Gluud LL, et al. Mortality in randomized trials of antioxidant supplements for primary and secondary prevention: systematic review and meta-analysis. JAMA 2007;297:842–57.
53. Gray SP, Di Marco E, Okabe J, et al. NADPH oxidase 1 plays a key role in diabetes mellitus-accelerated atherosclerosis. Circulation 2013;127:1888–902.
54. Milman U, Blum S, Shapira C, et al. Vitamin E supplementation reduces cardiovascular events in a subgroup of middle-aged individuals with both type 2 diabetes mellitus and the haptoglobin 2-2 genotype: a prospective double-blinded clinical trial. Arterioscler Thromb Vasc Biol 2008;28:341–7.
55. Dikalov SI, Dikalova AE. Contribution of mitochondrial oxidative stress to hypertension. Curr Opin Nephrol Hypertens 2016;25:73–80.
56. Sacks FM, Svetkey LP, Vollmer WM, et al. Effects on blood pressure of reduced dietary sodium and the dietary approaches to stop hypertension (DASH) diet. Dash-sodium collaborative research group. N Engl J Med 2001;344:3–10.
57. Park E, Edirisinghe I, Choy YY, et al. Effects of grape seed extract beverage on blood pressure and metabolic indices in individuals with pre-hypertension: a randomised, double-blinded, two-arm, parallel, placebo-controlled trial. Br J Nutr 2016;115:226–38.
58. Wang D, Chen Y, Chabrashvili T, et al. Role of oxidative stress in endothelial dysfunction and enhanced responses to angiotensin II of afferent arterioles from rabbits infused with angiotensin II. J Am Soc Nephrol 2003;14:2783–9.

59. Fellner SK, Arendshorst WJ. Angiotensin II, reactive oxygen species, and Ca2+ signaling in afferent arterioles. Am J Physiol Renal Physiol 2005;289:F1012–9.
60. Chabrashvili T, Kitiyakara C, Blau J, et al. Effects of ANG II type 1 and 2 receptors on oxidative stress, renal NADPH oxidase, and SOD expression. Am J Physiol Regul Integr Comp Physiol 2003;285:R117–24.
61. Araujo M, Wilcox CS. Oxidative stress in hypertension: role of the kidney. Antioxid Redox Signal 2014;20(1):74–101.
62. Li L, Lai EY, Wellstein A, et al. Differential effects of superoxide and hydrogen peroxide on myogenic signaling, membrane potential, and contractions of mouse renal afferent arterioles. Am J Physiol Renal Physiol 2016;310:F1197–205.
63. Nagase M, Shibata S, Yoshida S, et al. Podocyte injury underlies the glomerulopathy of Dahl salt-hypertensive rats and is reversed by aldosterone blocker. Hypertension 2006;47:1084–93.
64. Meng S, Cason GW, Gannon AW, et al. Oxidative stress in Dahl salt-sensitive hypertension. Hypertension 2003;41:1346–52.
65. Raij L, Tian R, Wong JS, et al. Podocyte injury: the role of proteinuria, urinary plasminogen and oxidative stress. Am J Physiol Renal Physiol 2016. [Epub ahead of print].
66. Jia J, Ding G, Zhu J, et al. Angiotensin II infusion induces nephrin expression changes and podocyte apoptosis. Am J Nephrol 2008;28:500–7.
67. Ren Z, Liang W, Chen C, et al. Angiotensin II induces nephrin dephosphorylation and podocyte injury: role of caveolin-1. Cell Signal 2012;24:443–50.
68. Hua P, Feng W, Rezonzew G, et al. The transcription factor ETS-1 regulates angiotensin II-stimulated fibronectin production in mesangial cells. Am J Physiol Renal Physiol 2012;302:F1418–29.
69. Wang H, Chen X, Su Y, et al. p47(phox) contributes to albuminuria and kidney fibrosis in mice. Kidney Int 2015;87:948–62.
70. Banday AA, Lokhandwala MF. Loss of biphasic effect on Na/K-ATPase activity by angiotensin II involves defective angiotensin type 1 receptor-nitric oxide signaling. Hypertension 2008;52:1099–105.
71. Han W, Li H, Villar VA, et al. Lipid rafts keep NADPH oxidase in the inactive state in human renal proximal tubule cells. Hypertension 2008;51:481–7.
72. Banday AA, Fazili FR, Lokhandwala MF. Oxidative stress causes renal dopamine D1 receptor dysfunction and hypertension via mechanisms that involve nuclear factor-kappaB and protein kinase C. J Am Soc Nephrol 2007;18:1446–57.
73. Banday AA, Lau YS, Lokhandwala MF. Oxidative stress causes renal dopamine D1 receptor dysfunction and salt-sensitive hypertension in Sprague-Dawley rats. Hypertension 2008;51:367–75.
74. Deng A, Baylis C. Locally produced EDRF controls preglomerular resistance and ultrafiltration coefficient. Am J Physiol 1993;264:F212–5.
75. Vallon V, Traynor T, Barajas L, et al. Feedback control of glomerular vascular tone in neuronal nitric oxide synthase knockout mice. J Am Soc Nephrol 2001;12:1599–606.
76. Liu R, Ren Y, Garvin JL, et al. Superoxide enhances tubuloglomerular feedback by constricting the afferent arteriole. Kidney Int 2004;66:268–74.
77. Nouri P, Gill P, Li M, et al. p22phox in the macula densa regulates single nephron GFR during angiotensin II infusion in rats. Am J Physiol Heart Circ Physiol 2007;292:H1685–9.
78. Sun Y, Zhang JN, Zhao D, et al. Role of the epithelial sodium channel in salt-sensitive hypertension. Acta Pharmacol Sin 2011;32:789–97.

79. Sun P, Yue P, Wang WH. Angiotensin II stimulates epithelial sodium channels in the cortical collecting duct of the rat kidney. Am J Physiol Renal Physiol 2012; 302:F679–87.
80. Yu L, Bao HF, Self JL, et al. Aldosterone-induced increases in superoxide production counters nitric oxide inhibition of epithelial Na channel activity in A6 distal nephron cells. Am J Physiol Renal Physiol 2007;293:F1666–77.
81. Ilatovskaya DV, Pavlov TS, Levchenko V, et al. ROS production as a common mechanism of ENaC regulation by EGF, insulin, and IGF-1. Am J Physiol Cell Physiol 2013;304:C102–11.
82. Wu F, Park F, Cowley AW Jr, et al. Quantification of nitric oxide synthase activity in microdissected segments of the rat kidney. Am J Physiol 1999;276:F874–81.
83. Dickhout JG, Mori T, Cowley AW Jr. Tubulovascular nitric oxide crosstalk: buffering of angiotensin II–induced medullary vasoconstriction. Circ Res 2002;91: 487–93.
84. Mattson DL, Roman RJ, Cowley AW Jr. Role of nitric oxide in renal papillary blood flow and sodium excretion. Hypertension 1992;19:766–9.
85. Mori T, Cowley AW Jr. Angiotensin II-NAD(P)H oxidase-stimulated superoxide modifies tubulovascular nitric oxide cross-talk in renal outer medulla. Hypertension 2003;42:588–93.
86. Beltowski J, Marciniak A, Jamroz-Wisniewska A, et al. Nitric oxide–superoxide cooperation in the regulation of renal Na(+),K(+)-ATPase. Acta Biochim Pol 2004;51:933–42.
87. Silva GB, Ortiz PA, Hong NJ, et al. Superoxide stimulates NaCl absorption in the thick ascending limb via activation of protein kinase C. Hypertension 2006;48: 467–72.
88. Silva GB, Garvin JL. Angiotensin II-dependent hypertension increases Na transport-related oxygen consumption by the thick ascending limb. Hypertension 2008;52:1091–8.
89. Garvin JL, Herrera M, Ortiz PA. Regulation of renal NaCl transport by nitric oxide, endothelin, and ATP: clinical implications. Annu Rev Physiol 2011;73: 359–76.
90. Garvin JL, Hong NJ. Nitric oxide inhibits sodium/hydrogen exchange activity in the thick ascending limb. Am J Physiol 1999;277:F377–82.
91. Ohsaki Y, O'Connor P, Mori T, et al. Increase of sodium delivery stimulates the mitochondrial respiratory chain H2O2 production in rat renal medullary thick ascending limb. Am J Physiol Renal Physiol 2012;302:F95–102.
92. Guyenet PG. The sympathetic control of blood pressure. Nat Rev Neurosci 2006;7:335–46.
93. Peterson JR, Sharma RV, Davisson RL. Reactive oxygen species in the neuropathogenesis of hypertension. Curr Hypertens Rep 2006;8:232–41.
94. Gordon FJ, Haywood JR, Brody MJ, et al. Effect of lesions of the anteroventral third ventricle (AV3V) on the development of hypertension in spontaneously hypertensive rats. Hypertension 1982;4:387–93.
95. Brody MJ. Central nervous system and mechanisms of hypertension. Clin Physiol Biochem 1988;6:230–9.
96. Whyte DG, Johnson AK. Thermoregulatory role of periventricular tissue surrounding the anteroventral third ventricle (AV3V) during acute heat stress in the rat. Clin Exp Pharmacol Physiol 2005;32:457–61.
97. Zimmerman MC, Lazartigues E, Lang JA, et al. Superoxide mediates the actions of angiotensin II in the central nervous system. Circ Res 2002;91:1038–45.

98. Zimmerman MC, Lazartigues E, Sharma RV, et al. Hypertension caused by angiotensin II infusion involves increased superoxide production in the central nervous system. Circ Res 2004;95:210–6.

99. Zimmerman MC, Sharma RV, Davisson RL. Superoxide mediates angiotensin II–induced influx of extracellular calcium in neural cells. Hypertension 2005;45:717–23.

100. Peterson JR, Burmeister MA, Tian X, et al. Genetic silencing of Nox2 and Nox4 reveals differential roles of these NADPH oxidase homologues in the vasopressor and dipsogenic effects of brain angiotensin II. Hypertension 2009;54:1106–14.

101. Lob HE, Schultz D, Marvar PJ, et al. Role of the NADPH oxidases in the subfornical organ in angiotensin II–induced hypertension. Hypertension 2013;61:382–7.

102. Erdos B, Broxson CS, King MA, et al. Acute pressor effect of central angiotensin II is mediated by NAD(P)H-oxidase-dependent production of superoxide in the hypothalamic cardiovascular regulatory nuclei. J Hypertens 2006;24:109–16.

103. Wang G, Anrather J, Huang J, et al. NADPH oxidase contributes to angiotensin II signaling in the nucleus tractus solitarius. J Neurosci 2004;24:5516–24.

104. Nozoe M, Hirooka Y, Koga Y, et al. Inhibition of Rac1-derived reactive oxygen species in nucleus tractus solitarius decreases blood pressure and heart rate in stroke-prone spontaneously hypertensive rats. Hypertension 2007;50:62–8.

105. Ostrowski TD, Hasser EM, Heesch CM, et al. H(2)O(2) induces delayed hyperexcitability in nucleus tractus solitarii neurons. Neuroscience 2014;262:53–69.

106. Wang G, Coleman CG, Glass MJ, et al. Angiotensin II type 2 receptor-coupled nitric oxide production modulates free radical availability and voltage-gated Ca2+ currents in NTS neurons. Am J Physiol Regul Integr Comp Physiol 2012;302:R1076–83.

107. Guyenet PG, Darnall RA, Riley TA. Rostral ventrolateral medulla and sympathorespiratory integration in rats. Am J Physiol 1990;259:R1063–74.

108. Kishi T, Hirooka Y, Kimura Y, et al. Overexpression of eNOS in RVLM improves impaired baroreflex control of heart rate in SHRSP. Rostral ventrolateral medulla. Stroke-prone spontaneously hypertensive rats. Hypertension 2003;41:255–60.

109. Kishi T, Hirooka Y, Kimura Y, et al. Increased reactive oxygen species in rostral ventrolateral medulla contribute to neural mechanisms of hypertension in stroke-prone spontaneously hypertensive rats. Circulation 2004;109:2357–62.

110. Li Z, Mao HZ, Abboud FM, et al. Oxygen-derived free radicals contribute to baroreceptor dysfunction in atherosclerotic rabbits. Circ Res 1996;79:802–11.

111. Grassi G, Seravalle G, Brambilla G, et al. The sympathetic nervous system and new nonpharmacologic approaches to treating hypertension: a focus on renal denervation. Can J Cardiol 2012;28:311–7.

112. Wang D, Jose P, Wilcox CS. Beta(1) Receptors protect the renal afferent arteriole of angiotensin-infused rabbits from norepinephrine-induced oxidative stress. J Am Soc Nephrol 2006;17:3347–54.

113. Boivin V, Jahns R, Gambaryan S, et al. Immunofluorescent imaging of beta 1- and beta 2-adrenergic receptors in rat kidney. Kidney Int 2001;59:515–31.

114. DiBona GF, Esler M. Translational medicine: the antihypertensive effect of renal denervation. Am J Physiol Regul Integr Comp Physiol 2010;298:R245–53.

115. Johns EJ, Kopp UC, DiBona GF. Neural control of renal function. Compr Physiol 2011;1:731–67.

116. Chan SH, Tai MH, Li CY, et al. Reduction in molecular synthesis or enzyme activity of superoxide dismutases and catalase contributes to oxidative stress and

neurogenic hypertension in spontaneously hypertensive rats. Free Radic Biol Med 2006;40:2028–39.

117. Ye S, Zhong H, Yanamadala S, et al. Oxidative stress mediates the stimulation of sympathetic nerve activity in the phenol renal injury model of hypertension. Hypertension 2006;48:309–15.

118. Campese VM, Ye S. A vitamin-E-fortified diet reduces oxidative stress, sympathetic nerve activity, and hypertension in the phenol-renal injury model in rats. J Am Soc Hypertens 2007;1:242–50.

119. Cai H, Li Z, Dikalov S, et al. NAD(P)H oxidase-derived hydrogen peroxide mediates endothelial nitric oxide production in response to angiotensin II. J Biol Chem 2002;277:48311–7.

120. Beswick RA, Dorrance AM, Leite R, et al. NADH/NADPH oxidase and enhanced superoxide production in the mineralocorticoid hypertensive rat. Hypertension 2001;38:1107–11.

121. Suzuki H, Swei A, Zweifach BW, et al. In vivo evidence for microvascular oxidative stress in spontaneously hypertensive rats. Hydroethidine microfluorography. Hypertension 1995;25:1083–9.

122. Zhou X, Bohlen HG, Miller SJ, et al. NAD(P)H oxidase-derived peroxide mediates elevated basal and impaired flow-induced NO production in SHR mesenteric arteries in vivo. Am J Physiol Heart Circ Physiol 2008;295:H1008–16.

123. Swei A, Lacy F, DeLano FA, et al. Oxidative stress in the Dahl hypertensive rat. Hypertension 1997;30:1628–33.

124. Zhang C, Hein TW, Wang W, et al. Upregulation of vascular arginase in hypertension decreases nitric oxide-mediated dilation of coronary arterioles. Hypertension 2004;44:935–43.

125. Chandra S, Romero MJ, Shatanawi A, et al. Oxidative species increase arginase activity in endothelial cells through the RhoA/Rho kinase pathway. Br J Pharmacol 2012;165:506–19.

126. Ortiz MC, Sanabria E, Manriquez MC, et al. Role of endothelin and isoprostanes in slow pressor responses to angiotensin II. Hypertension 2001;37:505–10.

127. Minuz P, Patrignani P, Gaino S, et al. Increased oxidative stress and platelet activation in patients with hypertension and renovascular disease. Circulation 2002;106:2800–5.

128. Folkow B, Grimby G, Thulesius O. Adaptive structural changes of the vascular walls in hypertension and their relation to the control of the peripheral resistance. Acta Physiol Scand 1958;44:255–72.

129. Zafari AM, Ushio-Fukai M, Akers M, et al. Role of NADH/NADPH oxidase-derived H2O2 in angiotensin II–induced vascular hypertrophy. Hypertension 1998;32:488–95.

130. Laude K, Cai H, Fink B, et al. Hemodynamic and biochemical adaptations to vascular smooth muscle overexpression of p22phox in mice. Am J Physiol Heart Circ Physiol 2005;288:H7–12.

131. Patel R, Cardneau JD, Colles SM, et al. Synthetic smooth muscle cell phenotype is associated with increased nicotinamide adenine dinucleotide phosphate oxidase activity: effect on collagen secretion. J Vasc Surg 2006;43:364–71.

132. Virdis A, Neves MF, Amiri F, et al. Role of NAD(P)H oxidase on vascular alterations in angiotensin II–infused mice. J Hypertens 2004;22:535–42.

133. Lijnen P, Papparella I, Petrov V, et al. Angiotensin II-stimulated collagen production in cardiac fibroblasts is mediated by reactive oxygen species. J Hypertens 2006;24:757–66.

134. Zaw KK, Yokoyama Y, Abe M, et al. Catalase restores the altered mRNA expression of collagen and matrix metalloproteinases by dermal fibroblasts exposed to reactive oxygen species. Eur J Dermatol 2006;16:375–9.

135. Park JB, Intengan HD, Schiffrin EL. Reduction of resistance artery stiffness by treatment with the AT(1)-receptor antagonist losartan in essential hypertension. J Renin Angiotensin Aldosterone Syst 2000;1:40–5.

136. Schiffrin EL. Vascular stiffening and arterial compliance. Implications for systolic blood pressure. Am J Hypertens 2004;17:39S–48S.

137. Kals J, Kampus P, Kals M, et al. Inflammation and oxidative stress are associated differently with endothelial function and arterial stiffness in healthy subjects and in patients with atherosclerosis. Scand J Clin Lab Invest 2008;68:594–601.

138. Stephen EA, Venkatasubramaniam A, Good TA, et al. The effect of oxidation on the mechanical response and microstructure of porcine aortas. J Biomed Mater Res A 2014;102(9):3255–62.

139. Soskel NT, Watanabe S, Sandberg LB. Mechanisms of lung injury in the copper-deficient hamster model of emphysema. Chest 1984;85:70S–3S.

140. Prysyazhna O, Rudyk O, Eaton P. Single atom substitution in mouse protein kinase G eliminates oxidant sensing to cause hypertension. Nat Med 2012;18: 286–90.

141. Liu Y, Bubolz AH, Mendoza S, et al. H2O2 is the transferrable factor mediating flow-induced dilation in human coronary arterioles. Circ Res 2011;108:566–73.

142. Kohler R, Heyken WT, Heinau P, et al. Evidence for a functional role of endothelial transient receptor potential V4 in shear stress-induced vasodilatation. Arterioscler Thromb Vasc Biol 2006;26:1495–502.

143. Fleming I, Michaelis UR, Bredenkotter D, et al. Endothelium-derived hyperpolarizing factor synthase (cytochrome P450 2C9) is a functionally significant source of reactive oxygen species in coronary arteries. Circ Res 2001;88:44–51.

144. Zheng X, Zinkevich NS, Gebremedhin D, et al. Arachidonic acid-induced dilation in human coronary arterioles: convergence of signaling mechanisms on endothelial TRPV4-mediated Ca2+ entry. J Am Heart Assoc 2013;2:e000080.

145. Cai H, Li Z, Davis ME, et al. Akt-dependent phosphorylation of serine 1179 and mitogen-activated protein kinase kinase/extracellular signal-regulated kinase 1/2 cooperatively mediate activation of the endothelial nitric-oxide synthase by hydrogen peroxide. Mol Pharmacol 2003;63:325–31.

146. Drummond GR, Cai H, Davis ME, et al. Transcriptional and posttranscriptional regulation of endothelial nitric oxide synthase expression by hydrogen peroxide. Circ Res 2000;86:347–54.

147. Landmesser U, Harrison DG. Oxidative stress and vascular damage in hypertension. Coron Artery Dis 2001;12:455–61.

148. Theuer J, Dechend R, Muller DN, et al. Angiotensin II induced inflammation in the kidney and in the heart of double transgenic rats. BMC Cardiovasc Disord 2002;2:3.

149. Liu J, Yang F, Yang XP, et al. NAD(P)H oxidase mediates angiotensin II–induced vascular macrophage infiltration and medial hypertrophy. Arterioscler Thromb Vasc Biol 2003;23:776–82.

150. Vaziri ND, Rodriguez-Iturbe B. Mechanisms of disease: oxidative stress and inflammation in the pathogenesis of hypertension. Nat Clin Pract Nephrol 2006;2:582–93.

151. Liao TD, Yang XP, Liu YH, et al. Role of inflammation in the development of renal damage and dysfunction in angiotensin II–induced hypertension. Hypertension 2008;52:256–63.

152. Sesso HD, Buring JE, Rifai N, et al. C-reactive protein and the risk of developing hypertension. JAMA 2003;290:2945–51.
153. Preston RA, Ledford M, Materson BJ, et al. Effects of severe, uncontrolled hypertension on endothelial activation: soluble vascular cell adhesion molecule-1, soluble intercellular adhesion molecule-1 and von Willebrand factor. J Hypertens 2002;20:871–7.
154. Guzik TJ, Hoch NE, Brown KA, et al. Role of the T cell in the genesis of angiotensin II induced hypertension and vascular dysfunction. J Exp Med 2007;204: 2449–60.
155. Crowley SD, Frey CW, Gould SK, et al. Stimulation of lymphocyte responses by angiotensin II promotes kidney injury in hypertension. Am J Physiol Renal Physiol 2008;295:F515–24.
156. Mattson DL, Lund H, Guo C, et al. Genetic mutation of recombination activating gene 1 in Dahl salt-sensitive rats attenuates hypertension and renal damage. Am J Physiol Regul Integr Comp Physiol 2013;304:R407–14.
157. Madhur MS, Lob HE, McCann LA, et al. Interleukin 17 promotes angiotensin II–induced hypertension and vascular dysfunction. Hypertension 2010;55:500–7.
158. Cornelius DC, Hogg JP, Scott J, et al. Administration of interleukin-17 soluble receptor c suppresses TH17 cells, oxidative stress, and hypertension in response to placental ischemia during pregnancy. Hypertension 2013;62(6):1068–73.
159. Nguyen H, Chiasson VL, Chatterjee P, et al. Interleukin-17 causes Rho-kinase-mediated endothelial dysfunction and hypertension. Cardiovasc Res 2013;97: 696–704.
160. Norlander AE, Saleh MA, Kamat NV, et al. Interleukin-17A regulates renal sodium transporters and renal injury in angiotensin II–induced hypertension. Hypertension 2016;68:167–74.
161. Wu J, Thabet SR, Kirabo A, et al. Promote aortic stiffening in hypertension through activation of p38 mitogen-activated protein kinase. Circ Res 2014;114:616–25.
162. Wu J, Saleh MA, Kirabo A, et al. Immune activation caused by vascular oxidation promotes fibrosis and hypertension. J Clin Invest 2016;126:50–67.
163. Ganta CK, Lu N, Helwig BG, et al. Central angiotensin II-enhanced splenic cytokine gene expression is mediated by the sympathetic nervous system. Am J Physiol Heart Circ Physiol 2005;289:H1683–91.

What Have We Learned from the Genetics of Hypertension?

Friedrich C. Luft, MD

KEYWORDS

- Genetics • Blood pressure • Hypertension • Mendelian
- Genomewide association studies

KEY POINTS

- Twin studies show that about half the risk of hypertension development is inherited.
- Mendelian hypertension has elucidated astounding basic pathways contributing to hypertension over (presumably) dietary salt intake or directly through increased peripheral vascular resistance.
- The Mendelian mutations exercise large effects on blood pressure. The genetics of hypertension-producing tumors underscores the point. Inversely, studying the entire human genome for sources signaling blood pressure has yielded many signals with small effects.
- Thus far, few loci have been validated or translated into targets. Both genetic strategies are necessary, and much remains to be done.

INTRODUCTION

Beginning titles with questions is risky. A weakness is that the readership could quickly conclude: "It's a question! So evidently not much has been learned." A debate ensued early on in the 20th century involving Mendelian (1 or few genes) genetic inheritance or multifactorial genetic inheritance of blood pressure.[1] We need not pick up on the winners and losers of that argument here.[2] We know since the first studies in monozygotic and dizygotic twins that the genetic components influencing blood pressure lie by about 50% (genetic variance), largely including the mechanistic components of blood pressure control.[3] The residual (other half) could be attributed to environment, behavior, and the vicissitudes of life.[4] This figure has changed but little. Many genetic mechanisms are responsible for hypertension in most hypertensive individuals.[5] The arguments between Platt[1] and Pickering[2] seem mundane today but they nevertheless

Disclosures: None.
Charité Medical Faculty, Experimental and Clinical Research Center, Max-Delbrück Center for Molecular Medicine, Lindenbergerweg 80, Berlin 13125, Germany
E-mail address: friedrich.luft@charite.de

Med Clin N Am 101 (2017) 195–206
http://dx.doi.org/10.1016/j.mcna.2016.08.015
0025-7125/17/© 2016 Elsevier Inc. All rights reserved.

medical.theclinics.com

pursue us and still have a major impact on how resources are distributed.[6] The entire debate would remain an academic exercise were it not for molecular biological methods that allow both ideas to be tested.

THE PLATTONISTS

The clinician/scientist Robert Platt believed that blood pressure was heritable as a Mendelian (autosomal-dominant) trait.[1] He drew his conclusions from studying families. In his day, he could not go further. In comparison, Platt's modern followers have matters relatively easy. And they have found numerous genes that have major (20–50 mm Hg) influences on arterial blood pressure. The affected individuals have a substantial risk of hypertensive complications. This line of pursuit has resulted in a mechanistic bonanza.

Lifton and colleagues[7] found that a chimeric 11 β-hydroxylase/aldosterone synthase gene (CYP11B1/CYP11B2) causes glucocorticoid-remediable aldosteronism and human hypertension. The regulatory region of the chimeric gene is influenced by adrenocorticotropic hormone; however, the product is the mineralocorticoid aldosterone. This condition had been recognized years earlier and the genetics appreciated, but the mechanism was unknown. As a result of this work, mineralocorticoid-induced hypertension was elucidated. Moreover, because the mechanism clearly involved increased sodium reabsorption, the genetics of "salt-sensitive" hypertension seemed to be more established. Next was the observation that a mutation truncating the carboxy terminus of the γ subunit of the epithelial sodium channel (ENaC) is the cause of Liddle's syndrome.[8] The truncated subunit activates channel activity, as channel degradation (ubiquitination) does not occur.[9] ENaC subunits are ubiquitinated by the NEDD4. Failure of this process can also result in salt-sensitive hypertension through hyperactivity of ENaC in the distal nephron. The finding clarified the genetic salt-sensitive hypertension first described by Grant Liddle years earlier.[8] Moreover, through the careful molecular studies of Rossier and colleagues[10] and researchers worldwide, a vista on sodium transport was opened. Thereafter came the finding that an activating mineralocorticoid receptor mutation in a woman with hypertension caused much worse hypertension during pregnancy. This novel finding implicated the mineralocorticoid receptor directly in the development of genetic hypertension.[11]

White[12] drew attention to inherited forms of mineralocorticoid-associated hypertension that appeared already in childhood. Deficiencies of steroid 11 β-hydroxylase or 17 α-hydroxylase are types of congenital adrenal hyperplasia, the autosomal recessive inability to synthesize cortisol. These 2 defects often cause hypertension because of cortisol-precursor overproduction. The precursors are then metabolized to agents activating the mineralocorticoid receptor. Such disorders result from mutations in the CYP11B1 and CYP17 genes. Apparent mineralocorticoid excess results from loss of functional ligand specificity of the mineralocorticoid receptor caused by a deficiency of the renal 11 β-hydroxysteroid dehydrogenase-2 (11-β HSD2) isozyme. This enzyme normally metabolizes cortisol to cortisone to prevent cortisol from occupying the mineralocorticoid receptor.[13] Phenotypically, these forms of genetic hypertension featured low plasma renin activity, hypokalemia, and a degree of metabolic alkalosis. The phenotype is mimicked by licorice gluttony.

A genetic syndrome also known years earlier and described in part by Gordon features hypertension, mild metabolic acidosis, and hyperkalemia.[14] The condition is perhaps more appropriately termed *pseudohypoaldosteronism type II*. Initially, 2 genes were found causing this condition, both encoding with-no-lysine kinases (WNKs). *WNK1* and *WNK4* both encode members of the WNK serine-threonine kinase family. Disease-causing mutations in *WNK1* are large intronic deletions that increase WNK1 expression. The mutations in *WNK4* are missense. These mutations cluster in a short, highly conserved segment of the encoded protein. Both proteins localize to the distal nephron, a renal segment involved in sodium-positive (Na^+), potassium-positive (K^+), and pH homeostasis. WNK1 is cytoplasmic, whereas WNK4 localizes to tight junctions.[15] The *WNK* findings ushered in a major entire field of research, clearly not confined to hypertension. WNKs are everywhere. For us, the function in the distal nephron of the kidney would seem most important. Genetic findings, particularly on ENaC and WNK, have had ramifications far beyond blood pressure regulatory mechanisms.[16]

The importance of these rare and easily treated Mendelian hypertension forms lies in the pathways uncovered by this research.[17] In the kidney, the WNK pathways, via protein odd-skipped–related 1 and STE20/SPS1-related proline/alanine-rich kinase,[18] are responsible for the sodium-chloride cotransporter, sodium-potassium-2 chloride transporter, the renal ENaC, and renal outer-medullary potassium channel regulation.[19] Pseudohypoaldosteronism type II is also caused by heterozygous mutation in the cullin-3 (*CUL3*) gene on chromosome 2q36. Boyden and colleagues[20] used exome sequencing to identify mutations in kelch-like 3 (*KLHL3*) or *CUL3* in pseudohypoaldosteronism type II patients from 41 unrelated families. *KLHL3* mutations were either recessive or dominant, whereas *CUL3* mutations were dominant and generally de novo. Ohta and colleagues[21] subsequently immunoprecipitated KLHL3 and found that KLHL3 was strongly associated with WNK isoforms and CUL3 but not with other components of the pathway regulating sodium chloride cotransporter. Their results suggested that the CUL3-KLHL3 E3 ligase complex regulates blood pressure via interaction with and ubiquitination of WNK isoforms. Their study showed how mutations disrupting the ability of an E3 ligase to interact with and ubiquitinate a critical cellular substrate such as WNK isoforms can trigger hypertension. These Mendelian syndromes provided strong support for the idea that a high salt intake is largely responsible for hypertension (**Fig. 1**). None of these Mendelian syndromes were specifically tested for salt sensitivity by means of protocols for that purpose. However, because all directly involve salt reabsorption along the distal nephron and collecting duct, the salt-sensitivity explanation seems irrefutable. Nevertheless, some skeptics suggest otherwise.[22]

Autosomal hypertension with type E brachydactyly (HTNB) is not related to salt reabsorption. In affected persons, blood pressure increases with increasing age by 50 mm Hg at age 50 years.[23] In HTNB, age-dependent elevation in blood pressure is invariably inherited together with brachydactyly. A volume-expansion, volume-contraction protocol was used to show a salt-resistant form of hypertension.[24] An increased fibroblast growth rate, neurovascular contact at the rostral ventrolateral medulla, altered baroreflex blood pressure regulation, and death from stroke before age 50 years when untreated also characterize the syndrome.[25] In vitro analyses of mesenchymal stem cell–derived vascular smooth muscle cells (VSMCs) and chondrocytes provided insights into molecular pathogenesis. We reported 6 missense mutations in *PDE3A* (encoding phosphodiesterase 3A) in 6 unrelated families with HTNB.[26] The mutations increased protein kinase A–mediated PDE3A phosphorylation and resulted in gain of function, with increased cAMP-hydrolytic activity and enhanced cell proliferation. Levels of phosphorylated vasodilator-stimulated phosphoprotein were diminished, and parathyroid hormone–related peptide (PTHrP) levels were dysregulated. In earlier studies, the current authors found that PTHLH, the gene encoding parathyroid hormone–related peptide, was responsible for brachydactyly type E.[27] The authors suggest that the identified *PDE3A* mutations cause the syndrome

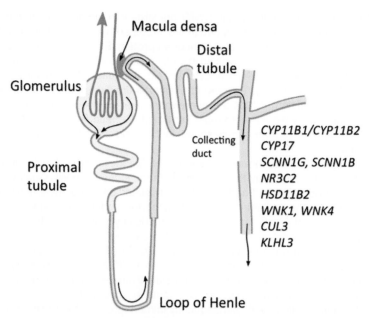

Fig. 1. A nephron with genes causing Mendelian hypertension related to increased Na⁺ reabsorption in the distal tubule and collecting duct. Glucocorticoid-remediable aldosteronism involves *CYP11B1* and *CYP11B2*. Steroid-17α-Hydroxylase is encoded by *CYP17*. The ENaCγ and ENaCβ subunits are encoded by *SCNN1G* and *SCNN1B*. *NR3C2* encodes the mineralocorticoid receptor. HSD11B2 encodes 11-β hydoxysteroid dehydrogenase-2. The WNKs are encoded by *WNK1* and *WNK4*. Cullin-3 and Kelch-3 are encoded by *CUL3* and *KLHL3*.

(**Fig. 2**). The authors conducted clinical studies of vascular function, cardiac functional imaging, platelet function in affected and nonaffected persons, and cell-based assays. Large-vessel and cardiac functions indeed seem to be preserved. The platelet studies found normal platelet function. Cell-based studies found that available pharmacologic PDE3A inhibitors suppress the mutant isoforms. However, increasing cyclic guanosine monophosphate to indirectly inhibit the enzyme seemed to have particular utility. VSMC-expressed PDE3A deserves scrutiny as a therapeutic target for the treatment of hypertension.[28] These observations served to further define the syndrome and to set the directions of further research.

Ji and colleagues[29] conducted larger genetic investigations in collaboration to verify the importance of Mendelian findings. The Lifton group raised a compelling argument regarding rare, independent mutations in renal salt handling genes and their contributions to blood pressure variation. They implicated many rare alleles that alter renal salt handling in blood pressure variation in the general population and identified alleles with health benefits that are nonetheless under purifying selection. Their findings have implications for the genetic architecture of hypertension and other common complex traits.

THE HYPERTENSION/ONCOLOGISTS

Cancers epitomize genetics. Not rarely, germline mutations are responsible for cancer. Invariably, somatic mutations are present in malignant tumors and a major

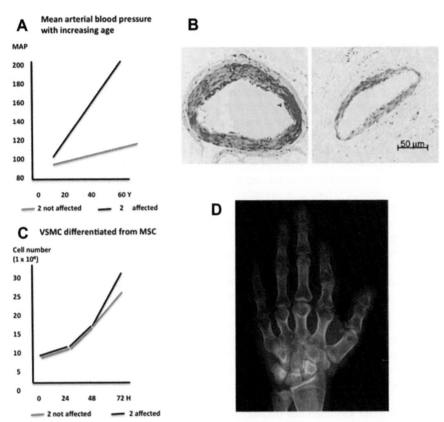

Fig. 2. Consequences of gain-of-function mutations in *PDE3A* are shown.[26] (*A*) Mean arterial blood pressure increases with age in affected and nonaffected persons. (*B*) Two small-vessel biopsies in young people hardly yet differing in blood pressure indicate VSMC proliferation. (*C*) Mesenchymal stem cell–derived VSMC exhibit increased proliferation. (*D*) Brachydactyly type E. *PTHLH* and *PDE3A* were expressed in fingertips during development, and PTRrP was dysregulated.

industry is directed at finding such mutations and suppressing their actions.[30] Interestingly, so-called "benign" tumors also involve mutations, commonly somatic.[31] Ruling out secondary forms of hypertension is a major clinical sport within our specialty. The activity is directed at finding pheochromocytoma (PCC) or aldosterone-producing adenomas; both are tumors and are thought to be generally benign.

In Europe, one-third of PCCs result from a genetic, commonly Mendelian-inherited, origin. The details of this amazing adventure story cannot be repeated here.[32] Within the PCCs reside also the paragangliomas (PGLs). The problem is well worked out.[33] Genetic mutations are mainly classified into 2 major clusters. Cluster 1 mutations are involved with the pseudohypoxic pathway. These mutations comprise *PHD2*, *VHL*, *SDHx*, *IDH*, *HIF2A*, *MDH2*, and fumarate hydratase *(FH)*-mutated PCC/PGL. Cluster 2 mutations are associated with abnormal activation of kinase signaling pathways and include mutations of *RET*, *NF1*, *KIF1Bβ*, *MAX*, *and TMEM127*. In addition, *VHL*, *SDHx* (cluster 1 genes), *RET*, and *NF1* (cluster 2 genes) germline mutations are involved in the neuronal precursor cell pathway in the pathogeneses of PCC/PGL. Also, *GDNF, H-ras, K-ras, GNAS, CDKN2A (p16), p53, BAP1, BRCA1* and *2,*

ATRX, and *KMT2D* mutations have roles in the development of PCC/PGLs. Overall, known genetic mutations account for the pathogenesis of approximately 60% of PCC/PGLs. Genetic mutations, pathologic parameters, and biochemical markers are used for better prediction of the outcome of patients with this group of tumors. Immunohistochemistry and gene sequencing can ensure a more effective detection, prediction of malignant potential, and treatment of PCC/PCLs. The bottom line is the importance of a family history (drawing a family tree) and considering any patient with PCC a candidate for a genetic syndrome.

The second clinical cause of secondary hypertension is primary aldosteronism (PA) generally caused by aldosterone-producing tumors (APA). This story is similarly amazing to the PCC story just told and cannot be recapitulated here in any detail. PA is the most common form of secondary hypertension with an estimated prevalence of approximately 10% (perhaps overstated) in referred patients. The 2 major causes of PA are APA and bilateral adrenal hyperplasia, accounting together for approximately 95% of cases. The findings of Scholl and colleagues[34] and Scholl and Lifton[35] are convincing. These investigators recently reported that either of 2 somatic gain-of-function mutations in the inward rectifier potassium channel KCNJ5 (Kir3.4) is present in approximately 40% of APAs. The mutations alter the channel's selectivity filter. Mutant channels gain permeability to sodium, resulting in cellular depolarization and activation of voltage-gated calcium channels. The resulting calcium influx is sufficient to produce aldosterone secretion and cell proliferation, accounting for APA development. Germline KCNJ5 mutations also result in either of 2 autosomal-dominant syndromes featuring early-onset primary aldosteronism. Mutations identical or similar to those found in APAs result in massive bilateral adrenal hyperplasia. A different mutation at the same position produces a less-severe syndrome without adrenal hyperplasia because this mutation results in Na-dependent cell lethality caused by a drastic increase in Na conductance. The identification of recurrent and somatic mutations in genes coding for ion channels (KCNJ5 and CACNA1D) and ATPases (ATP1A1 and ATP2B3) allowed highlighting the central role of calcium signaling in autonomous aldosterone production by the adrenal gland.

THE DISCIPLES OF SIR GEORGE

To my knowledge, George Pickering is the only clinician/scientist investigating hypertension that has been knighted. His accomplishments were many, and his dabbling into the genetics of hypertension was a side issue. He and his disciples (residents, fellows, and other servants) recruited a patient sample including hypertensive and control persons. They then recruited relatives of the patients and the controls. After careful measurements of blood pressure, this large collective was stratified in terms of age by decades from 10 to 79 years. Overlapping frequency distributions of blood pressure were observed, underscoring genetic influences but eliminating the possibility that they were dealing with a Mendelian trait.[36–39] Instead, many genes in any given individual would influence blood pressure and, if the constellation were perhaps unfavorable, increase the propensity to hypertension. Association (case-control) studies were used to test genetic variants, commonly in angiotensinogen-converting enzyme (ACE). Initially, variants in single genes, such as the one encoding ACE (*DCP1*), harbored an insertion-deletion Alu repeat in the gene (intron 16). An Alu element is a short stretch of DNA originally characterized by the action of the Alu (*Arthrobacter luteus*) restriction endonuclease. This ACE polymorphism in *DCP1* is a record holder in genetic studies. Association studies involving this allele number in the thousands, across every phenotype that can be imagined (about 5000 have been reported).

Next, the approach was greatly magnified to include single-nucleotide polymorphism (SNP) variants across the entire genome in thousands of cases and controls. Such heroic efforts demanded the recruitment of epidemiologists (Framingham for instance) that had such cohorts at their disposal. Confirmation cohorts were soon demanded so that consortia and networks were necessary to pursue such studies. To date, close to 300 genomewide association studies (GWAS) have been reported on blood pressure and hypertension alone. Many gene loci influencing blood pressure have been identified (too numerous to discuss here), each with a small effect on blood pressure, far less than in Mendelian syndromes.

More than 1 billion people worldwide have hypertension ($\geq$140 mm Hg systolic blood pressure or $\geq$90 mm Hg diastolic blood pressure). Even small increments in blood pressure are associated with an increased risk of cardiovascular events. An international consortium used a multistage design in 200,000 individuals of European descent, identified 16 novel loci: 6 of these loci contain genes previously known or suspected to regulate blood pressure (*GUCY1A3-GUCY1B3, NPR3-C5orf23, ADM, FURIN-FES, GOSR2, GNAS-EDN3*); the other 10 loci provide new clues to blood pressure physiology. A genetic risk score based on 29 genomewide significant variants was associated with hypertension.[40]

Another example of this daunting research is analysis of the Atherosclerosis Risk in Communities cohort. Salfati and colleagues[41] used data on 6,365,596 and 9,578,528 genotyped and imputed common SNPs in 8901 European-ancestry and 2860 African-ancestry Atherosclerosis Risk in Communities participants, respectively, and then used a mixed linear model for analyses. First, the investigators found that for blood pressure measurements, the heritability was approximately 20%/approximately 50% and approximately 27%/ approximately 39% for systolic/diastolic blood pressure in European-ancestry and African-ancestry individuals. These findings are not that much off from those of twin studies. Second, the investigators observed that common variants with allele frequency greater than 10% recapitulate most of the blood-pressure heritability in their data. Third, most blood pressure heritability varied by chromosome depending on the chromosome's length and was largely concentrated in noncoding genomic regions annotated as DNaseI hypersensitive sites. Fourth, most heritability arose from loci not harboring currently known cardiovascular and renal genes. Because 97% of the genome consists of noncoding genomic regions, the findings are not unexpected. The authors concluded that GWAS and admixture mapping have identified approximately 50 loci associated with blood pressure and hypertension, yet they account for only a small fraction ($\sim$2%) of the heritability. The implication is that we have yet to find the other 48%.

GWAS has introduced integrative network analysis. For instance, Huan and colleagues[42] integrated blood pressure GWAS with whole-blood mRNA expression profiles in 3679 individuals using network approaches. Blood pressure transcriptomic signatures at the single-gene and the coexpression network module levels were identified. The authors found 4 coexpression modules as potentially causal based on genetic inference because expression-related SNPs for their corresponding genes showed enrichment for blood pressure GWAS signals. Genes from the 4 modules were further projected onto predefined molecular interaction networks, revealing key drivers. The investigators were able to validated the lymphocyte adaptor protein LNK (gene better known as *SH2B3*), one of the top key drivers, using Sh2b3(−/−) mice. They found that a significant number of genes predicted to be regulated by *SH2B3* in gene networks are perturbed in *Sh2b3*(−/−) mice. The mice showed an exaggerated pressor response to angiotensin II infusion. *SH2B3* is one of the few genes found in GWAS that has been corroborated as mechanistically hypertension relevant in independent molecular genetic research.[43]

Hypertension GWAS studies increase in complexity. A recent transancestry GWAS identified 12 genetic loci influencing blood pressure and implicated a role for DNA methylation.[44] The investigators found sentinel SNPs enriched for association with DNA methylation at multiple cytosine-phosphatidyl-guanine (CpG) sites suggesting that, at some of the loci identified, DNA methylation may lie on the regulatory pathway linking sequence variation to blood pressure. The authors were particularly interested in this study, as *PDE3A* was one of the loci identified (**Fig. 3**). Generally, GWAS have not identified the loci of the Mendelian syndromes described earlier. HTNB is a definite exception, raising the expectation that PDE3A is relevant to essential hypertension by influencing peripheral vascular resistance.

THE EPIGENETICISTS

Epigenetics is defined as the transmission of gene expression patterns and chromosome remodeling from 1 cell generation to the next, which do not rely on differences in DNA sequence. The topic was briefly introduced in the GWAS study above, examining DNA methylation and CpG sites.[44] The CpG sites or CpG islands are regions of DNA in which a cytosine nucleotide is followed by a guanine nucleotide in the linear sequence

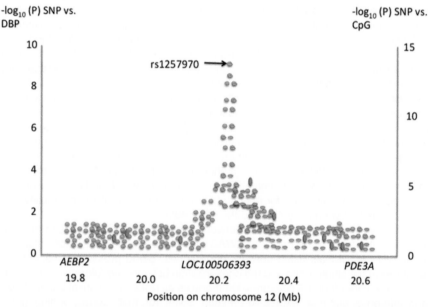

Fig. 3. The interpretation of genomewide association results can be greatly facilitated by visualization of regional association plots. Regional plots for the 2 newly identified loci were associated with diastolic blood pressure (DBP) as adapted from Kato et al.[44] Associations of SNPs with DBP in the transancestry GWAS (*blue markers*; n = 99,994) and of sentinel SNPs with methylation at nearby CpG sites (*red markers*; n = 2664) are shown. The identities of the sentinel SNP and most closely associated CpG site are provided. The authors set the threshold for genomewide significance as $P = 1 \times 10^{-9}$ to provide a conservative Bonferroni correction for testing ~2.1 million SNPs against the blood pressure phenotypes. LOC100506393 is probably a long-noncoding RNA.

of bases along its 5' → 3' direction. CpG is shorthand for 5'—C—phosphate—G—3', namely, cytosine and guanine separated by only one phosphate; phosphate links any 2 nucleosides together in DNA. DNA methylation occurs at CpG dinucleotides and is responsible for inhibition of transcription. Histones are another regulatory site. Histones are highly alkaline proteins found in eukaryotic cell nuclei that package and order the DNA into structural units called nucleosomes. Hyperacetylation of the histones correlates with transcriptional activation, whereas deacetylation is associated with transcriptional inactivation (**Fig. 4**).

Epigenetic modification is recognized as an essential process in biology but is now being investigated for its role in the development of specific pathologic conditions, including hypertension.[45] Epigenetic research will provide insights into the pathogenesis of blood pressure regulation that cannot be explained by classic Mendelian inheritance or be elucidated by conventional GWAS. The major epigenetic features of mammalian cells include DNA methylation, posttranslational histone modifications, and RNA-based mechanisms including those controlled by small noncoding micro RNAs (miRNAs). The miRNAs are a family of small noncoding RNAs that are important posttranscriptional regulators of gene expression. Another important aspect of epigenetic mechanisms is that they are potentially reversible and may be influenced by nutritional-environmental factors and through gene-environment interactions. Studies

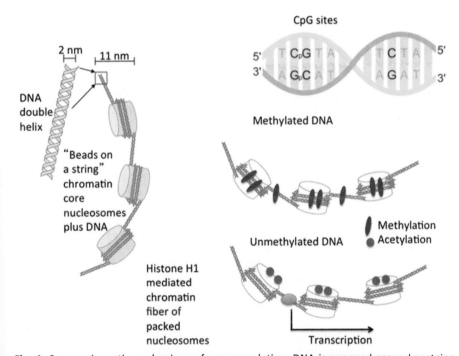

Fig. 4. Some epigenetic mechanisms of gene regulation. DNA is wrapped around proteins called histones. Histones can be acetylated and deacetylated by appropriate enzymes. Hyperacetylation of the histones correlates with transcriptional activation, whereas deacetylation is associated with transcriptional inactivation. DNA methylation occurs at CpG dinucleotides and is responsible for inhibition of transcription. Some epigenetic alterations can be reversed by pharmacologic agents, such as histone deacetylase inhibitors.

on epigenetic modulations could help us understand the mechanisms involved in essential hypertension and further prevent the condition's progression.

As mentioned earlier, 97% of the genome does not code for protein. It is now known that most of this sequence encodes RNA, not only miRNA but long noncoding RNA, and circular RNA. These RNA transcripts act as competing endogenous RNAs or natural microRNA sponges.[46] They evidently communicate with and coregulate each other by competing for binding to shared miRNAs. Understanding this novel RNA crosstalk will lead to significant insight into gene regulatory networks and have implications in human development and chronic conditions such as hypertension (and the other 97% of everything else).

SUMMARY

Twenty-five years ago, Corvol and colleagues[47] speculated that the development of molecular genetics would establish a link between high blood pressure and specific phenotypes. They suggested several strategies that could be used for the genetic study of arterial hypertension: linkage studies in informative families, population association studies, analysis of subjects with contrasted predisposition to high blood pressure, and the affected sib-pair method. They predicted that loci implicated in blood pressure regulation would be detected. They suggested 2 main approaches. One approach would be based on the study of candidate genes, genes whose products are known to participate in blood pressure regulation, such as those of the renin-angiotensin system. The other approach would involve testing a series of markers distributed randomly throughout the genome to establish a link between increased blood pressure and a particular region of the genome. These predictions were prescient and have been amply confirmed. Dzau and colleagues[48] went further to predict the potential of transgenic animals in the study of regulation of gene expression in the whole animal and the contribution of selective genes to hypertension. This prediction, outside of our framework here, has also been far superseded. Indeed, molecular genetics has been the lynchpin in basic hypertension-related research and promises to remain so in the future.

REFERENCES

1. Platt R. Heredity in hypertension. Q J Med 1947;16:311.
2. Pickering G. Hyperpiesis: high blood-pressure without evident cause: essential hypertension. Br Med J 1965;2:1021–1026 concl.
3. Grim CE, Miller JZ, Luft FC, et al. Genetic influences on renin, aldosterone, and the renal excretion of sodium and potassium following volume expansion and contraction in normal man. Hypertension 1979;1:583–90.
4. Luft FC, Miller JZ, Grim CE, et al. Salt sensitivity and resistance of blood pressure. Age and race as factors in physiological responses. Hypertension 1991;17: I102–8.
5. Pickering GW. The genetic component in high blood pressure. Triangle 1957;3: 59–66.
6. Zanchetti A. Platt versus pickering: an episode in recent medical history. By JD. Swales, editor. An essay review. Med Hist 1986;30:94–6.
7. Lifton RP, Dluhy RG, Powers M, et al. A chimaeric 11 beta-hydroxylase/aldosterone synthase gene causes glucocorticoid-remediable aldosteronism and human hypertension. Nature 1992;355:262–5.
8. Warnock DG. Liddle syndrome: an autosomal dominant form of human hypertension. Kidney Int 1998;53:18–24.

9. Hansson JH, Nelson-Williams C, Suzuki H, et al. Hypertension caused by a truncated epithelial sodium channel gamma subunit: genetic heterogeneity of liddle syndrome. Nat Genet 1995;11:76–82.

10. Vallet V, Chraibi A, Gaeggeler HP, et al. An epithelial serine protease activates the amiloride-sensitive sodium channel. Nature 1997;389:607–10.

11. Geller DS, Farhi A, Pinkerton N, et al. Activating mineralocorticoid receptor mutation in hypertension exacerbated by pregnancy. Science 2000;289:119–23.

12. White PC. Inherited forms of mineralocorticoid hypertension. Hypertension 1996; 28:927–36.

13. Mune T, Rogerson FM, Nikkila H, et al. Human hypertension caused by mutations in the kidney isozyme of 11 beta-hydroxysteroid dehydrogenase. Nat Genet 1995;10:394–9.

14. O'Shaughnessy KM. Gordon syndrome: a CONTINUING story. Pediatr Nephrol 2015;30:1903–8.

15. Wilson FH, Disse-Nicodeme S, Choate KA, et al. Human hypertension caused by mutations in WNK kinases. Science 2001;293:1107–12.

16. Kahle KT, Ring AM, Lifton RP. Molecular physiology of the WNK kinases. Annu Rev Physiol 2008;70:329–55.

17. Sohara E, Uchida S. Kelch-like 3/cullin 3 ubiquitin ligase complex and WNK signaling in salt-sensitive hypertension and electrolyte disorder. Nephrol Dial Transplant 2016;31(9):1417–24.

18. Rafiqi FH, Zuber AM, Glover M, et al. Role of the WNK-activated SPAK kinase in regulating blood pressure. EMBO Mol Med 2010;2:63–75.

19. Huang CL, Cheng CJ. A unifying mechanism for WNK kinase regulation of sodium-chloride cotransporter. Pflugers Arch 2015;467:2235–41.

20. Boyden LM, Choi M, Choate KA, et al. Mutations in kelch-like 3 and cullin 3 cause hypertension and electrolyte abnormalities. Nature 2012;482:98–102.

21. Ohta A, Schumacher FR, Mehellou Y, et al. The cul3-klhl3 e3 ligase complex mutated in gordon's hypertension syndrome interacts with and ubiquitylates WNK isoforms: Disease-causing mutations in klhl3 and WNK4 disrupt interaction. Biochem J 2013;451:111–22.

22. Kurtz TW, Dominiczak AF, DiCarlo SE, et al. Molecular-based mechanisms of mendelian forms of salt-dependent hypertension: questioning the prevailing theory. Hypertension 2015;65:932–41.

23. Schuster H, Wienker TE, Bahring S, et al. Severe autosomal dominant hypertension and brachydactyly in a unique turkish kindred maps to human chromosome 12. Nat Genet 1996;13:98–100.

24. Schuster H, Wienker TF, Toka HR, et al. Autosomal dominant hypertension and brachydactyly in a turkish kindred resembles essential hypertension. Hypertension 1996;28:1085–92.

25. Bahring S, Kann M, Neuenfeld Y, et al. Inversion region for hypertension and brachydactyly on chromosome 12p features multiple splicing and noncoding RNA. Hypertension 2008;51:426–31.

26. Maass PG, Aydin A, Luft FC, et al. Pde3a mutations cause autosomal dominant hypertension with brachydactyly. Nat Genet 2015;47:647–53.

27. Maass PG, Rump A, Schulz H, et al. A misplaced lncRNA causes brachydactyly in humans. J Clin Invest 2012;122:3990–4002.

28. Toka O, Tank J, Schachterle C, et al. Clinical effects of phosphodiesterase 3a mutations in inherited hypertension with brachydactyly. Hypertension 2015;66: 800–8.

29. Ji W, Foo JN, O'Roak BJ, et al. Rare independent mutations in renal salt handling genes contribute to blood pressure variation. Nat Genet 2008;40:592–9.
30. Aparicio S, Caldas C. The implications of clonal genome evolution for cancer medicine. N Engl J Med 2013;368:842–51.
31. Bulun SE. Uterine fibroids. N Engl J Med 2013;369:1344–55.
32. Neumann HP, Vortmeyer A, Schmidt D, et al. Evidence of men-2 in the original description of classic pheochromocytoma. N Engl J Med 2007;357:1311–5.
33. Pillai S, Gopalan V, Smith RA, et al. Updates on the genetics and the clinical impacts on phaeochromocytoma and paraganglioma in the new era. Crit Rev Oncol Hematol 2016;100:190–208.
34. Scholl UI, Goh G, Stolting G, et al. Somatic and germline cacna1d calcium channel mutations in aldosterone-producing adenomas and primary aldosteronism. Nat Genet 2013;45:1050–4.
35. Scholl UI, Lifton RP. New insights into aldosterone-producing adenomas and hereditary aldosteronism: Mutations in the k+ channel kcnj5. Curr Opin Nephrol Hypertens 2013;22:141–7.
36. Hamilton M, Pickering GW, Roberts JA, et al. The aetiology of essential hypertension. I. The arterial pressure in the general population. Clin Sci 1954;13:11–35.
37. Hamilton M, Pickering GW, Roberts JA, et al. The aetiology of essential hypertension. II. Scores for arterial blood pressures adjusted for differences in age and sex. Clin Sci 1954;13:37–49.
38. Pickering GW, Roberts JA, Sowry GS. The aetiology of essential hypertension. 3. The effect of correcting for arm circumference on the growth rate of arterial pressure with age. Clin Sci 1954;13:267–71.
39. Hamilton M, Pickering GW, Roberts JA, et al. The aetiology of essential hypertension. 4. The role of inheritance. Clin Sci 1954;13:273–304.
40. International Consortium for Blood Pressure Genome-Wide Association Studies, Ehret GB, Munroe PB, Rice KM, et al. Genetic variants in novel pathways influence blood pressure and cardiovascular disease risk. Nature 2011;478:103–9.
41. Salfati E, Morrison AC, Boerwinkle E, et al. Direct estimates of the genomic contributions to blood pressure heritability within a population-based cohort (ARIC). PLoS One 2015;10:e0133031.
42. Huan T, Meng Q, Saleh MA, et al. Integrative network analysis reveals molecular mechanisms of blood pressure regulation. Mol Syst Biol 2015;11:799.
43. Saleh MA, McMaster WG, Wu J, et al. Lymphocyte adaptor protein lnk deficiency exacerbates hypertension and end-organ inflammation. J Clin Invest 2015;125:1189–202.
44. Kato N, Loh M, Takeuchi F, et al. Trans-ancestry genome-wide association study identifies 12 genetic loci influencing blood pressure and implicates a role for DNA methylation. Nat Genet 2015;47:1282–93.
45. Scherrer U, Rimoldi SF, Sartori C, et al. Fetal programming and epigenetic mechanisms in arterial hypertension. Curr Opin Cardiol 2015;30:393–7.
46. Tay Y, Rinn J, Pandolfi PP. The multilayered complexity of cerna crosstalk and competition. Nature 2014;505:344–52.
47. Corvol P, Jeunemaitre X, Plouin PF, et al. The application of molecular genetics to the study of familial arterial hypertension. Clin Exp Hypertens A 1989;11:1053–73.
48. Dzau VJ, Paul M, Nakamura N, et al. Role of molecular biology in hypertension research. State of the art lecture. Hypertension 1989;13:731–40.

The Kidney in Hypertension

Hillel Sternlicht, MD, George L. Bakris, MD*

KEYWORDS

- Renal • Hypertension • Kidney • Outcomes • Diabetes

KEY POINTS

- Hypertension is the second most common cause of kidney disease.
- Nephropathy progression in those with an estimated glomerular filtration rate of less than 60 mL/min/1.73 m^2 has slowed from a decline of 8 to 2 mL/min/year.
- Goal blood pressure is well below 140/90 mm Hg.

EPIDEMIOLOGY OF CHRONIC KIDNEY DISEASE

According to the Kidney Disease Outcome Quality Initiative guidelines, chronic kidney disease (CKD) is a glomerular filtration rate (GFR) of less than 60 mL/min/1.73 m^2 for longer than 3 months or other markers of kidney damage such as structural (ie, parenchymal, anatomic) or functional (ie, proteinuria, hematuria) abnormalities.[1] Although historically the Cockcroft–Gault equation has been used to calculate GFR, the more recent Modification of Diet in Renal Disease (MDRD) and CKD Epidemiology Collaboration formulas have proven more accurate, particularly with GFRs less (MDRD) or more (CKD Epidemiology Collaboration) than 60 mL/min/1.73 m^2.[2] With these equations and the severity of albuminuria, levels of kidney function and the risk of progression of kidney disease can be ascertained (**Table 1**).[3] Using data from the 13,000 individuals participating in National Health and Nutrition Examination Surveys from 1999 to 2004, 13% of those 20 years of age or older suffer from CKD as determined by the MDRD equation, with stage 3 disease being the most prevalent (7.8%; **Table 2**).[4]

Disclosure Statement: Dr H. Sternlicht has no conflicts of interest. Dr G.L. Bakris is the principal investigator on an international outcome trial of diabetic nephropathy (FIDELIO) funded by Bayer and serves on the Steering Committees of two other nephropathy outcomes studies CREDENCE and SONAR funded by Janssen and AbbVie respectively. He is a Special Government Employee of the Food and Drug Administration and CMS. Consultant-Bayer, Medtronic, Relypsa, AbbVie, Janssen, Boehringer-Ingelheim, Astra Zeneca, NxStage.

Section of Endocrinology, Diabetes and Metabolism, Department of Medicine, ASH Comprehensive Hypertension Center, The University of Chicago Medicine, 5841 South Maryland Avenue, MC 1027, Chicago, IL 60637, USA

* Corresponding author.

E-mail address: gbakris@medicine.bsd.uchicago.edu

Med Clin N Am 101 (2017) 207–217
http://dx.doi.org/10.1016/j.mcna.2016.08.001

medical.theclinics.com

Table 1
Relative risk of progression to ESRD by eGFR (mL/min/1.73 m^2) and level of albuminuria

eGFR	ACR <10	ACR 10–30	ACR 30–300	ACR >300
>105	Reference	Reference	7.8	18
90–105	Reference	Reference	11	20
75–90	Reference	Reference	3.8	48
60–75	Reference	Reference	7.4	67
45–60	5.2	22	40	147
30–45	56	74	294	763
15–30	433	1044	1056	2286

Abbreviations: ACR, albumin to creatinine ratio; eGFR, estimated glomerular filtration rate.
   Data from Levey AS, de Jong PE, Coresh J, et al. The definition, classification, and prognosis of chronic kidney disease: a KDIGO Controversies Conference report. Kidney Int 2011;80(1):17–28.

PATHOPHYSIOLOGY OF HYPERTENSION BASED ON KIDNEY DISEASE STATUS

In its simplest form, hypertension is the product of systemic vascular resistance and cardiac output (cardiac output = heart rate × stroke volume). Although numerous mechanisms have been implicated, the principal driver of increases in blood pressure involve the interwoven disorders of pressure natriuresis/salt sensitivity, dysregulation of the sympathetic and renal–angiotensin–aldosterone systems (RAAS), endothelial dysfunction, and pathologic arterial stiffness.[5] Pressure natriuresis refers to enhanced renal sodium excretion in response to increases in blood pressure such that sodium balance, and by extension blood pressure, returns to its previous state of equilibrium. In salt-sensitive states such as advanced age or CKD, salt handling is impaired, resulting in an expansion of extracellular volume, increased systemic vascular resistance, and ultimately overt hypertension (**Fig. 1**).[6] Sympathetic nervous system activation, manifest by increases in systemic catecholamine levels, leads to vasoconstriction, endothelial dysfunction, and a salt avid state.[7,8] Activation of the RAAS, specifically via the angiotensin II type 1 receptor, results in smooth muscle vasoconstriction, sodium retention, upregulation of aldosterone synthesis, fibrosis, and vascular injury.[9] At the level of the endothelium, the interplay of nitric oxide, endothelin-1, and oxidative stress figure prominently in blood pressure homeostasis. Endothelial production of the vasoactive peptide nitric oxide results in vascular smooth muscle relaxation, a process stimulated by flow (ie, blood pressure) induced shear stress.[10] However, nitric

Table 2
Prevalence of CKD by stage among US adults

CKD Stage	Prevalence (%)
1	1.8
2	3.2
3	7.7
4	0.4
5	NA

Abbreviation: CKD, chronic kidney disease.
   Data from Coresh J, Selvin E, Stevens LA, et al. Prevalence of chronic kidney disease in the United States. JAMA 2007;298(17):2038–47.

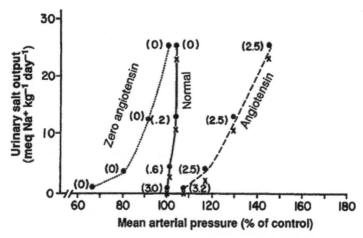

Fig. 1. Mean arterial pressure as a function of urinary salt excretion in the presence and absence of angiotensin. (*Adapted from* Guyton AC. Arterial pressure and hypertension. Philadelphia: Saunders, 1980; with permission.)

oxide–mediated vasodilation is counteracted by endothelin-1, a vasoconstricting substance whose production is enhanced by activation of the aforementioned RAAS and sympathetic nervous systems. Further attenuating nitric oxide's hypotensive effect is the generation of reactive oxygen species by catecholamines, vascular distention, and RAAS activation. These free radicals are both proinflammatory and decrease nitric oxide bioavailability, ultimately promoting increases in blood pressure.[11] Finally, arterial stiffness, long considered a consequence of hypertension, may indeed antecede its onset. For example, owing to the pulsatile load associated with ventricular contraction, arteriolar elastin fibers are fractured and ultimately replaced by the less distensible collagen, further decreasing vascular compliance.[12]

HYPERTENSION AS A RISK FACTOR FOR CHRONIC KIDNEY DISEASE

Hypertension is an independent predictor of CKD progression and the second most common cause of end-stage renal disease (ESRD). Among the 12,000 patients followed for an average of 14 years in the Hypertension Screening and Treatment Program, rates of progression to dialysis were proportional to pretreatment blood pressure (**Fig. 2**) with risk ratios of 1.9 for those with systolic pressures of 165 to 180 mm Hg and 4.6 for those with values greater than 180 mm Hg.[13] These results are consistent with the subsequent post hoc analysis of the Multiple Risk Factor Intervention Trial data, a 25-year study of 13,000 individuals evaluating the effects of lifestyle interventions on the incidence of cardiovascular disease. Individuals progressing to ESRD had higher systolic (142 vs 135 mm Hg) and diastolic (93 mm Hg vs 91 mm Hg) blood pressure at study entry; for every increase in systolic pressure of 10 mm Hg, participants reached ESRD at a 30% higher rate.[14]

Whereas these papers analyzed hypertensive cohorts with and without kidney disease, studies limited to individuals with CKD (attributable to diabetes or other causes), found even more striking associations between levels of blood pressure and progression to ESRD. A prospective evaluation of 220 patients with CKD 3 (mean GFR, 33 mL/min/1.73 m²) found the 7-year incidence of ESRD to be 7.2% among those with achieved systolic pressures of less than 130 mm Hg, 28% among those with

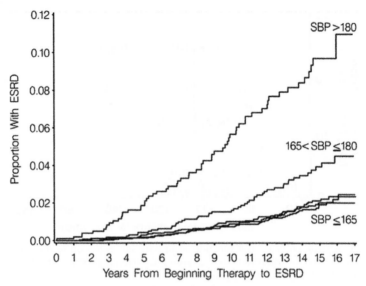

Fig. 2. Rates of end-stage renal disease (ESRD) after first treatment visit, stratified by pretreatment systolic blood pressure (SBP). (*From* Perry HM, Miller JP, Fornoff JR, et al. Early predictors of 15-year end-stage renal disease in hypertensive patients. Hypertension 1995;25(4 Pt 1):591; with permission.)

pressures between 130 and 150 mm Hg, and 71% among those with values of greater than 150 mm Hg.[15] Among more than 4000 patients with a mean GFR of 22 mL/min/ 1.73 m² (CKD stage 4) retrospectively evaluated over a 2.5-year period, the GFR decreased at a rate of greater than 5.0 mL/min/1.73 m² in those with achieved blood pressures of 145/80 mm Hg compared with decreases in GFR of less than 2.2 mL/min/ 1.73 m² in those with pressures of 137/74 mm Hg.[16] Among the 1500 patients in The Reduction of Endpoints in non–insulin-dependent diabetes mellitus with the RENAAL trials (Angiotensin II Antagonist Losartan; mean creatinine, 1.9 mg/dL), the hazard ratio for progression to ESRD (based on last systolic blood pressure before the onset of ESRD) over 3.5 years of follow-up was 1.5 for those with systolic pressures between 140 to 159 mm Hg, 3.0 for those with systolic pressures of 160 to 179 mm Hg, and 4.6 for those with systolic pressures in excess of 180 mm Hg.[17]

PREVENTION OF CHRONIC KIDNEY DISEASE PROGRESSION: BLOOD PRESSURE GOALS

Although there is ample evidence to link poor blood pressure control to the progression of CKD, studies evaluating specific blood pressure targets among nondiabetic CKD cohorts have largely been negative; prospective trials among those with diabetic nephropathy are lacking. In the MDRD study consisting of 1600 patients with nondiabetic nephropathy (mean GFR, 39 mL/min/1.73 m²; mean proteinuria, 1.1 g/d), those randomized to tight mean arterial pressures (MAP; achieved MAP, 91 mm Hg [≈125/ 75 mm Hg]) failed to have slower rates of GFR decline (cumulative 11.5 mL/min/ 1.73 m²) after 3 years than participants allocated to the usual blood pressure arm (achieved MAP, 96 mm Hg [≈130/80 mm Hg]). However, in the subset of patients with greater than 3 g/d of proteinuria, GFR decline was slower (6.7 vs 10.2 mL/min/ 1.73 m²) among those achieving lower blood pressure targets.[18] Upon study completion at 3 years, individuals were followed for an additional 6 years, during which time neither blood pressure was measured nor a target pressure specified. Nonetheless, those randomized to the lower target were one-third less likely to progress to ESRD, a result driven by benefits realized among those with at least 1 g/d of proteinuria.[19]

The subsequent African American Study of Kidney Disease (AASK) was undertaken with a similar premise. Nearly 1100 black patients with kidney disease (mean GFR, 46 mL/min/1.73 m^2; mean proteinuria, 600 mg/d) in the absence of diabetes achieved a blood pressure goal of either 128/78 mm Hg or 141/85 mm Hg. Four years later, GFR worsened at a rate of 2.1 mL/min/1.73 m^2 per year regardless of arm or whether an angiotensin-converting enzyme inhibitor (ACEi), calcium channel blocker (CCB), or beta-blocker was used as an antihypertensive.[20] In aggregate, the results of these studies indicate that control of blood pressure to less than 130 to 140/80 to 85 mm Hg fails to further slow progression of nondiabetic CKD; however, there may be a modest benefit in those with the most advanced disease, that is, those with CKD 3 or greater and more than 2 g/d of proteinuria.

Despite the extensive literature available to guide antihypertensive agent selection among those with diabetic nephropathy, large high-quality prospective trials evaluating blood pressure targets with respect to CKD progression are lacking. In a trial randomizing 130 patients with type 1 diabetes with nephropathy (mean GFR, 63 mL/min/1.73 m^2; mean proteinuria, 1.1 g/d), those achieving a MAP of 92 mm Hg (~120/80 mm Hg) experienced a similar rate of GFR decline as those with measured MAPs of 98 mm Hg (~130/80 mm Hg) after 2 years of follow-up.[21]

In the ABCD trial (Appropriate Blood Pressure Control), consisting of 500 normotensive subjects with type 2 diabetes (one-third of whom had nephropathy) followed for 5 years, those achieving intensive (128/75 mm Hg) blood pressure control had no slower a rate of GFR decline than those achieving a more conservative blood pressure (137/81 mm Hg) goal.[22] In aggregate, there are 3 statistically powered studies demonstrating no additional benefit with respect to CKD progression with achieved blood pressures of less than 130/80 mm Hg. A notable caveat, if post hoc analysis are considered admissible, are those with 1 or more grams of proteinuria. However, data from SPRINT (Systolic Blood Pressure Intervention Trial) clearly indicate a reduced risk of cardiovascular events in people with CKD from nondiabetic causes who achieve an estimated office blood pressure between 125 and 132 mm Hg.[23,24]

PROTEINURIA AND THE KIDNEY

The presence of albuminuria indicates an increase in glomerular permeability and, when present in quantities greater than 300 mg/d ("macro" or "very high" albuminuria), signifies glomerular injury. In contradistinction, "micro" or "high" albuminuria indicates between 30 and 300 mg/d of urinary albumin loss.

Because very high albuminuria often precedes increases in creatinine, it has become an important modifiable risk factor for kidney disease progression. For example, in the aforementioned AASK trial, for every 2-fold increase in baseline proteinuria, the risk of progression to ESRD increased by 80%.[25] Conversely, reductions in very high albuminuria are associated with improved renal outcomes (**Fig. 3**). However, the agent used to achieve decreases in urinary protein excretion seems to be as important as the reductions achieved, particularly when proteinuria is greater than 300 mg/d.

In the ACCOMPLISH study (Avoiding Cardiovascular Events through Combination Therapy in Patients Living with Systolic Hypertension), the secondary endpoint of progression to ESRD was less common in benazepril/amlodipine–treated patients despite higher rates of high albuminuria.[26] Although decreases of very high

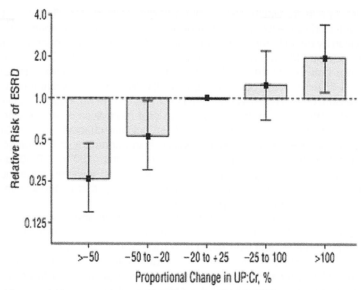

Fig. 3. Relationship between change in albuminuria at 6 months and risk of end-stage renal disease (ESRD). (*From* Lea J, Greene T, Hebert L, et al. The relationship between magnitude of proteinuria reduction and risk of end-stage renal disease: results of the African American Study of Kidney Disease and hypertension. Arch Intern Med 2005;165(8):950; with permission.)

albuminuria are commonly associated with slower CKD progression, changes in albuminuria have not been validated by the Food and Drug Administration as a surrogate for changes in GFR.

SELECTION OF ANTIHYPERTENSIVE THERAPY

Broadly speaking, thiazidelike diuretics, RAAS blockers, and CCBs remain the cornerstones of therapy for hypertensives with or without kidney disease. Given the salt-avid state characteristic of CKD, diuretics are critical to restoring euvolemia, even among those without physical examination findings consistent with volume excess. Among those with very high albuminuria of any etiology, a large body of literature supports the use of either ACEi or angiotensin receptor blocker (ARB) therapy to slow the progression of CKD.

Among the 350 patients with IgA nephropathy in the REIN-2 trial (Ramipril Efficacy in Nephropathy-2), those assigned to ramipril had a slower rate of GFR decline (0.52 mL/min/1.73 m^2) compared with placebo (0.88 mL/min/1.73 m^2) over 36 months of follow-up.[27] The Captopril trial, which enrolled 500 participants with diabetic nephropathy, showed that ACEi therapy resulted in a decline in creatinine clearance of 11% per year compared with 17% per year among placebo treated patients with diabetic nephropathy.[21] Comparable results were achieved with the ARB irbesartan in a population with diabetic nephropathy. Among the 1700 enrolled, patients treated with irbesartan were one-third less likely to have a doubling of their serum creatinine (vs placebo) over 2.5 years of follow-up.[28] Equally impressive results were achieved in the Reduction of Endpoints in NIDDM with the RENAAL, which found that among the 1500 participants treated for 3.5 years, those in the losartan arm were 15% less likely to suffer a doubling of serum creatinine compared with placebo.[29]

In light of the above beneficial effects of ACEi or ARB therapy on renal outcomes, trials evaluating the effects their combination were conducted. In 3 separate trials involving about 25,000 patients, the ALTITUDE Trial (Aliskerin Trial in Type 2 Diabetes Using Cardiorenal Endpoints), the ONTARGET trial (Ongoing Telmisartan Alone or in Combination with Ramipril Global Endpoint Trial), and the VA NEPHRON-D (Veterans Affairs Nephropathy in Diabetes), found that dual therapy, while lowering levels of albuminuria more than ACEi or ARB monotherapy, resulted in higher rates of acute kidney injury, hypotension, and hyperkalemia than those randomized to single agent treatment.[30–32]

Although CCBs do not have the level of evidence available for RAAS blockers, they are safe and effective antihypertensives in those with CKD. Moreover, nondihydropyridine CCBs (diltiazem and verapamil) offer additional antiproteinuric effects when compared with the dihydropyridine subclass.[33] Nonetheless, decreases in proteinuria reduction with nondihydropyridine CCBs have not been properly studied to assess their effects on CKD progression. Animal data suggest a beneficial effect similar to RAS blockers on morphologic changes in the kidney by diltiazem but not as protective.[34] As such, dihydropyridine CCBs be accompanied by a RAAS blocker when used among those with high albuminuria.[17] Conversely, nondihydropyridine CCBs may be used without a RAAS blocker if the patient is not a candidate for the latter.[17]

Data regarding the effectiveness of β-blockers as among hypertensives with CKD is limited. Among patients in the AASK trial, those randomized to the metoprolol arm experienced rates of CKD progression comparable with those allocated to the amlodipine arm with both inferior to ACEi therapy.[35] Accordingly, such agents are generally reserved for those with cardiac indications or among those requiring multiple classes to achieve blood pressure control. However, a recent study in dialysis patients demonstrated a mortality risk reduction with a β-blocker and not an ACEi.[36]

As of late, there has been renewed interest in aldosterone antagonists such as spironolactone and eplerenone. These agents demonstrate efficacy in cases of "resistant" hypertension and further reduce albuminuria in those treated with ACEi or ARB monotherapy.[37,38] Physiologic plausibility of their utility lies in their ability to prevent the "aldosterone escape" that occurs after sustained therapy with either ACEi or ARBs.[39] The PATHWAY-2 trial (Spironolactone versus Placebo, Bisoprolol, and Doxazosin to Determine the Optimal Treatment for Drug Resistant Hypertension) randomized roughly 325 patients with a mean home blood pressure of 148/84 mm Hg despite ACEi, CCB, and diuretic therapy to either spironolactone, bisoprolol, or doxazosin. Spironolactone therapy resulted in an 8.7-mm Hg reduction in home systolic blood pressure compared with placebo and a 4.3-mm Hg further reduction than either doxazosin or bisoprolol (**Fig. 4**).[37]

Evidence supporting spironolactone's use for proteinuria suppression have been published in both those with and without diabetic nephropathy. Among 75 patients with persistent diabetic nephropathy (mean GFR, 65 mL/min/1.73 m^2; mean albuminuria, 1 g/d) despite lisinopril, spironolactone was superior to losartan with respect to further urine protein reduction.[38] Comparable outcomes have been noted with the selective mineralocorticoid receptor blocker eplerenone.[40]

The principal obstacle to the widespread use of aldosterone antagonists remains hyperkalemia, an adverse event particularly common among those with diabetic nephropathy. Studies shows that those on ACEi or ARB therapy have a 3- to 8-fold greater risk of hyperkalemia if their pretreatment GFR is less than 45 mL/min/1.73 m^2 and pretreatment potassium is in excess of 4.5 mEq/L.[41] Finerenone, a nonsteroidal mineralocorticoid antagonist, was evaluated in the ARTS-DN (Mineralocorticoid Receptor Antagonist Tolerability Study-Diabetic Nephropathy) with this

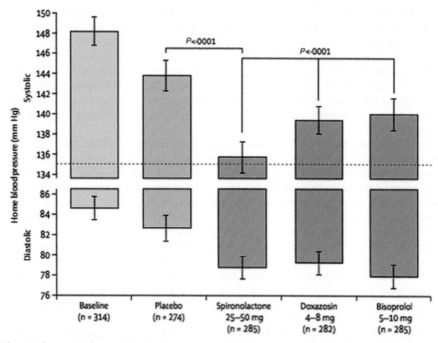

Fig. 4. Changes in home blood pressure among those treated with placebo, spironolactone, bisoprolol, or doxazosin. (*From* Williams B, MacDonald TM, Morant S, et al. Spironolactone versus placebo, bisoprolol, and doxazosin to determine the optimal treatment for drug-resistant hypertension (PATHWAY-2): a randomised, double-blind, crossover trial. Lancet 2015;386(10008):2063; with permission.)

endpoint in mind. Among the more than 800 participants (GFR, 65–70 mL/min/1.73 m^2; albuminuria, 180 mg/d) randomized to ACEi or ARB monotherapy plus finerenone or placebo, only 6% of participants exceeded a serum potassium of 5.6 mEq/L, all while achieving a 40% reduction in albuminuria.[42]

Apart from diuretics and the cation exchange resin sodium polystyrene sulfonate, there were historically few treatment options available to prevent hyperkalemia; as such, application of aldosterone antagonist therapy was limited. Recently, 2 novel cation exchange compounds, patiromer and zirconium cyclosilicate (ZS-9), have been developed. Patiromer is currently approved by the Food and Drug Administration, whereas ZS-9 has not. Mechanistically, both agents bind enteric potassium preventing systemic absorption in a manner similar to sodium polystyrene; however, ZS-9 is sodium based and patiromer is paired with calcium.

In 2 double-blind, placebo-controlled trials involving more than 1000 patients, the HARMONIZE (Hyperkalemia Randomized Intervention Multi-dose ZS-9 Maintenance) and a trial by Packham and colleagues, the selective sodium and hydrogen exchanger ZS-9 was compared with placebo for 2 to 4 weeks. In both trials, the majority of patients had diabetes (60%), CKD stage 3 (75%), and were on RAAS therapy (75%). The percentage of patients on diuretics was not reported. Baseline potassium was between 5.3 to 5.6m Eq/L. Reductions in potassium were dose dependent with absolute reductions up to 1.2 mEq/L. Adverse effects between groups were identical apart edema, which was more commonly encountered as ZS-9 dose rose (6% on high-dose therapy).[43,44]

In the AMETHYST-DN trial, 300 individuals with diabetic nephropathy were administered patiromer. One-half of study patients were on RAAS blockers and 40% on diuretic therapy. Reductions in potassium were again dose dependent with decreases of up to 1.0 mEq/L noted. The most common adverse event was constipation, occurring in 5% to 10% of patients.[45] Based on these results, the OPAL-HK study was undertaken to evaluate the efficacy of patiromer among those with advanced CKD (mean GFR, 35–40 mL/min/1.73 m^2) on RAAS inhibitors. The cohort was 60% diabetic and 50% were on diuretics. After a 1-month period where all 225 patients were placed on patiromer, those whose potassium decreased were then randomized to continuation of therapy or placebo. In contrast with an increase in potassium of 0.7 mEq/L in those switched to placebo, potassium remained within the normal range among those on resin therapy.[46] In aggregate, these apparently well-tolerated novel therapies should allow for wider application of both ACE/ARB and aldosterone antagonist therapy. They will also permit trials testing the lowest GFR, up to which RAAS blockers continue to offer renal protection.

REFERENCES

1. Foundation NK. K/DOQI clinical practice guidelines for chronic kidney disease: evaluation, classification, and stratification. Am J Kidney Dis 2002;39(2 Suppl 1):S1–266.
2. Levey AS, Stevens LA, Schmid CH, et al. A new equation to estimate glomerular filtration rate. Ann Intern Med 2009;150(9):604–12.
3. Levey AS, de Jong PE, Coresh J, et al. The definition, classification, and prognosis of chronic kidney disease: a KDIGO controversies conference report. Kidney Int 2011;80(1):17–28.
4. Coresh J, Selvin E, Stevens LA, et al. Prevalence of chronic kidney disease in the United States. JAMA 2007;298(17):2038–47.
5. Skorecki K, Cheroot G, Marsden P. Brenner and Rector's the kidney. 10th edition. Philadelphia: Elsevier; 2016.
6. Guyton AC. Blood pressure control–special role of the kidneys and body fluids. Science 1991;252(5014):1813–6.
7. Mancia G, Grassi G. The autonomic nervous system and hypertension. Circ Res 2014;114(11):1804–14.
8. Grassi G, Cattaneo BM, Seravalle G, et al. Baroreflex control of sympathetic nerve activity in essential and secondary hypertension. Hypertension 1998;31(1):68–72.
9. Crowley SD, Gurley SB, Herrera MJ, et al. Angiotensin II causes hypertension and cardiac hypertrophy through its receptors in the kidney. Proc Natl Acad Sci U S A 2006;103(47):17985–90.
10. Spieker LE, Flammer AJ, Lüscher TF. The vascular endothelium in hypertension. Handb Exp Pharmacol 2006;176(Pt 2):249–83.
11. Dharmashankar K, Widlansky ME. Vascular endothelial function and hypertension: insights and directions. Curr Hypertens Rep 2010;12(6):448–55.
12. Quinn U, Tomlinson LA, Cockcroft JR. Arterial stiffness. JRSM Cardiovasc Dis 2012;1(6):1–8.
13. Perry HM Jr, Miller JP, Fornoff JR, et al. Early predictors of 15-year end-stage renal disease in hypertensive patients. Hypertension 1995;25(4 Pt 1):587–94.
14. Ishani A, Grandits GA, Grimm RH, et al. Association of single measurements of dipstick proteinuria, estimated glomerular filtration rate, and hematocrit with 25-year incidence of end-stage renal disease in the multiple risk factor intervention trial. J Am Soc Nephrol 2006;17(5):1444–52.

15. Agarwal R. Blood pressure components and the risk for end-stage renal disease and death in chronic kidney disease. Clin J Am Soc Nephrol 2009;4(4):830–7.
16. Levin A, Djurdjev O, Beaulieu M, et al. Variability and risk factors for kidney disease progression and death following attainment of stage 4 CKD in a referred cohort. Am J Kidney Dis 2008;52(4):661–71.
17. Bakris GL, Weir MR, Shanifar S, et al. Effects of blood pressure level on progression of diabetic nephropathy: results from the RENAAL study. Arch Intern Med 2003;163(13):1555–65.
18. Klahr S, Levey AS, Beck GJ, et al. The effects of dietary protein restriction and blood-pressure control on the progression of chronic renal disease. Modification of Diet in Renal Disease Study Group. N Engl J Med 1994;330(13):877–84.
19. Sarnak MJ, Greene T, Wang X, et al. The effect of a lower target blood pressure on the progression of kidney disease: long-term follow-up of the modification of diet in renal disease study. Ann Intern Med 2005;142(5):342–51.
20. Appel LJ, Wright JT, Greene T, et al. Long-term effects of renin-angiotensin system-blocking therapy and a low blood pressure goal on progression of hypertensive chronic kidney disease in African Americans. Arch Intern Med 2008;168(8): 832–9.
21. Lewis JB, Berl T, Bain RP, et al. Effect of intensive blood pressure control on the course of type 1 diabetic nephropathy. Collaborative Study Group. Am J Kidney Dis 1999;34(5):809–17.
22. Schrier RW, Estacio RO, Esler A, et al. Effects of aggressive blood pressure control in normotensive type 2 diabetic patients on albuminuria, retinopathy and strokes. Kidney Int 2002;61(3):1086–97.
23. SPRINT Research Group, Wright JT Jr, Williamson JD, et al. A Randomized Trial of Intensive versus Standard Blood-Pressure Control. N Engl J Med 2015;373(22): 2103–16.
24. Laffin LJ, Bakris GL. Update on blood pressure goals in diabetes mellitus. Curr Cardiol Rep 2015;17(6):37.
25. Lea J, Greene T, Hebert L, et al. The relationship between magnitude of proteinuria reduction and risk of end-stage renal disease: results of the African American Study of Kidney Disease and hypertension. Arch Intern Med 2005;165(8):947–53.
26. Bakris GL, Sarafidis PA, Weir MR, et al. Renal outcomes with different fixed-dose combination therapies in patients with hypertension at high risk for cardiovascular events (ACCOMPLISH): a prespecified secondary analysis of a randomised controlled trial. Lancet 2010;375(9721):1173–81.
27. Ruggenenti P, Perna A, Loriga G, et al. Blood-pressure control for renoprotection in patients with non-diabetic chronic renal disease (REIN-2): multicentre, randomised controlled trial. Lancet 2005;365(9463):939–46.
28. Lewis EJ, Hunsicker LG, Clarke WR, et al. Renoprotective effect of the angiotensin-receptor antagonist irbesartan in patients with nephropathy due to type 2 diabetes. N Engl J Med 2001;345(12):851–60.
29. Brenner BM, Cooper ME, de Zeeuw D, et al. Effects of losartan on renal and cardiovascular outcomes in patients with type 2 diabetes and nephropathy. N Engl J Med 2001;345(12):861–9.
30. Fried LF, Emanuele N, Zhang JH, et al. Combined angiotensin inhibition for the treatment of diabetic nephropathy. N Engl J Med 2013;369(20):1892–903.
31. Parving HH, Brenner BM, McMurray JJ, et al. Cardiorenal end points in a trial of aliskiren for type 2 diabetes. N Engl J Med 2012;367(23):2204–13.
32. Yusuf S, Teo KK, Pogue J, et al. Telmisartan, ramipril, or both in patients at high risk for vascular events. N Engl J Med 2008;358(15):1547–59.

33. Bakris GL, Weir MR, Secic M, et al. Differential effects of calcium antagonist sub-classes on markers of nephropathy progression. Kidney Int 2004;65(6): 1991–2002.
34. Gaber L, Walton C, Brown S, et al. Effects of different antihypertensive treatments on morphologic progression of diabetic nephropathy in uninephrectomized dogs. Kidney Int 1994;46(1):161–9.
35. Wright JT, Bakris G, Greene T, et al. Effect of blood pressure lowering and anti-hypertensive drug class on progression of hypertensive kidney disease: results from the AASK trial. JAMA 2002;288(19):2421–31.
36. Agarwal R, Sinha AD, Pappas MK, et al. Hypertension in hemodialysis patients treated with atenolol or lisinopril: a randomized controlled trial. Nephrol Dial Transplant 2014;29(3):672–81.
37. Williams B, MacDonald TM, Morant S, et al. Spironolactone versus placebo, biso-prolol, and doxazosin to determine the optimal treatment for drug-resistant hyper-tension (PATHWAY-2): a randomised, double-blind, crossover trial. Lancet 2015; 386(10008):2059–68.
38. Mehdi UF, Adams-Huet B, Raskin P, et al. Addition of angiotensin receptor blockade or mineralocorticoid antagonism to maximal angiotensin-converting enzyme inhibition in diabetic nephropathy. J Am Soc Nephrol 2009;20(12): 2641–50.
39. Bakris GL, Siomos M, Richardson D, et al. ACE inhibition or angiotensin receptor blockade: impact on potassium in renal failure. VAL-K Study Group. Kidney Int 2000;58(5):2084–92.
40. Epstein M, Williams GH, Weinberger M, et al. Selective aldosterone blockade with eplerenone reduces albuminuria in patients with type 2 diabetes. Clin J Am Soc Nephrol 2006;1(5):940–51.
41. Lazich I, Bakris GL. Prediction and management of hyperkalemia across the spectrum of chronic kidney disease. Semin Nephrol 2014;34(3):333–9.
42. Bakris GL, Agarwal R, Chan JC, et al. Effect of finerenone on albuminuria in pa-tients with diabetic nephropathy: a randomized clinical trial. JAMA 2015;314(9): 884–94.
43. Kosiborod M, Rasmussen HS, Lavin P, et al. Effect of sodium zirconium cyclosi-licate on potassium lowering for 28 days among outpatients with hyperkalemia: the HARMONIZE randomized clinical trial. JAMA 2014;312(21):2223–33.
44. Packham DK, Rasmussen HS, Lavin PT, et al. Sodium zirconium cyclosilicate in hyperkalemia. N Engl J Med 2015;372(3):222–31.
45. Bakris GL, Pitt B, Weir MR, et al. Effect of patiromer on serum potassium level in patients with hyperkalemia and diabetic kidney disease: the AMETHYST-DN ran-domized clinical trial. JAMA 2015;314(2):151–61.
46. Weir MR, Bakris GL, Bushinsky DA, et al. Patiromer in patients with kidney dis-ease and hyperkalemia receiving RAAS inhibitors. N Engl J Med 2015;372(3): 211–21.

Guidelines for the Management of Hypertension

Aram V. Chobanian, MD

KEYWORDS

- Hypertension • Antihypertensive therapy • SPRINT study • Blood pressure goals
- Management of hypertension

KEY POINTS

- This article summarizes pertinent data from clinical trials on the effects of antihypertensive therapy on cardiovascular complications.
- Prior definitions of hypertension and blood pressure goals of therapy are discussed, and differences between national and international guidelines on such goals are summarized.
- The results of the SPRINT study are summarized, and the impact of this study on future goals of treatment is discussed.
- New recommendations are provided on blood pressure goals, and the effects such goals might have on clinical practice are discussed.

INTRODUCTION

Actuarial data indicated almost a century ago that elevated blood pressure (BP) shortened life expectancy,[1] but it was not until many years later that much attention was given to lowering BP because of fear of compromising perfusion to vital organs.[2] However, a few pioneers, such as Walter Kempner, who used extreme dietary measures; Reginald Smithwick, who used surgical lumbodorsal sympathectomy; and my mentor, Robert Wilkins, using drug therapy, began to study the effects of BP lowering in persons with marked elevations and demonstrated that reducing BP was in fact well-tolerated by most.[3–5] Such observations led to a rapid expansion of efforts by the pharmaceutical industry to develop new therapies for hypertension. The advances made since then have been truly remarkable. Several effective and well-tolerated antihypertensive drugs were introduced (**Box 1**), and clinical trials were performed to study their effects in hypertensive persons. Initially, "proof of principle" studies were carried out in persons with malignant hypertension (whose life expectancy if untreated averages 6–12 months) and showed major benefits in preventing congestive heart failure, renal failure, and hemorrhagic strokes, and in prolonging life.[6] The landmark Veterans Administration

Department of Medicine, Boston University School of Medicine, Boston University, 72 East Concord Street, E-7, Boston, MA 02118, USA
E-mail address: achob@bu.edu

Med Clin N Am 101 (2017) 219–227
http://dx.doi.org/10.1016/j.mcna.2016.08.016
0025-7125/17/© 2016 Elsevier Inc. All rights reserved.

medical.theclinics.com

Box 1
Advances in the treatment of hypertension

Decade and Therapy

1940s
  Potassium thiocyanate
  Kempner diet
  Surgical sympathectomy

1950s
  Rauwolfia serpentina
  Ganglionic blockers
  Veratrum alkaloids
  Hydralazine
  Guanethidine
  Thiazide diuretics

1960s
  Alpha-2 adrenergic receptor agonists
  Spironolactone
  Beta adrenergic receptor antagonists

1970s
  Alpha-1 receptor antagonists
  Angiotensin-converting enzyme inhibitors

1980s
  Calcium channel blocking drugs

1990s
  Angiotensin receptor antagonists

2000s
  Renin inhibitors
  Renal sympathetic denervation (experimental)

Adapted from Chobanian AV. The Shattuck Lecture. The hypertension paradox–more uncontrolled disease despite improved therapy. N Engl J Med 2009;361:878–87; with permission.

Cooperative Trials then demonstrated benefits of treatment in those with diastolic BP (DBP) in the 115 to 129 mm Hg range and subsequently in the 90 to 114 range.[7,8]

After epidemiologic data demonstrated that systolic BP (SBP) was a more important cardiovascular disease (CVD) risk factor than DBP after age 50, placebo-controlled trials were performed to investigate the benefits of decreasing SBP in older persons with isolated systolic hypertension. Notable in this regard were the Systolic Hypertension in the Elderly Program (SHEP) in which reducing SBP to lower than 160 mm Hg with chlorthalidone-based therapy was associated with reductions in incidences of stroke and cardiac diseases,[9] and also the Systolic Hypertension in Europe Trial (Syst-Eur), which showed broadly similar benefits but with nitrendipine-based treatment.[10] These and various other studies demonstrated that BP reduction in persons with hypertension can reduce the incidence of stroke, coronary heart disease (CHD), congestive heart failure (CHF), and chronic renal disease, and that such benefits can be obtained independent of age, gender, race, ethnicity, socioeconomic status, severity of hypertension, or the presence or absence of target organ damage.[11]

DEFINITION OF HYPERTENSION

The definition of hypertension has changed over the past several years. BP on a population-wide basis is a continuous variable with a Gaussian distribution and without any clear point that would denote abnormality. The relationship between both SBP and DBP and CVD risk also appears continuous. In a large observational study involving approximately 1 million individuals, mortality from heart disease and stroke increased almost linearly from BP levels as low as 115/75 mm Hg with an approximate doubling of risk for every 20/10 mm Hg increase above that level.[12] The definition of hypertension has reflected in part the level above which the benefits of treatment outweigh the risks, so it is not surprising that as more effective and safer drugs became available, the definition changed. In the late 1950s, when thiazide diuretics first were introduced, hypertension was not well defined but generally was considered to be associated with BP levels greater than 180/100 mm Hg. Succeeding decades brought lower values (**Table 1**).[11,13] Most current definitions denote hypertension as SBP ≥140 mm Hg and/or DBP ≥90 mm Hg.

In prior classifications of BP, other categories were included, such as mild, moderate, and severe hypertension; isolated systolic hypertension; and high normal BP. The current classification, which was introduced in the Seventh Joint National Committee (JNC-7) Report in 2003, simplifies previous versions (**Table 2**).[11] Only 2 levels of severity of hypertension are designated to reflect the view that any BP level ≥160/100 mm Hg deserves aggressive therapy. A new category of "prehypertension," as defined by BP levels between 120 and 139/80 to 89 mm Hg was introduced to identify individuals who could benefit most from lifestyle changes that would reduce BP or delay its age-associated transition to hypertension.

TREATMENT APPROACHES
Lifestyle Modifications

The adoption of certain healthy lifestyles is recommended for all persons with hypertension, whether or not they are receiving drug therapy. The most important of these nondrug approaches are weight control, exercise, dietary sodium restriction, moderation of alcohol intake, and use of the Dietary Approaches to Stop Hypertension (DASH) eating plan, which emphasizes intake of fruits, vegetables, complex carbohydrates, legumes, and low-fat dairy products.[14] Most persons with stage 1 hypertension can be treated initially with lifestyle modifications, and drug therapy can be delayed for 4 to 6 months until the effects become apparent.

Drug Treatment

Thiazide-type diuretics, beta blockers (BB), angiotensin-converting enzyme inhibitors (ACEI), angiotensin receptor blockers (ARB), and calcium channel blockers (CCB) are the most useful classes of antihypertensive drugs, having been shown in clinical trials to reduce CVD complications.[11] The average BP reduction with each of these classes is comparable at recommended dosages, although differences in response can exist in individual patients. More than one-half of hypertensive persons will require 2 or more antihypertensive medications to achieve goal BP, so fixed-drug combinations are also useful.

Table 1
Definitions of hypertension 1950 to the present

Period	Hypertension BP Level
1950s and 1960s	>180/100 mm Hg
1970s–1984	≥160/95 mm Hg
1985–present	≥140/90 mm Hg

Table 2 Current classification of blood pressure in adults			
Classification	SBP, mm Hg		DBP, mm Hg
Normal	<120	and	<80
Prehypertension	129–139	and/or	80–89
Stage 1 hypertension	140–159	and/or	90–99
Stage 2 hypertension	≥160	and/or	≥100

From Chobanian AV, Bakris GL, Black HR, et al. Seventh report of the Joint National Committee on prevention, detection, evaluation, and treatment of high blood pressure. Hypertension 2003;42(6):1206–52; with permission.

Several studies have been performed to determine whether any particular antihypertensive drug class or combination of drugs is superior to any other, but in general, only slight differences in clinical outcomes between the drug classes has been shown as long as equivalent reductions in BP are achieved.[15] However, in the Losartan Intervention for Endpoint Reduction in Hypertension (LIFE) study, losartan-based therapy was found to be superior to atenolol-based treatment.[16] Additional studies also suggested that BBs were not as effective in reducing stroke as other antihypertensive medications, so BBs are not recommended for initial treatment unless a compelling indication exists for their use.[15]

Compelling indications for selection of specific drug classes include use of ACEIs and ARBs in patients with chronic renal disease, diabetes, heart failure, and post–myocardial infarction; and BBs in those with angina pectoris, arrhythmias, post–myocardial infarction, and heart failure.[11]

A treatment algorithm for hypertension is shown in **Fig. 1**. As noted, in stage 1 hypertension (SBP 140–159 mm Hg and/or DBP 90–99 mm Hg), treatment can be initiated with lifestyle modifications and drugs added if goal BP is not reached. As already indicated, the initial selection of either a diuretic, ACEI, CCB, or ARB is appropriate depending on physician experience and patient acceptance or the presence of a compelling indication. A second, and if needed, a third drug from a different class can be added, although a combination of an ACEI and ARB is not indicated. Doses should be optimized and adherence to therapy assessed if the response is still insufficient.

With stage 2 hypertension (BP ≥160/100 mm Hg), the initial approach, although broadly similar to that indicated for stage 1 hypertension, should be more aggressive. Drug treatment should not be delayed and can be started with 2 drugs or a combination preparation. Should goal BP not be attained after concurrent use of 3 antihypertensive medications, then the addition of an aldosterone antagonist to the regimen is particularly useful to control the refractory hypertension. Poor adherence to therapy, insufficient dosages of medications, and possible salt retention should be ruled out. Such refractory patients also should be evaluated for secondary causes of hypertension, including use of recreational drugs and excessive intake of alcohol.

BLOOD PRESSURE GOALS OF ANTIHYPERTENSIVE THERAPY

A DBP goal of lower than 90 mm Hg has been considered appropriate for most adults, but the target for SBP has been more controversial. In the SHEP trial, the reduction of SBP from pretreatment levels of ≥160 mm Hg to 143 mm Hg with active treatment and to 155 mm Hg with placebo was associated with a 36% reduction in stroke incidence

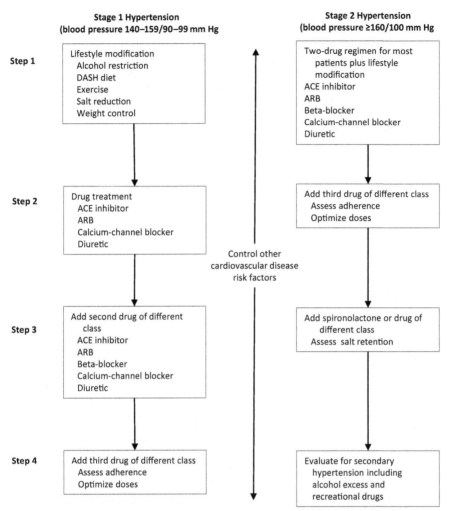

Fig. 1. Algorithm for management of hypertension. (*Adapted from* Chobanian AV. The Shattuck Lecture. The hypertension paradox – more uncontrolled disease despite improved therapy. N Engl J Med 2009;361:878–87; with permission.)

and 54% in heart failure with drug treatment.[9] The Hypertension in the Very Elderly Trial focused on those older than 80 with systolic hypertension who were treated with either a placebo or a combination of an ACEI and a thiazide-type diuretic.[17] Reduction of SBP to an average of 143 mm Hg with medications was associated with a significant reduction in CVD events.

Many hypertension treatment guidelines have been published in the past few years. How these have addressed the treatment goals is worth reviewing because of the lack of agreement existing between them. As examples, the National Institute for Clinical Excellence (NICE) has recommended drug therapy for those with SBP ≥140 mm Hg who are diabetic or who have a history of chronic renal disease or CVD. However, in those at low risk for CVD, only lifestyle changes are advocated by NICE unless SBP is ≥160 mm Hg.[18] The joint European Society of Hypertension/European Society of

Cardiology committee has recommended an SBP goal of lower than 140 mm Hg, except in those older than 80, in whom the recommended goal is 140 to 150 mm Hg.[19] In the American Society of Hypertension and International Society of Hypertension joint report, a goal of 150/90 mm Hg is advocated for those ≥80 years of age.[20] The report by members of the JNC-8 Committee originally appointed by the National Heart, Lung, and Blood Institute (NHLBI) but later disenfranchised by it added to the confusion. Unlike prior JNC groups, JNC-8 focused primarily on data obtained from randomized controlled clinical trials rather than considering the totality of clinical evidence as had been done by prior JNC groups. The JNC-8 Report advocated a target BP of lower than 140/90 mm Hg in those younger than 60 and lower than 150/90 mm Hg in persons 60 years or older.[21] However, the Committee was divided on increasing the goal for the older age group, so much so that a minority report was also published by a subgroup of the Committee advocating a target of lower than 140/90 mm Hg in those older than 60.[22]

SYSTOLIC BLOOD PRESSURE INTERVENTION TRIAL

All of the treatment goals noted previously probably need to be reconsidered now because of the recently published findings from the Systolic Blood Pressure Intervention Trial (SPRINT).[23,24] SPRINT was a randomized, controlled, open-labeled study funded by the NHLBI that involved more than 9300 individuals 50 years of age and older who had SBP in the 130 to 180 mm Hg range. They either had evidence of prior CVD events or were at high risk for CVD. Persons with diabetes were excluded because another NHLBI-funded study with a similar protocol, the ACCORD trial, dealt exclusively with diabetic persons.[25] Other exclusions in SPRINT included individuals with a history of stroke or those who were not ambulatory or who were confined to institutions. Office BP measurements were made after a period of rest with an automated device. The main objective of SPRINT was to determine whether lowering SBP to lower than 120 mm Hg (intensive therapy) caused a lower incidence of CVD events than when SBP was lowered to lower than 140 mm Hg (standard therapy). The selection of antihypertensive medications was left to the discretion of the clinician, although chlorthalidone was preferred as the thiazide-type diuretic and amlodipine as the preferred CCB, consistent with the use of these 2 drugs in other recent NHLBI-sponsored trials. As shown in **Table 3**, impressive benefits were observed in the intensive group, which had a 25% lower incidence of composite primary events (myocardial infarction, other coronary syndromes, CHF, stroke, or death from CVD). In addition, total mortality was 27% lower with intensive as compared with standard therapy. Because of these remarkable findings, the study was terminated prematurely after an average follow-up of 3.3 years. In a subgroup analysis of individuals 75 years or older included in the trial, the results were comparable to those observed in the total SPRINT cohort with a 34% lower incidence of the primary outcome and a 33% lower total mortality with intensive therapy.[24] Of interest with respect to prior concerns about the risk of lowering DBP excessively in the elderly was the finding that CHD incidence in the SPRINT elderly group was significantly lower with intensive therapy, even though DBP was reduced to an average level of 62 mm Hg or 5 mm Hg lower than that achieved with standard therapy.

The safety data available currently for SPRINT have been somewhat reassuring in that no major problems have been reported as yet with intensive treatment except for slight increases in incidence of hypotension, syncope, electrolyte abnormalities, and acute changes in renal function. Additional information about these and other potential problems including the effects of treatment on cognitive function will be important to examine before the full significance of the study can be determined.

Table 3	
Benefits of intensive versus standard therapy in SPRINT	
Outcome	Relative Risk Reduction
Composite primary endpoint	−25%
Secondary endpoints	
Myocardial infarction	−17%
Heart failure	−38%
Death from cardiovascular causes	−43%
Death from all causes	−27%

Adapted from SPRINT Research Group, Wright JT Jr, Williamson JD, Whelton PK, et al. A randomized trial of intensive versus standard blood-pressure control. N Engl J Med 2015;373:2103–16.

Because of the exclusion criteria used, the SPRINT findings are not applicable to persons with diabetes or prior stroke. The ACCORD study of individuals with type 2 diabetes failed to show a reduction in the composite primary endpoint with intensive BP lowering.[25] However, there was a significant decrease in stroke incidence in this group and a nonsignificant reduction in primary events. It has been speculated that because ACCORD involved a much smaller group than SPRINT, it was not powered sufficiently to detect a significant effect on primary outcomes.[23]

NEW RECOMMENDATIONS ON BLOOD PRESSURE GOALS

The SPRINT findings require a reassessment of the goals, notwithstanding the fact that subjects recruited into SPRINT were probably not representative of those seen in clinical practice who typically have more concurrent illnesses and are on more other medications. In addition, the office BP measurements in SPRINT were made under relatively basal conditions, and the values recorded and used for treatment decisions were probably less than if obtained in busy office settings in which a "white coat" effect would be more likely. Nevertheless, the SPRINT findings are so impressive that they cannot be disregarded.

What should we now conclude regarding BP goals? For most hypertensive adults younger than age 50, I think that a BP goal of 120 to 125/80 to 85 mm Hg is reasonable based on the available data from both clinical trials and epidemiologic and observational studies. For most nondiabetic persons 50 to 74 years of age, including those with CVD or chronic renal disease, an SBP goal of lower than 130 mm Hg seems appropriate (although a somewhat lower goal may be indicated in those with CHF). A goal of lower than 120 mm Hg in the 50-year to 74-year age group would not be appropriate despite the SPRINT data because the SBP actually achieved with intensive therapy in SPRINT averaged 123 and not lower than 120 mm Hg and because of the possible measurement issues noted previously.

In the 75 years of age or older group, although a goal of lower than 130 mm Hg might be reasonable for many, I would advocate a stepwise approach to achieving such a target to minimize adverse events. An initial SBP goal of lower than 140 mm Hg is appropriate and perhaps adequate in some, but if well-tolerated, a further titration to lower than 130 mm Hg could be considered. However, there should not be any urgency in pursuing this goal. Such patients should be monitored closely for adverse effects, such as orthostatic hypotension, syncope, and changes in cognition and renal function. Treatment of nonambulatory, institutionalized, or frail persons should be managed on an individual basis.

Currently, using the lower than 140/90 mm Hg goal level, slightly more than 50% of hypertensive persons in the United States would be considered as controlled.[26]

Lowering the SBP goal to lower than 130 mm Hg would mean that between one-half to two-thirds of hypertensive persons are inadequately treated. The impact on clinical practice could be considerable. Additional antihypertensive medications would need to be used in some, and closer monitoring of patients and more frequent clinic visits might be required. It therefore becomes even more important to use nurse practitioners, physician assistants, and other nonphysician personnel, as well as treatment algorithms, and other approaches to optimize follow-up care.

PUBLIC HEALTH CONSIDERATIONS

The prevention and management of hypertension remains a major public health problem in the United States and the rest of the world. Although the major focus of this article has been on drug treatment and treatment goals, measures to prevent or slow the onset of hypertension should not be disregarded, as the prevalence of hypertension continues to increase steadily worldwide. In 1988, its prevalence in the United States was estimated at 57 million,[11] and currently the estimates are between 75 and 78 million. Changes in lifestyles, although difficult to achieve, could not only slow the rate of development of hypertension but have the additional benefit of reducing other cardiovascular risk factors as well. Unfortunately, such preventive measures continue to receive relatively low priority in this country, where the major emphasis is still being placed on drug treatment of established disease.

Despite many remaining uncertainties regarding the management of hypertension, the progress made to date in achieving its control and reducing its complications has been one of the major success stories in medicine in the past half century. Hopefully, a similar degree of progress can be made in the future to prevent hypertension.

REFERENCES

1. Hunter A, Rogers OH. Mortality study of impaired lives. Actuarial Soc 1923;24:338.
2. Perera GA. Hypertensive vascular disease; description and natural history. J Chronic Dis 1955;1:33–42.
3. Kempner W. Treatment of hypertensive vascular disease with rice diet. Am J Med 1948;26:545–77.
4. Smithwick RH. The surgical treatment of hypertension. N Y State J Med 1944;44:1693–708.
5. Wilkins RW. New drug therapies in arterial hypertension. Ann Intern Med 1952;37:1144–55.
6. Dustan H, Schneckloth RE, Corcoran AC, et al. The effectiveness of long-term treatment of malignant hypertension. Circulation 1958;18:644–51.
7. Veterans Administration Cooperative Study Group on Antihypertensive Agents. Effects of treatment on morbidity in hypertension. Results in patients with diastolic blood pressures averaging 115 through 129 mm Hg. JAMA 1967;202:1028–34.
8. Veterans Administration Cooperative Study Group on Antihypertensive Agents. Effects of treatment on morbidity in hypertension. II. Results in patients with diastolic blood pressure averaging 90 through 114 mm Hg. JAMA 1970;213:1143–52.
9. Prevention of stroke by antihypertensive drug treatment in older persons with isolated systolic hypertension. Final results of the Systolic Hypertension in the Elderly Program (SHEP). SHEP Cooperative Research Group. JAMA 1991;265:3255–64.
10. Staessen J, Fagard R, Thijs L, et al. Randomised double-blind comparison of placebo and active treatment for older patients with isolated systolic hypertension. Lancet 1997;350:757–64.

11. Chobanian AV, Bakris GL, Black HR, et al, National High Blood Pressure Education Program Coordinating Committee. The seventh report of the Joint National Committee on the prevention, detection, evaluation and treatment of high blood pressure. Hypertension 2003;42:1206–52.

12. Lewington S, Clarke R, Qizilbash N, et al. Age-specific relevance of usual blood pressure to vascular mortality. Lancet 2002;360:1903–13.

13. Final Report of the Subcommittee on Definition and Prevalence of the 1984 Joint National Committee. Hypertension prevalence and the status of awareness, treatment and control in the United States. Hypertension 1985;7:457–68.

14. Sacks FM, Svetkey LP, Vollmer WM, et al. Effects on blood pressure of reduced dietary sodium and the Dietary Approaches to Stop Hypertension (DASH) diet. DASH-Sodium Collaborative Research Group. N Engl J Med 2001;344:3–10.

15. Chobanian AV. The hypertension paradox–more uncontrolled disease despite improved therapy. N Engl J Med 2009;361:878–87.

16. Dahlöf B, Devereux RB, Kjeldsen SE, et al, LIFE Study Group. Cardiovascular morbidity and mortality in the Losartan Intervention For Endpoint reduction in hypertension study (LIFE): a randomized trial against atenolol. Lancet 2002;359:995–1003.

17. Beckett NS, Peters R, Fletcher AE, et al. Treatment of hypertension in patients 80 years of age or older. N Engl J Med 2008;358:1887–98.

18. National Institute for Health and Clinical Excellence. Hypertension: clinical management of hypertension in adults. Available at: http://www.nice.org.uk/guidance/cg127. Accessed June 2, 2016.

19. Mancia G, Fagard R, Narkiewicz K, et al. Guidelines for the management of arterial hypertension: the Task Force for the management of arterial hypertension of the European Society of Hypertension (ESH) and the European Society of Cardiology (ESC). J Hypertens 2013;31:1281–357.

20. Weber MA, Schffrin EL, White WB, et al. Clinical practice guidelines for the management of hypertension in the community: a statement by the American Society of Hypertension and the International Society of Hypertension. J Clin Hypertens 2014;32:3–15.

21. James PA, Oparil S, Carter BL, et al. 2014 evidence-based guideline for the management of high blood pressure in adults. Report from the panel members appointed to the Eighth Joint National Committee (JNC 8). JAMA 2014;311:507–20.

22. Wright JT, Fine LJ, Lackland DT, et al. Evidence supporting a systolic blood pressure goal of less than 150 mmHg in patients aged 60 years or older: the minority view. Ann Intern Med 2014;160:499–503.

23. SPRINT Research Group, Wright JT, Williamson JD, Whelton PK, et al. A randomized trial of intensive versus standard blood-pressure control. N Engl J Med 2015;373:2103–16.

24. Williamson JD, Supiano MA, Applegate WB, et al. Intensive versus standard blood pressure control and cardiovascular disease outcomes among adults age 75 and older. JAMA 2016;315(24):2673–82.

25. Cushman WC, Evans GW, Byington RP, et al. Effects of intensive blood-pressure control in type 2 diabetes mellitus (ACCORD). N Engl J Med 2010;362:1575–85.

26. Go AS, Mozaffarian D, Roger VL, et al, American Heart Association Statistics Committee and Stroke Statistics Subcommittee. Executive summary: heart disease and stroke statistics—2014 update: a report from the American Heart Association. Circulation 2014;129:399–410.

Adherence to Antihypertensive Therapy

Erin Peacock, PhD, MPH[a], Marie Krousel-Wood, MD, MSPH[a,b,c,]*

KEYWORDS

- Medication adherence • Hypertension • Interventions

KEY POINTS

- Relatively modest changes in adherence can lead to clinically significant improvements in BP control and reductions in cardiovascular events.
- Interventions associated with improved adherence tend to use ongoing, sustained focus, repeated contacts, and multiple strategies for addressing medication-taking behaviors.
- Promising strategies to improve antihypertensive medication adherence include regimen simplification, reduction of out-of-pocket costs, use of allied health professionals in delivering interventions (including team-based collaborative care), and self-monitoring of BP.
- Research to understand the effects of emerging technology-mediated interventions, mechanisms underlying adherence behavior, and sex-race differences in determinants of low adherence and intervention effectiveness may enhance patient-specific approaches to improve adherence and disease control.

INTRODUCTION

On average, only 50% of adults adhere to chronic disease medications[1,2]; and in the case of high blood pressure (BP), lower levels of adherence are associated with worse BP control and adverse outcomes, including stroke, myocardial infarction, heart failure, and death.[3–5] Although effective medications that control BP and reduce the risk of stroke, renal, and cardiovascular disease are available, uncontrolled BP and low adherence to antihypertensive drugs persist as major public health and clinical challenges.[6,7] Research in the past decade has identified determinants of poor adherence and explored the impact of interventions to address barriers, improve adherence, and ultimately achieve BP control. Several approaches have proven successful, although no single intervention has emerged as superior in improving

Disclosure: See last page of article.
[a] Department of Medicine, Tulane University School of Medicine, 1430 Tulane Avenue, New Orleans, LA 70112, USA; [b] Department of Epidemiology, Tulane University School of Public Health and Tropical Medicine, 1440 Canal Street, New Orleans, LA 70112, USA; [c] Center for Health Research, Ochsner Clinic Foundation, 1514 Jefferson Highway, New Orleans, LA 70121, USA
* Corresponding author. Tulane University School of Medicine, 1430 Tulane Avenue, New Orleans, LA 70112.
E-mail addresses: mawood@tulane.edu; mawood@ochsner.org

Med Clin N Am 101 (2017) 229–245
http://dx.doi.org/10.1016/j.mcna.2016.08.005
0025-7125/17/© 2016 Elsevier Inc. All rights reserved.

adherence and lowering BP across all groups. As the lower systolic BP (SBP) treatment target (<120 mm Hg) suggested by the recent Systolic Blood Pressure Intervention Trial (SPRINT) results[8,9] is integrated into clinical practice guidelines,[10] new performance standards for BP control will likely emerge and greater attention will be given to improving patient adherence to prescribed therapies in an effort to achieve BP control using the lower target.

Modest changes in adherence can lead to clinically significant reductions in BP.[11] In turn, relatively small reductions in BP are associated with improvements in mortality[12–14]: a reduction in SBP of 3 mm Hg is associated with an 8% reduction in stroke mortality and a 5% reduction in mortality from coronary heart disease.[14] Thus, efforts that lead to even modest improvements on adherence can have an appreciable effect on health outcomes at the population level. The purpose of this article was to provide an overview of the current status and recent developments regarding interventions to improve adherence to antihypertensive medications for primary prevention of cardiovascular events.

TYPES OF INTERVENTIONS TO IMPROVE MEDICATION ADHERENCE

Interventions to promote medication adherence may target a number of identified patient-specific barriers: asymptomatic nature of hypertension[15,16]; depression[17–21]; comorbidities[20]; low health literacy[22–24]; medication complexity, cost, and concerns[25–28]; use of alternative medicine[29–31]; poor health care system perceptions[32]; perceived discrimination[26,33]; poor communication or provider-patient interaction[33–35]; medication side effects[34,36]; forgetfulness[37,38]; inadequate social support or coping[39,40]; caring for dependents[41]; and lack of motivation for self-care.[42] Interventions to target these factors can be classified as informational, behavioral, social, or combined.[43] *Informational interventions* use didactic or interactive approaches to educate and motivate patients and to increase understanding of their condition and its treatment.[43] *Behavioral interventions* move beyond the cognitive approaches of informational interventions to influence patient behaviors by shaping, reminding, or rewarding desired behaviors, whereas *social interventions* enlist family members or others in supporting medication adherence.[43] Finally, *combined interventions*, which are becoming increasingly common, include elements of more than one informational, behavioral, or social strategy. Strategies may vary in intensity, setting (eg, individual, group), mechanism of delivery (eg, face-to-face, technology-mediated), and required personnel (eg, physician, allied health professional, or lay individual) (**Table 1**).

When evaluating the effectiveness of interventions to improve adherence, consideration should be given to the adherence measure used. Validated objective (eg, pharmacy fill,[44,45] electronic monitoring[46]) and subjective (eg, self-report[37,38,47–50]) measures for assessing medication-taking behavior are available (**Table 2**). An effect size of d = 0.2 is considered small, d = 0.5 medium, and d = 0.8 large.[51] In a recent meta-analysis assessing the impact of adherence interventions, the largest effect sizes were found among studies using objective measures of adherence, including electronic event monitoring (d = 0.621), followed by pharmacy fill measures (d = 0.299) and pill counts (d = 0.299), whereas studies using subjective, self-report measures produced smaller effect sizes (d = 0.232).[11] This may be due, in part, to objective measures being less prone to the measurement noise associated with self-report measures, thereby rendering more precise estimates of adherence and easier differentiation between low and high adherence.[52] Given that different tools assess different aspects of behavior along the adherence cascade (**Fig. 1**), use of both objective and self-report measures to identify at-risk patients and target patient-specific needs to improve adherence may facilitate our ability to promote adherence and increase BP control.[5]

Table 1
Strategies for promoting medication adherence

Strategy	Description	Examples
Patient education	Didactic or interactive approaches to provide information and educate patients	• Face-to-face education session • Written or audiovisual education • Mailed instructional material
Social support	Enlistment of family members, friends, or other individuals to support patients in taking their medications as prescribed	• Lay health mentoring • Group support meetings • Family education
Patient motivation	Motivation of patients to take their medication as prescribed and removal of barriers that work against their motivation	• Motivational interviewing • Case management • Problem-solving • Decisional balance activities • Self-monitoring and feedback (see the next two rows)
Self-monitoring	Enlistment of patients to monitor their own BP or adherence	• Home or ambulatory BP monitoring • Home titration[90]
Feedback	Feedback to patients about their adherence or BP	• Telemonitoring of BP data • Rewards for meeting BP goals
Reminders	Reminders to patients to take their medications	• Calendars • Alarms • Pillboxes
Drug packaging	Changes in packaging of medications, intended to remind patients and/or give feedback about medication-taking behavior	• Pillboxes • Blister packaging • Adherence packets
Regimen simplification	Prescription changes or changes in dosage schedule to simplify the regimen	• Combination pills • Once-daily dosing
Reduction of out-of-pocket costs	Reduction of patient out-of-pocket drug costs	• Reduced medication copayments • Improved drug prescription coverage
Communication or interactions with provider	Improvements in patient-provider communication or interactions	• Communication skills training for patients and/or clinicians
Allied health providers and collaborative care	Enlistment of allied health care providers, individually or working as collaborative teams, to implement the intervention	• Pharmacist-delivered interventions • Nurse-delivered interventions • Team-based care

Abbreviation: BP, blood pressure

PROMISING STRATEGIES FOR IMPROVING ADHERENCE

Meta-analyses have linked several intervention characteristics to modest improvements in antihypertensive medication adherence (**Table 3**). Interventions that provide behavioral rather than informational support,[53] are delivered over a longer time

Table 2
Key medication adherence measures

Objective	Subjective
Pharmacy fill[6,17]	Morisky Medication Adherence Scale (MMAS), 4-item and 8-item versions[37,38,47]
• Medication Possession Ratio (MPR)	
• Proportion of Days Covered (PDC)[44,45]	• MMAS-4
Electronic monitoring[46]	• MMAS-8
Pill counts[46]	Krousel-Wood 4-item adherence tool (K-Wood-4)[48]
Direct measurement of drug concentration in blood[46]	Hill-Bone Compliance Scale[49]
	Medication Adherence Estimator[50]

frame,[11,53] and include more intervention components[11] have larger effects on adherence. With respect to health outcomes, larger intervention doses (measured by minutes per session and number of sessions) are more effective at improving BP.[55] Moreover, face-to-face versus mediated delivery of adherence interventions (eg, via mail) is associated with a larger decrease in diastolic BP (DBP), but not with a larger decrease in SBP[55] Taken together, these findings indicate that effective interventions to promote adherence and improve BP control are likely to require ongoing, sustained focus with repeated contacts and a combination of strategies that can be tailored to patients' needs. These intervention characteristics are well-aligned with current movement toward patient-centered approaches to the management of chronic diseases. When implementing and evaluating any intervention, and particularly those that are complex and multicomponent, it is critical to attend to feasibility and implementation fidelity, as the lack of effect found in some studies of multicomponent interventions may be due to poor adherence to the intervention.[56] Challenges associated with poor adherence to multiple components of complex interventions may be addressed by providing incentives for participation, automating aspects of the intervention (eg, wireless home BP monitoring devices that communicate automatically with clinicians and automated feedback provided to patients), or changing defaults to make it easier to make healthy choices (eg, 90-day instead of 30-day prescription refills).[56]

There are specific strategies that should be considered for inclusion in an antihypertensive medication adherence intervention. Regimen simplification, through once-daily dosing, has long been known to be effective at improving medication adherence.[28] Similarly, the use of combination pills may promote medication adherence: in a single study, multivariate odds ratio (OR) for achieving proportion of days covered (PDC) $\geq$80% at 6-month follow-up using single amlodipine/atorvastatin combination pill versus various combinations of separate pills ranged from 1.95 to 3.10 (all $P<.0001$).[57] There is low strength evidence supporting case management as an effective strategy for promoting adherence and improving BP

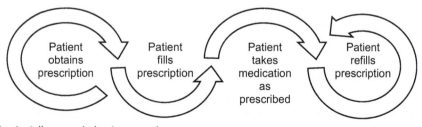

Fig. 1. Adherence behavior cascade.

Table 3
Comparing the effects of intervention characteristics on adherence and blood pressure

Effect on Adherence[a]	Effect on Blood Pressure[b]
Larger effect	Larger effect
• Longer vs shorter time frame (P<.001)	Systolic blood pressure
• More vs fewer intervention components (P<.001)	• Larger intervention dose (P = .021)
• Behavioral vs informational[53]	• Delivered in pharmacies (d = 0.360) vs other locations (d = 0.226) (P = .031)
• Delivered to patients (d = 0.316) vs health care providers (d = 0.107) (P = .030)	• Delivered to groups (d = 0.399) vs individuals/families (d = 0.228) (P = .029)
No difference in effect	Diastolic blood pressure
• Target adherence exclusively (d = 0.318) vs address additional health behaviors (d = 0.292) (P = .768)	• Larger intervention dose (P = .027)
	• Face-to-face (d = 0.221) vs mediated delivery (d = 0.060) (P<.05)
• Delivered in ambulatory care settings (d = 0.272) vs other setting (d = 0.282) (P = .938)	• Delivered in pharmacies (d = 0.356) vs other locations (d = 0.177) (P = .009)
• Delivered in pharmacies (d = 0.432) vs other locations (d = 0.290) (P = .405)	• Delivered to groups (d = 0.376) vs individuals/families (d = 0.179) (P = .018)
• Face-to-face (d = 0.319) vs mediated delivery (d = 0.259) (P = .400)	No difference in effect
• Theory-based (d = 0.335) vs not theory-based (d = 0.284) (P = .554)	Systolic blood pressure
• Larger intervention dose (i.e., no relationship between total minutes of intervention and effect size) (P = .534)	• Presence vs absence of behavior change theory
	• Face-to-face (d = 0.256) vs mediated delivery (d = 0.179) (P>.05)
	• Target patients/families vs health care providers
	• Delivered in ambulatory care settings vs home/community centers
	Diastolic blood pressure
	• Presence vs absence of behavior change theory
	• Target patients/families vs health care providers
	• Delivered in ambulatory care settings vs home/community centers

Where effect sizes and p-values are not listed, those data were not available from the source. No differences in effect may be due to small number of studies using these approaches.
  [a] All results from Conn et al 2015,[11] unless specified.
  [b] All results from Conn et al 2016.[55]

outcomes.[54] Finally, home BP telemonitoring[58] and habit-based interventions[55] have larger effects on health outcomes compared to other interventions, but evidence for larger effects on adherence is limited.[11,58]

Three additional promising interventions for improving medication adherence include reduction of out-of-pocket costs (**Table 4**), use of allied health professionals in promoting medication adherence (**Table 5**), and self-monitoring of BP (**Table 6**). Across several individual studies, reductions in patients' out-of-pocket drug costs (through reduced copayment rates[59,60] and introduction of drug insurance coverage)[61,62] were associated with significant improvements in adherence. Only 1 study, involving financial incentives equal to copayment expenditures, found no effect on adherence.[63] Evidence is limited regarding effects of reduced out-of-pocket costs on health outcomes.

Use of allied health professionals, particularly pharmacists, in interventions to improve medication adherence has proliferated in recent years. In interventions to

Table 4
Effectiveness of interventions to reduce out-of-pocket costs: evidence from individual studies

Study	Description of Intervention	Effect on Adherence[a]

Chernew et al,[59] 2008	Reduction of copayment rates for ACE inhibitors, ARBs, and beta-blockers	• MPR:
		  ○ +2.6% points for ACE inhibitors/ARBs ($P<.001$)
		  ○ +3.0% points for beta-blockers ($P<.001$)

Maciejewski et al,[60] 2010	Reduction of copayment rates	• MPR:
		  ○ +3.4% for diuretics ($P<.001$)
		  ○ +3.1% for ACE inhibitors ($P<.001$)
		  ○ +2.7% for beta-blockers ($P<.001$)
		  ○ +1.3% for calcium-channel blockers ($P<.05$)

Zhang et al,[61] 2010	Introduction of Medicare Part D coverage ($8/$20 copayments for generic/brand medications) to 3 intervention groups with following baseline conditions:
	1. No coverage
	2. Coverage with low quarterly drug spending cap
	3. Coverage with high quarterly drug spending cap
	[Comparison group had benefits similar to Part D coverage at baseline.]
		• MPR:
		  ○ +13.5% points for group with no coverage at baseline (95% CI 11.5–15.5)
		  ○ +2.6% points for group with low cap at baseline (95% CI 1.2–4.1)
		  ○ +2.5% points for group with high cap at baseline (95% CI 1.7–3.2)

Li et al,[62] 2012	Medicare Part D coverage gap, 3 intervention groups with following baseline conditions:
	1. No coverage
	2. Generic-only coverage
	3. Brand and generic coverage
	[Comparison group eligible for low-income subsidies during the gap.]
		• PDC <0.8 (low adherence)
		  ○ OR = 1.60 (95% CI 1.50–1.71) for group with no coverage at baseline
		  ○ OR = 1.50 (95% CI 1.30–1.73) for group with generic-only coverage at baseline
		  ○ OR = 1.00 (95% CI 0.88–1.15) for group with brand and generic coverage at baseline

Volpp et al,[63] 2014	Financial incentive equal to copayments for all antihypertensive medications, which effectively eliminated copayments	• MPR: ○ No effect ($P = .74$)

Abbreviations: ACE, angiotensin-converting enzyme; ARB, angiotensin receptor blocker; BP, blood pressure; CI, confidence interval; MPR, medication possession ratio; OR, odds ratio; PDC, proportion of days covered.

[a] Only Volpp et al assessed the effect of the intervention on BP outcomes; no effect was detected.

improve BP outcomes, pharmacists deliver education about hypertension and its treatment, identify prescribing and safety issues, and/or dispense lifestyle advice.[64] Several reviews and meta-analyses demonstrate associations between pharmacist-delivered interventions and improved BP outcomes.[54,55,64–67] In fact, a recent meta-analysis found that pharmacist-delivered interventions had the largest effect on BP

Table 5
Effectiveness of interventions involving allied health professionals (including collaborative care): summary of evidence from reviews and meta-analyses

Type of Intervention [Review/Meta-analysis]	Effects on Adherence	Effects on Blood Pressure
Nurse- and pharmacist-led care [Glynn et al,[65] 2010]	• Not assessed	• Mean difference SBP, range: −13 mm Hg to 0 mm Hg • Mean difference DBP, range: −8 mm Hg to 0 mm Hg
Pharmacist interventions [Morgado et al,[66] 2011]	• 44% of interventions increased adherence	• WMD SBP: −4.9 mm Hg, 95% CI −5.8 to −4.0 • WMD DBP: −2.6 mm Hg, 95% CI −3.5 to −1.7
Pharmacist-delivered face-to-face education; collaborative care [Viswanathan et al,[54] 2012][a]	• Pharmacist-delivered education: low strength evidence of benefit • Collaborative care: low strength evidence of no benefit	• Pharmacist-delivered education: decreased SBP and DBP (mean decrease not specified)
Multiprofessional informational, behavioral, and combined strategies [Mansoor et al,[69] 2013][a]	• Few informational or combined interventions improved adherence • All behavioral interventions improved adherence	• Most informational or combined interventions improved health outcomes, including BP • All behavioral interventions improved health outcomes, including BP
Team-based care interventions [Proia et al,[68] 2014]	• Insufficient information provided	• Median effect estimate SBP: −5.4 mm Hg, 95% CI −7.2 to −2.0 • Median effect estimate DBP: −1.8 mm Hg, 95% CI −3.2 to 0.7
Pharmacist-led interventions [Cheema et al,[64] 2014]	• OR (improved adherence) = 12.1, 95% CI 4.2–34.6	• WMD SBP: −6.1 mm Hg, 95% CI −8.4 to −3.8 • WMD DBP: −2.5 mm Hg, 95% CI −3.5 to −1.6
Pharmacist interventions [Santschi et al,[67] 2014]	• Not assessed	• WMD SBP: −7.6 mm Hg, 95% CI −9.0 to −6.3 • WMD DBP: −3.9 mm Hg, 95% CI −5.1 to −2.8
Pharmacist-delivered interventions; increased integration of care [Conn et al,[11] 2015]	• Pharmacist-delivered intervention (d = 0.356) vs not delivered by pharmacist (d = 0.277) (P = .327) • Studies that increased integration across providers (d = 0.185) vs studies without integration (d = 0.344) (P = .021)	Not assessed

(continued on next page)

Table 5 (continued)		
Type of Intervention [Review/Meta-analysis]	**Effects on Adherence**	**Effects on Blood Pressure**

Pharmacist, nurse, and physician interventionist [Conn et al,[55] 2016]	• Not assessed	• SBP
		  ○ Pharmacist d = 0.317 ($P<.001$)
		  ○ Nurse, advanced practice d = 0.298 ($P = .001$)
		  ○ Physician d = 0.218 ($P<.001$)
		  ○ Nurse, not advanced practice d = 0.142 ($P = .089$)
		• DBP
		  ○ Pharmacist d = 0.235 ($P<.001$)
		  ○ Nurse, advanced practice d = 0.224 ($P = .030$)
		  ○ Physician d = 0.199 ($P<.001$)
		  ○ Nurse, not advanced practice d = 0.149 ($P = .101$)

Abbreviations: BP, blood pressure; CI, confidence interval; DBP, diastolic blood pressure; SBP, systolic blood pressure; WMD, weighted mean difference.
[a] Specific data not reported in source

outcomes, followed by those delivered by advanced practice nurses, and then physicians.[55] Although it is clear that interventions delivered by pharmacists improve BP outcomes, there is a great deal of unexplained heterogeneity in effects[67] and it is uncertain if the effect on BP outcomes is mediated by improved adherence or by some other mechanism, as effects on adherence reported across reviews and meta-analyses are inconsistent.[11,54,64,66]

Team-based collaborative care is a specific type of intervention involving allied health professionals. Multiple reviews and meta-analyses have identified improved BP outcomes associated with collaborative care models[68,69]; there is, however, limited evidence supporting adherence as the mechanism leading to improved outcomes.[11,54,68] A recent meta-analysis found that studies focusing on increasing integration of patient care across providers had a significantly *smaller* effect on adherence than interventions that did not have a focus on integration.[11] These negative findings may be due to a failure to account for differences in effectiveness between multiprofessional behavioral and informational or combined interventions. Mansoor and colleagues[69] reported that multiprofessional behavioral interventions improved adherence while multiprofessional informational or combined interventions did not. Further research is needed to identify the best model and determine if multiprofessional interventions are superior to those delivered by a single professional.[69]

Across a number of systematic reviews and meta-analyses, self-monitoring of BP leads to improvements in BP outcomes,[52,53,65,70,71] although the mechanism for this effect remains unclear. Potential mechanisms include pharmacologic (increased medication and better adherence) and nonpharmacologic (healthier lifestyle) factors.[52]

Table 6
Effectiveness of self-monitoring of blood pressure: summary of evidence from reviews and meta-analyses

Review/Meta-analysis	Effects on Adherence	Effects on Blood Pressure
Glynn et al,[65] 2010	• Not assessed	• WMD SBP: −2.5 mm Hg, 95% CI −3.7 to −1.3 • WMD DBP: −1.8 mm Hg, 95% CI −2.4 to −1.2
Bray et al,[70] 2010	• Not assessed	• WMD SBP: −3.8 mm Hg, 95% CI −5.6 to −2.0 • WMD DBP: −1.5 mm Hg, 95% CI −2.0 to −0.9
van Dalem et al,[53] 2012	• Contradictory results (2 studies)	• Mean DBP: "significant decrease" (2 studies; data not reported)
Uhlig et al,[71] 2013	• "A few studies" found effect (data not reported)	Self-monitoring only • WMD SBP, 6 mo: −3.9 mm Hg, $P<.001$ • WMD DBP, 6 mo: −2.4 mm Hg, $P<.001$ • WMD SBP, 12 mo: −1.5 mm Hg, $P>.05$ • WMD DBP, 12 mo: −0.8 mm Hg, $P>.05$ Self-monitoring + additional support • Net difference SBP, range, 12 mo: −8.9 to −2.1 mm Hg • Net difference DBP, range, 12 mo: −4.4 to 0.0 mm Hg
Fletcher et al,[52] 2015	• d = 0.21 (95% CI 0.08–0.34)	• WMD SBP: −4.1 mm Hg, 95% CI −6.7 to −1.4 • WMD DBP: −2.0 mm Hg, 95% CI −2.9 to −1.1
Conn et al,[11] 2015	• Self-monitoring (d = 0.381) vs no self-monitoring (d = 0.261) ($P = .160$)	• Not assessed
Conn et al,[55] 2016	• Not assessed	• No difference in effect (effect sizes not reported)

Abbreviations: CI, confidence interval; DBP, diastolic blood pressure; SBP, systolic blood pressure; WMD, weighted mean difference.

The evidence for an effect of self-monitoring of BP on adherence is inconsistent,[11,53,71] but a recent meta-analysis of the effect of self-monitoring of BP found a "small but significant" effect on medication adherence.[52]

STRATEGIES WITH UNCERTAIN EFFICACY FOR IMPROVING ADHERENCE

The efficacy of other strategies to improve antihypertensive medication adherence remains uncertain. There is little evidence that, compared to other interventions, informational interventions, particularly those relying on written materials, or social support interventions are more effective at promoting antihypertensive medication adherence or improving health outcomes.[11,55] Data supporting the efficacy of particular behavioral interventions are also limited. Interventions using adherence problem-solving, decisional balance activities, and medication administration calendars are not associated with larger improvements in adherence.[11] Furthermore, adherence barrier management, rewards for adherence, and adherence goal setting are not associated with larger improvements in BP outcomes.[55] According to recent meta-analyses, when compared with other interventions, motivational interviewing, self-monitoring of medication administration/adherence, feedback about adherence, drug packaging, and efforts to improve communication between patients and providers are not associated with larger improvements in adherence and BP control.[11,55]

Although the research to date does not provide evidence that these interventions are more effective at improving adherence compared to other interventions, it is important to note that much of the research on intervention efficacy lacks methodological rigor, leading to low-quality evidence about which interventions are most effective. More high-quality studies on the effectiveness of various approaches for improving adherence and health outcomes are needed.

NEW FRONTIERS IN THE PROMOTION OF MEDICATION ADHERENCE

Technology-mediated interventions include both medical devices (eg, electronic drug monitors, pillboxes with alarms, home BP monitors, telehealth devices) and information and communication technologies (eg, computers, telephones, cell phones, e-mails, text messages), which may be used to support adherence through education and counseling, self-monitoring and feedback, or provision of reminders.[72] Research on the effectiveness of these interventions is under way. A recent review found inconsistent evidence for the effectiveness of technology-mediated interventions to promote medication adherence and improve health outcomes.[72] In contrast, a meta-analysis of Internet-based counseling demonstrated a mean reduction in SBP of 3.8 mm Hg ($P = .002$) and a mean reduction in diastolic BP (DBP) of 2.1 mm Hg ($P = .03$).[73] Another meta-analysis reported that mobile phone text messaging for adherence to medications for chronic disease led to a doubling of the odds of adherence in intervention compared with control participants (OR = 2.11, $P<.001$).[74] Notably, technology-mediated interventions are often just one component of complex, multicomponent interventions and it is difficult to isolate the effects of the technology piece.[72,73] High-quality studies with longer follow-up and objective adherence measures are needed to adequately explore the potential of technology-mediated interventions for improving adherence.

Interactive digital interventions, which include interventions accessed through a computer, smartphone, or other handheld device (eg, Web-based or computer programs, or apps for online or offline use) deserve further mention. Several characteristics of interactive digital interventions make them especially promising for the promotion of antihypertensive medication adherence. First, they are interactive, requiring input from users, which can be used to produce tailored content. Second, they can function without the need for input from a health professional, making them potentially cost-effective tools for delivering long-term, multiple-contact adherence support. Finally, once developed, these interventions are highly scalable, able to reach innumerable users for only marginal additional cost. A recent meta-analysis of interactive digital interventions demonstrated that interactive digital interventions are effective in lowering both SBP (weighted mean difference [WMD] −3.74 mm Hg, 95% confidence interval [CI] −5.28 to −2.19) and DBP (WMD −2.37 mm Hg, 95% CI −4.35 to −0.40) compared with usual care.[75] Few studies in the review included medication adherence as an outcome measure. Despite the promising results, little is known about the sustainability, long-term effectiveness, and active components of these interventions; thus, the evidence is not robust enough to warrant a policy or practice change at this time.[75] A recent content analysis of 166 medication adherence apps found that the extent to which established behavior change techniques are used in adherence apps is limited.[76] Future research incorporating advances in behavior change theory, and practice will likely guide development in this emerging area.

GAPS IN OUR KNOWLEDGE ABOUT PROMOTING MEDICATION ADHERENCE

Despite evidence supporting the efficacy of a range of promising interventions, gaps in knowledge remain. A 2014 Cochrane review of interventions to promote medication adherence suggests, "It is possible that interventions to date are not very effective because we do not understand in sufficient detail exactly what the adherence problems are."[77] For example, unconscious, self-protective "hidden motives"[78] that render patients "immune to change" their medication-taking behavior have recently been identified and may be contributing to nonadherence to antihypertensive medications. Work is under way to fill the gaps in our understanding of these novel barriers: tools to identify individuals with hidden motives for nonadherence are being developed, and interventions to overturn nonadherence mindsets are being designed and tested. These efforts will yield insights into psychological processes underlying nonadherence and may provide a novel approach for improving adherence, BP control, and quality of life in people with hypertension.

Although it is certain that more work is needed to understand the barriers to and underlying mechanisms for adherence, there is also a need to implement and evaluate interventions that address well-established barriers to adherence. For example, a number of studies and a meta-analysis have demonstrated that low adherence to medications is associated with depression and stressful life events.[17–19,39] In one study, adjustment by depressive symptoms attenuated the association between social support and antihypertensive medication adherence.[18] Yet, with the exception of a trial that found that integrated management of hypertension and depression led to improvements in medication adherence and health outcomes,[79] few intervention trials have focused on addressing these barriers. In addition, although some work suggests that depression leads to low adherence through the mechanism of low self-efficacy,[80,81] additional research is needed to understand the mechanisms linking depression to low adherence so that targeted interventions can be developed.

In addition, work is needed to uncover sex and race differences in determinants of low adherence and effects of interventions to improve adherence. Racial and ethnic disparities in adherence rates are well-documented[82–84]; however, little is known about the root causes. Sex differences in determinants of adherence have been identified.[34] These efforts at achieving a nuanced understanding of how the relationships between adherence and its determinants are moderated by demographic and other factors will help us to tailor interventions to meet the varied needs of diverse patients. A consideration of demographic differences should be applied to intervention trials as well: a recent meta-analysis found that effect sizes of antihypertensive adherence interventions were larger for older, female, and moderate-to high-income participants, signaling the need to explore alternative interventions for younger, male, and low-income participants.[11] In general, there are major gaps in our understanding about how best to tailor interventions to meet the needs of patients with adherence problems, different types of nonadherence (eg, intentional vs unintentional), and different preferences for delivery (eg, technology-mediated vs face-to-face).[11,85,86]

Finally, further work is needed to fully understand the link between antihypertensive medication adherence and cardiovascular outcomes. Although several studies to date have identified a significant association between adherence and cardiovascular outcomes, including myocardial infarction, heart failure, stroke, and death,[5] further work is needed to explore an association between adherence and other outcomes, such as diastolic dysfunction, a condition in which abnormalities in mechanical function of the heart are present during diastole. Hypertension may lead to diastolic dysfunction even in the absence of systolic dysfunction.[87] Diastolic heart failure accounts for approximately 40% to 60% of patients with chronic heart failure; the prognosis for these patients may be similar to that of patients with systolic heart failure.[88] Appropriate treatment of hypertension together with high patient medication adherence may be key to preventing onset of diastolic dysfunction and other cardiovascular diseases.

SUMMARY

Adherence to antihypertensive medication remains a key modifiable factor in the management of hypertension, an important, preventable risk factor for cardiovascular disease and death.[89] Timely attention in clinical and research settings to identifying and addressing barriers to low medication adherence and uncontrolled BP for the general population may interrupt the costly cycle of this chronic disease and prevent the declines in quality of life associated with the consequences of uncontrolled hypertension.

DISCLOSURES

The authors have no commercial or financial conflicts of interest to disclose. This work was supported in part by 1 U54 GM104940 from the National Institute of General Medical Sciences of the National Institutes of Health (NIH), which funds the Louisiana Clinical and Translational Science Center. Dr. Krousel-Wood also received funding from the NIH for the following grants: 5K12HD043451; U54TR001368-01; 1P20GM109036-01A1. The content is solely the responsibility of the authors and does not necessarily represent the official views of the National Institutes of Health.

REFERENCES

1. Haynes RB, McDonald HP, Garg AX. Helping patients follow prescribed treatment: clinical applications. JAMA 2002;288(22):2880–3.
2. Kronish IM, Ye S. Adherence to cardiovascular medications: lessons learned and future directions. Prog Cardiovasc Dis 2013;55(6):590–600.
3. DiMatteo MR, Giordani PJ, Lepper HS, et al. Patient adherence and medical treatment outcomes: a meta-analysis. Med Care 2002;40(9):794–811.
4. Ho PM, Bryson CL, Rumsfeld JS. Medication adherence: its importance in cardiovascular outcomes. Circulation 2009;119(23):3028–35.
5. Krousel-Wood M, Holt E, Joyce C, et al. Differences in cardiovascular disease risk when antihypertensive medication adherence is assessed by pharmacy fill versus self-report: the Cohort Study of Medication Adherence among Older Adults (CoSMO). J Hypertens 2015;33(2):412–20.
6. Krousel-Wood M, Thomas S, Muntner P, et al. Medication adherence: a key factor in achieving blood pressure control and good clinical outcomes in hypertensive patients. Curr Opin Cardiol 2004;19(4):357–62.
7. Krousel-Wood MA, Muntner P, Islam T, et al. Barriers to and determinants of medication adherence in hypertension management: perspective of the cohort study

of medication adherence among older adults. Med Clin North Am 2009;93(3): 753–69.

8. Wright JT Jr, Williamson JD, Whelton PK, et al. A randomized trial of intensive versus standard blood-pressure control. N Engl J Med 2015;373(22):2103–16.

9. Williamson JD, Supiano MA, Applegate WB, et al. Intensive vs standard blood pressure control and cardiovascular disease outcomes in adults aged >/=75 years: a randomized clinical trial. JAMA 2016;315(24):2673–82.

10. Leung AA, Nerenberg K, Daskalopoulou SS, et al. Hypertension Canada's 2016 Canadian hypertension education program guidelines for blood pressure measurement, diagnosis, assessment of risk, prevention, and treatment of hypertension. Can J Cardiol 2016;32(5):569–88.

11. Conn VS, Ruppar TM, Chase JA, et al. Interventions to improve medication adherence in hypertensive patients: systematic review and meta-analysis. Curr Hypertens Rep 2015;17(12):94.

12. Cook NR, Cohen J, Hebert PR, et al. Implications of small reductions in diastolic blood pressure for primary prevention. Arch Intern Med 1995;155(7):701–9.

13. Stamler J, Stamler R, Neaton JD. Blood pressure, systolic and diastolic, and cardiovascular risks. US population data. Arch Intern Med 1993;153(5):598–615.

14. Collins R, Peto R, MacMahon S, et al. Blood pressure, stroke, and coronary heart disease. Part 2, short-term reductions in blood pressure: overview of randomised drug trials in their epidemiological context. Lancet 1990;335(8693):827–38.

15. Ogedegbe G, Harrison M, Robbins L, et al. Reasons patients do or do not take their blood pressure medications. Ethn Dis 2004;14(1):158.

16. Ogedegbe G, Harrison M, Robbins L, et al. Barriers and facilitators of medication adherence in hypertensive African Americans: a qualitative study. Ethn Dis 2004; 14(1):3–12.

17. Krousel-Wood MA, Frohlich ED. Hypertension and depression: coexisting barriers to medication adherence. J Clin Hypertens (Greenwich) 2010;12(7):481–6.

18. Krousel-Wood M, Islam T, Muntner P, et al. Association of depression with antihypertensive medication adherence in older adults: cross-sectional and longitudinal findings from CoSMO. Ann Behav Med 2010;40(3):248–57.

19. Grenard JL, Munjas BA, Adams JL, et al. Depression and medication adherence in the treatment of chronic diseases in the United States: a meta-analysis. J Gen Intern Med 2011;26(10):1175–82.

20. Wang PS, Avorn J, Brookhart MA, et al. Effects of noncardiovascular comorbidities on antihypertensive use in elderly hypertensives. Hypertension 2005;46(2): 273–9.

21. Wang PS, Bohn RL, Knight E, et al. Noncompliance with antihypertensive medications: the impact of depressive symptoms and psychosocial factors. J Gen Intern Med 2002;17(7):504–11.

22. Egan BM, Lackland DT, Cutler NE. Awareness, knowledge, and attitudes of older Americans about high blood pressure: implications for health care policy, education, and research. Arch Intern Med 2003;163(6):681–7.

23. Egan BM, Zhao Y, Axon RN. US trends in prevalence, awareness, treatment, and control of hypertension, 1988-2008. JAMA 2010;303(20):2043–50.

24. Ogedegbe G, Mancuso CA, Allegrante JP. Expectations of blood pressure management in hypertensive African-American patients: a qualitative study. J Natl Med Assoc 2004;96(4):442–9.

25. Briesacher BA, Gurwitz JH, Soumerai SB. Patients at-risk for cost-related medication nonadherence: a review of the literature. J Gen Intern Med 2007;22(6): 864–71.

26. Kronish IM, Diefenbach MA, Edmondson DE, et al. Key barriers to medication adherence in survivors of strokes and transient ischemic attacks. J Gen Intern Med 2013;28(5):675–82.

27. Edmondson D, Horowitz CR, Goldfinger JZ, et al. Concerns about medications mediate the association of posttraumatic stress disorder with adherence to medication in stroke survivors. Br J Health Psychol 2013;18(4):799–813.

28. Iskedjian M, Einarson TR, MacKeigan LD, et al. Relationship between daily dose frequency and adherence to antihypertensive pharmacotherapy: evidence from a meta-analysis. Clin Ther 2002;24(2):302–16.

29. Brown CM, Barner JC, Richards KM, et al. Patterns of complementary and alternative medicine use in African Americans. J Altern Complement Med 2007;13(7):751–8.

30. Gohar F, Greenfield SM, Beevers DG, et al. Self-care and adherence to medication: a survey in the hypertension outpatient clinic. BMC Complement Altern Med 2008;8:4.

31. Krousel-Wood MA, Muntner P, Joyce CJ, et al. Adverse effects of complementary and alternative medicine on antihypertensive medication adherence: findings from the cohort study of medication adherence among older adults. J Am Geriatr Soc 2010;58(1):54–61.

32. World Health Organization. Adherence to long-term therapies: Evidence for action. 2003.

33. Hagiwara N, Penner LA, Gonzalez R, et al. Racial attitudes, physician-patient talk time ratio, and adherence in racially discordant medical interactions. Soc Sci Med 2013;87:123–31.

34. Holt E, Joyce C, Dornelles A, et al. Sex differences in barriers to antihypertensive medication adherence: findings from the cohort study of medication adherence among older adults. J Am Geriatr Soc 2013;61(4):558–64.

35. Lutfey K. On practices of 'good doctoring': reconsidering the relationship between provider roles and patient adherence. Sociol Health Illn 2005;27(4):421–47.

36. Gregoire JP, Moisan J, Guibert R, et al. Tolerability of antihypertensive drugs in a community-based setting. Clin Ther 2001;23(5):715–26.

37. Morisky DE, Ang A, Krousel-Wood MA, et al. Predictive validity of a medication adherence measure in an outpatient setting. J Clin Hypertens 2008;10:348–54.

38. Morisky DE, Green LW, Levine DM. Concurrent and predictive validity of a self-reported measure of medication adherence. Med Care 1986;24(1):67–74.

39. Holt EW, Muntner P, Joyce C, et al. Life events, coping, and antihypertensive medication adherence among older adults: the cohort study of medication adherence among older adults. Am J Epidemiol 2012;176(Suppl 7):S64–71.

40. Fongwa MN, Evangelista LS, Hays RD, et al. Adherence treatment factors in hypertensive African American women. Vasc Health Risk Manag 2008;4(1):157–66.

41. Hyre AD, Krousel-Wood MA, Muntner P, et al. Prevalence and predictors of poor antihypertensive medication adherence in an urban health clinic setting. J Clin Hypertens (Greenwich) 2007;9(3):179–86.

42. Rollnick S, Miller WR, Butler C. Motivational interviewing in health care: helping patients change behavior. New York: Guilford Press; 2008.

43. Kripalani S, Yao X, Haynes RB. Interventions to enhance medication adherence in chronic medical conditions: a systematic review. Arch Intern Med 2007;167(6):540–50.

44. Nau DP. Proportion of days covered (PDC) as a preferred method of measuring medication adherence. Springfield (VA): Pharmacy Quality Alliance; 2012.

45. Choudhry NK, Shrank WH, Levin RL, et al. Measuring concurrent adherence to multiple related medications. Am J Manag Care 2009;15(7):457–64.
46. Farmer KC. Methods for measuring and monitoring medication regimen adherence in clinical trials and clinical practice. Clin Ther 1999;21(6):1074–90 [discussion: 1073].
47. Krousel-Wood M, Islam T, Webber LS, et al. New medication adherence scale versus pharmacy fill rates in seniors with hypertension. Am J Manag Care 2009;15(1):59–66.
48. Krousel-Wood M, Joyce C, Holt EW, et al. Development and evaluation of a self-report tool to predict low pharmacy refill adherence in elderly patients with uncontrolled hypertension. Pharmacotherapy 2013;33(8):798–811.
49. Kim MT, Hill MN, Bone LR, et al. Development and testing of the Hill-Bone Compliance to High Blood Pressure Therapy Scale. Prog Cardiovasc Nurs 2000;15(3):90–6.
50. McHorney CA. The Adherence Estimator: a brief, proximal screener for patient propensity to adhere to prescription medications for chronic disease. Curr Med Res Opin 2009;25(1):215–38.
51. Cohen J. Statistical power analysis for the behavioral sciences (revised edition). New York: Academic Press; 1977.
52. Fletcher BR, Hartmann-Boyce J, Hinton L, et al. The effect of self-monitoring of blood pressure on medication adherence and lifestyle factors: a systematic review and meta-analysis. Am J Hypertens 2015;28(10):1209–21.
53. van Dalem J, Krass I, Aslani P. Interventions promoting adherence to cardiovascular medicines. Int J Clin Pharm 2012;34(2):295–311.
54. Viswanathan M, Golin CE, Jones CD, et al. Interventions to improve adherence to self-administered medications for chronic diseases in the United States: a systematic review. Ann Intern Med 2012;157(11):785–95.
55. Conn VS, Ruppar TM, Chase JD. Blood pressure outcomes of medication adherence interventions: systematic review and meta-analysis. J Behav Med 2016. [Epub ahead of print].
56. Volpp KG. The counseling African Americans to control hypertension study and ways to enhance the next wave of behavioral interventions. Circulation 2014;129(20):2002–4.
57. Patel BV, Leslie RS, Thiebaud P, et al. Adherence with single-pill amlodipine/atorvastatin vs a two-pill regimen. Vasc Health Risk Manag 2008;4(3):673–81.
58. Omboni S, Gazzola T, Carabelli G, et al. Clinical usefulness and cost effectiveness of home blood pressure telemonitoring: meta-analysis of randomized controlled studies. J Hypertens 2013;31(3):455–67 [discussion: 467–58].
59. Chernew ME, Shah MR, Wegh A, et al. Impact of decreasing copayments on medication adherence within a disease management environment. Health Aff (Millwood) 2008;27(1):103–12.
60. Maciejewski ML, Farley JF, Parker J, et al. Copayment reductions generate greater medication adherence in targeted patients. Health Aff (Millwood) 2010;29(11):2002–8.
61. Zhang Y, Lave JR, Donohue JM, et al. The impact of Medicare Part D on medication adherence among older adults enrolled in Medicare-Advantage products. Med Care 2010;48(5):409–17.
62. Li P, McElligott S, Bergquist H, et al. Effect of the Medicare Part D coverage gap on medication use among patients with hypertension and hyperlipidemia. Ann Intern Med 2012;156(11):776–84, w-263, w-264, w-265, w-266, w-267, w-268, w-269.

63. Volpp K, Troxel A, Long J, et al. A randomized controlled trial of co-payment elimination: the CHORD trial. Am J Manag Care 2014;21(8):e455–64.
64. Cheema E, Sutcliffe P, Singer DR. The impact of interventions by pharmacists in community pharmacies on control of hypertension: a systematic review and meta-analysis of randomized controlled trials. Br J Clin Pharmacol 2014;78(6): 1238–47.
65. Glynn LG, Murphy AW, Smith SM, et al. Interventions used to improve control of blood pressure in patients with hypertension. Cochrane Database Syst Rev 2010;(3):CD005182.
66. Morgado MP, Morgado SR, Mendes LC, et al. Pharmacist interventions to enhance blood pressure control and adherence to antihypertensive therapy: review and meta-analysis. Am J Health Syst Pharm 2011;68(3):241–53.
67. Santschi V, Chiolero A, Colosimo AL, et al. Improving blood pressure control through pharmacist interventions: a meta-analysis of randomized controlled trials. J Am Heart Assoc 2014;3(2):e000718.
68. Proia KK, Thota AB, Njie GJ, et al. Team-based care and improved blood pressure control: a community guide systematic review. Am J Prev Med 2014;47(1): 86–99.
69. Mansoor SM, Krass I, Aslani P. Multiprofessional interventions to improve patient adherence to cardiovascular medications. J Cardiovasc Pharmacol Ther 2013; 18(1):19–30.
70. Bray EP, Holder R, Mant J, et al. Does self-monitoring reduce blood pressure? Meta-analysis with meta-regression of randomized controlled trials. Ann Med 2010;42(5):371–86.
71. Uhlig K, Patel K, Ip S, et al. Self-measured blood pressure monitoring in the management of hypertension: a systematic review and meta-analysis. Ann Intern Med 2013;159(3):185–94.
72. Mistry N, Keepanasseril A, Wilczynski NL, et al. Technology-mediated interventions for enhancing medication adherence. J Am Med Inform Assoc 2015; 22(e1):e177–93.
73. Liu S, Dunford SD, Leung YW, et al. Reducing blood pressure with Internet-based interventions: a meta-analysis. Can J Cardiol 2013;29(5):613–21.
74. Thakkar J, Kurup R, Laba TL, et al. Mobile telephone text messaging for medication adherence in chronic disease: a meta-analysis. JAMA Intern Med 2016; 176(3):340–9.
75. McLean G, Band R, Saunderson K, et al. Digital interventions to promote self-management in adults with hypertension systematic review and meta-analysis. J Hypertens 2016;34(4):600–12.
76. Morrissey EC, Corbett TK, Walsh JC, et al. Behavior change techniques in apps for medication adherence: a content analysis. Am J Prev Med 2016;50(5): e143–6.
77. Nieuwlaat R, Wilczynski N, Navarro T, et al. Interventions for enhancing medication adherence. Cochrane Database Syst Rev 2014;(11):CD000011.
78. Krousel-Wood M, Kegan R, Whelton PK, et al. Immunity-to-change: are hidden motives underlying patient nonadherence to chronic disease medications? Am J Med Sci 2014;348(2):121–8.
79. Bogner HR, de Vries HF. Integration of depression and hypertension treatment: a pilot, randomized controlled trial. Ann Fam Med 2008;6(4):295–301.
80. Chao J, Nau DP, Aikens JE, et al. The mediating role of health beliefs in the relationship between depressive symptoms and medication adherence in persons with diabetes. Res Social Adm Pharm 2005;1(4):508–25.

81. Schoenthaler A, Ogedegbe G, Allegrante JP. Self-efficacy mediates the relationship between depressive symptoms and medication adherence among hypertensive African Americans. Health Educ Behav 2009;36(1):127–37.

82. Gellad WF, Haas JS, Safran DG. Race/ethnicity and nonadherence to prescription medications among seniors: results of a national study. J Gen Intern Med 2007; 22(11):1572–8.

83. Holmes HM, Luo R, Hanlon JT, et al. Ethnic disparities in adherence to antihypertensive medications of medicare part D beneficiaries. J Am Geriatr Soc 2012; 60(7):1298–303.

84. Ishisaka DY, Jukes T, Romanelli RJ, et al. Disparities in adherence to and persistence with antihypertensive regimens: an exploratory analysis from a community-based provider network. J Am Soc Hypertens 2012;6(3):201–9.

85. Conn VS, Ruppar TM, Enriquez M, et al. Medication adherence interventions that target subjects with adherence problems: systematic review and meta-analysis. Res Social Adm Pharm 2016;12(2):218–46.

86. Hugtenburg JG, Timmers L, Elders PJ, et al. Definitions, variants, and causes of nonadherence with medication: a challenge for tailored interventions. Patient Prefer Adherence 2013;7:675–82.

87. Vasan RS, Larson MG, Benjamin EJ, et al. Congestive heart failure in subjects with normal versus reduced left ventricular ejection fraction: prevalence and mortality in a population-based cohort. J Am Coll Cardiol 1999;33(7):1948–55.

88. Senni M, Redfield MM. Heart failure with preserved systolic function. A different natural history? J Am Coll Cardiol 2001;38(5):1277–82.

89. Farley TA, Dalal MA, Mostashari F, et al. Deaths preventable in the U.S. by improvements in use of clinical preventive services. Am J Prev Med 2010;38(6): 600–9.

90. Margolius D, Bodenheimer T, Bennett H, et al. Health coaching to improve hypertension treatment in a low-income, minority population. Ann Fam Med 2012;10(3): 199–205.

Index

Note: Page numbers of article titles are in **boldface** type.

Med Clin N Am 101 (2017) 247–261
http://dx.doi.org/10.1016/S0025-7125(16)37378-3
0025-7125/17

Moving?

Make sure your subscription moves with you!

To notify us of your new address, find your **Clinics Account Number** (located on your mailing label above your name), and contact customer service at:

Email: journalscustomerservice-usa@elsevier.com

800-654-2452 (subscribers in the U.S. & Canada)
314-447-8871 (subscribers outside of the U.S. & Canada)

Fax number: 314-447-8029

Elsevier Health Sciences Division
Subscription Customer Service
3251 Riverport Lane
Maryland Heights, MO 63043

*To ensure uninterrupted delivery of your subscription, please notify us at least 4 weeks in advance of move.

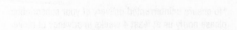

Printed and bound by CPI Group (UK) Ltd, Croydon, CR0 4YY

07/10/2024

01040506-0005